Dopaminergic System: Evolution from Biological to Clinical Aspects

Dopaminergic System: Evolution from Biological to Clinical Aspects

This document arises from "Dopaminergic System: Its Evolution from Biology to Clinical Aspects," a meeting cosponsored by WHO and AIREN held in Paris 22–24 November 1999.

Edited by C. Liana Bolis, Luca Pani, and Julio Licinio

World Health Organization Geneva

AIREN
Association Internationale pour la Recherche et l'Enseignement en Neurosciences

LIPPINCOTT WILLIAMS & WILKINS HEALTHCARE

Acquisitions Editor: Anne Sydor
Supervising Editor: Jennifer Kullgren
Purchasing Manager, Clinical and Healthcare: Jennifer Jett
Compositor: Lippincott Williams & Wilkins Healthcare
Printer: Edwards Brothers

530 Walnut Street,
Philadelphia, PA 19106 USA
www.lww.com

Printed in the USA

Library of Congress Cataloging-in-Publication Data
ISBN: 0-7817-3266-2

Care has been taken to confirm the accuracy of the information presented and to describe generally accepted practices. However, the authors, editors, and publisher are not responsible for errors or omissions or for any consequences from application of the information in this book and make no warranty, expressed or implied, with respect to the currency, completeness, or accuracy of the contents of the publication. Application of this information in a particular situation remains the professional responsibility of the practitioner.

The authors, editors, and publisher have exerted every effort to ensure that drug selection and dosage set forth in this text are in accordance with current recommendations and practice at the time of publication. However, in view of ongoing research, changes in government regulations, and the constant flow of information relating to drug therapy and drug reactions, the reader is urged to check the package insert for each drug for any change in indications and dosage and for added warnings and precautions. This is particularly important when the recommended agent is a new or infrequently employed drug.

Some drugs and medical devices presented in this publication have Food and Drug Administration clearance for limited use in restricted research settings. It is the responsibility of health care providers to ascertain the Food and Drug Administration status of each drug or device planned for use in their clinical practice.

00
1 2 3 4 5 6 7 8 9 10

CONTENTS

Preface

The study of dopamine neurotransmission is of great importance in understanding the biology and mechanisms of treatment of several human diseases. This was recognized by the awarding of the 2000 Nobel Prize in Medicine or Physiology to Arvid Carlsson, Paul Greengard, and Eric Kandel for the work of Arvid Carlsson on dopamine.

Dopamine was discovered in 1958 as a major neurotransmitter in the corpus striatum that participates in the brain regulation of motor behavior. Dopamine is synthesized from the amino acid tyrosine by the key enzyme tyrosine hydroxylase. The conversion of tyrosine to L-3,4-dihydroxyphenylalanine (L-DOPA) is the rate-limiting step in the synthesis of dopamine. L-DOPA is then converted to dopamine by aromatic L-amino acid decarboxylase. Once dopamine is synthesized and released, it binds to pre- and postsynaptic receptors. An important mechanism that regulates the amount of dopamine bioavailability is the existence of a specific dopamine transporter. In the last three decades multiple receptors have been identified that may be distinguished genetically, biochemically, and pharmacologically by selective agonists and antagonists

The Association Internationale pour la Recherche et l'Enseignement en Neurosciences organized a meeting cosponsored with the World Health Organization at the Pasteur Institute in Paris on 22–24 November 1999 to cover the evolution of our understanding of dopaminergic systems. *Dopaminergic Systems: Evolution from Biology to Clinical Aspects* is written by contributors who are recognized experts and who participated in this meeting. Our main feature is the integration of various perspectives from basic science and the implications of these perspectives for human disorders such as schizophrenia, reward systems, motor diseases, and dysthymia. Additionally, factors that contribute to dopaminergic neurotransmission include levels of stress, prenatal conditions, nutrition, and drugs.

Our contributors have different backgrounds and areas of expertise. Such multidisciplinary effort is needed to understand the complexities of dopaminergic function in health, disease, and therapeutics. To our knowledge, this book is the first effort to integrate diverse perspectives on dopamine from basic science and clinical medicine.

Our objectives in creating this book follow:

- To bring together a multidisciplinary group of experts to discuss the latest developments in the biology of dopaminergic transmission;
- To integrate knowledge on dopaminergic function from molecular biology, transgenic studies, biochemistry, imaging, behavior, genetics, and interactions with other transmitter systems;
- To integrate basic science and clinical experience in psychiatry and neurology;
- To ascertain how progress in research on dopaminergic function affects basic investigation, patient-oriented research, and clinical medicine;
- To identify gaps in our knowledge and to indicate directions for future work.

A particular feature of this book is its timeliness. The chapters were written, reviewed, and published in 2000, thus ensuring that this volume will reach the intended public in time to be topical and current. Our readership includes advanced students, researchers, and clinicians interested in the role of dopamine in biology, human disease, and therapeutics.

The complexities of dopaminergic function are such that the field can only be fully covered by experts in several preclinical and clinical disciplines. We hope that this book will stimulate further multidisciplinary efforts aimed at integrating basic science and clinical aspects of dopaminergic function. It is crucial that scientists and clinicians gather in forums that facilitate dialogue, cooperation, and collaboration. This book provides the current status of such integrative work on dopaminergic systems.

C. Liana Bolis
Julio Licinio
October 2000

Contributors

Anissa Abi-Dargham
Department of Psychiatry
College of Physicians and Surgeons
Columbia University
New York State Psychiatric Institute
New York, New York

Mayada Akil
Department of Psychiatry
University of Pittsburgh
Pittsburgh, Pennsylvania
Current affiliation:
Clinical Brain Disorders Branch
National Institute of Mental Health
National Institutes of Health
Bethesda, Maryland

Shiro Aoyama
Institute of Genetics and
Molecular and Cellular Biology
Illkirch Cedex CU de Strasbourg, France
Current affiliation: Pharmaceutical Research Institute
Kyowa Hakko Kogyo
Shizuoka, Japan

Francine M. Benes
Laboratory for Structural Neuroscience
McLean Hospital
Belmont, Massachusetts
Department of Psychiatry and
Program in Neuroscience
Harvard Medical School
Boston, Massachusetts

Jonathan Benjamin
Faculty of Health Sciences
Ben Gurion University of the Negev
Beersheva, Israel

C. Liana Bolis
Association Internationale pour la Recherche et l'Enseignement en Neurosciences
World Health Organization Collaborating Centre for Research and Training in Neuroscience
Geneva, Switzerland

Emiliana Borrelli
Institute of Genetics and
Molecular and Cellular Biology
Illkirch Cedex CU de Strasbourg, France

Paola Devoto
"B. Brodie" Department of Neuroscience
University of Cagliari
Cagliari, Italy

Richard P. Ebstein
Research Laboratory
S. Herzog Memorial Hospital
Jerusalem, Israel

Jianhua Fan
Institute of Mental Health
Beijing Medical University
Beijing, China

R. Frussa-Filho
Department of Pharmacology
School of Medicine
Federal University of São Paulo
São Paulo, Brazil

Gian Luigi Gessa
Center for Neuropharmacology and
"B. B. Brodie" Department of Neuroscience
Consiglio Nazionale delle Ricerche
University of Cagliari
Cagliari, Italy

Inga Gritsenko
Research Laboratory
S. Herzog Memorial Hospital
Jerusalem, Israel

Lamine Gueye
Service de Neurologie
Centre Hospitalier
Laboratory of Physiology
Faculty of Medicine
University of Dakar
Dakar, Senegal

Jonas Hannestad
Department of Psychiatry and
Neuropsychiatric Institute
School of Medicine
University of California Los Angeles
Los Angeles, California

Daniel J. Healy
Mental Health Research Institute
Department of Psychiatry
University of Michigan
Ann Arbor, Michigan

Jarmo Hietala
Department of Psychiatry
Turku University Central Hospital
Department of Pharmacology and
Clinical Pharmacology
University of Turku
Turku, Finland

Xianzhang Hu
Institute of Mental Health
Beijing Medical University
Beijing, China

James L. Kennedy
Neurogenetics Section
Clarke Division
Centre for Addiction and Mental Health
University of Toronto
Toronto, Ontario, Canada

Minoru Kobayashi
Institute of Genetics and
Molecular and Cellular Biology
Illkirch Cedex CU de Strasbourg, France
Moshe Kotler
Beersheva Mental Health Center
Faculty of Health Sciences
Ben-Gurion University of the Negev
Beersheva, Israel

Marc Laruelle
Department of Psychiatry
College of Physicians and Surgeons
Columbia University
New York State Psychiatric Institute
New York, New York

David A. Lewis
Departments of Psychiatry and Neuroscience
University of Pittsburgh
Pittsburgh, Pennsylvania

Julio Licinio
Department of Psychiatry and
Neuropsychiatric Institute
School of Medicine
University of California Los Angeles
Los Angeles, California

Livia Martucci
Neurogenetics Section
Clarke Division
Centre for Addiction and Mental Health
University of Toronto
Toronto, Ontario
Canada

Carole Mathis
Institute of Genetics and
Molecular and Cellular Biology
Illkirch Cedex CU de Strasbourg, France

James H. Meador-Woodruff
Mental Health Research Institute
Department of Psychiatry
University of Michigan
Ann Arbor, Michigan

Ibrahima Pierre Ndiaye
Service de Neurologie
Centre Hospitalier
University of Fann Dakar
Dakar Fann, Senegal

J. Palermo-Neto
Applied Pharmacology and Toxicology
Laboratory
School of Veterinary Medicine
University of São Paulo
São Paulo, Brazil

Luca Pani
Center for Neuropharmacology and
"B. B. Brodie" Department of Neuroscience
Consiglio Nazionale delle Ricerche
University of Cagliari
Cagliari, Italy

Joseph N. Pierri
Department of Psychiatry
University of Pittsburgh
Pittsburgh, Pennsylvania

Anna Porcella
Center for Neuropharmacology and
"B. B. Brodie" Department of Neuroscience
Consiglio Nazionale delle Ricerche
University of Cagliari
Cagliari, Italy

Werner J. Schmidt
Department of Neuropharmacology
University of Tübingen
Tübingen, Germany

Yucun Shen
Institute of Mental Health
Beijing Medical University
Beijing, China

Robert E. Smith
Mental Health Research Institute
Department of Psychiatry
University of Michigan
Ann Arbor, Michigan

Erkka Syvälahti
Department of Psychiatry
Turku University Central Hospital
Department of Pharmacology and
Clinical Pharmacology
University of Turku
Turku, Finland

Elisabeth Trouche
Laboratory of Cellular and Functional
Neurobiology
Centre National de la Recherche Scientifique
Marseilles, France

Feng Wei
Institute of Mental Health
Beijing Medical University
Beijing, China

Xiangyang Zhang
Institute of Mental Health
Beijing Medical University
Beijing, China

Dongfeng Zhou
Institute of Mental Health
Beijing Medical University
Beijing, China

Rulun Zhou
Institute of Mental Health
Beijing Medical University
Beijing, China

1.

Hypothesis Testing

Dopaminergic System, Environmental Pressure, and Evolutionary Mismatch

Luca Pani, Anna Porcella, and Gian Luigi Gessa

In the distant future I see open fields for far more important researches. Psychology will be based on a new foundation, that of the necessary acquirement of each mental power and capacity by gradation.

—Charles Darwin (1859)

One of Darwin's most striking intuitions appears in the closing pages of his famous work, where he foresaw the implications of the theory of natural selection for interpreting the psychopathology of the human brain, a view shared today by most scientists researching evolution of the brain (Divac, 1995; Wilson, 1993). The

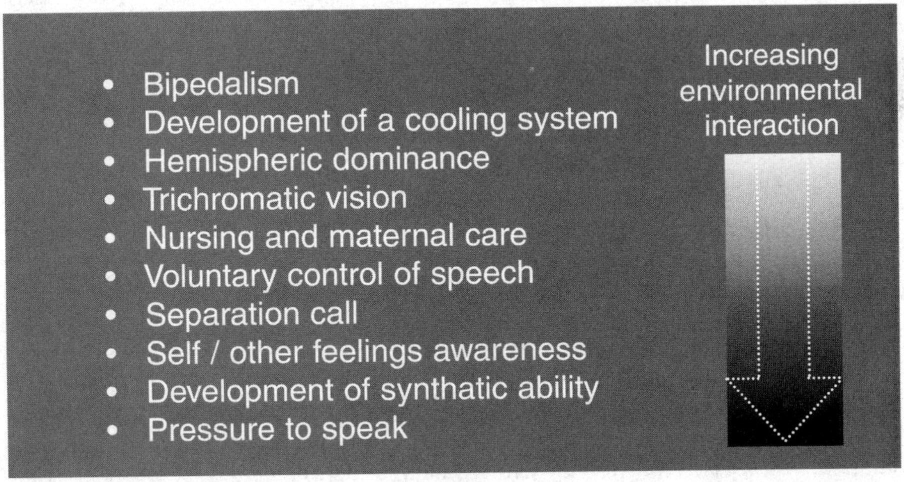

FIG. 1-1. Some crucial steps in evolution of the human brain. Evolution of the central nervous system has been characterized by increasing psychomotor interaction with the external world. The same stimuli shaped both a powerful limbic system eagerly reactive to the environment and a system susceptible to changes emanating from that environment.

steps considered essential from early mammals to humans show an increasing motor (Greenfield, 1994) and cognitive-emotional interaction (Povinelli and Preuss, 1995) with the external world (Fig. 1-1). This environmental pressure, in turn, requires development of a neuronal system that can cope with the signals and stimuli coming from the brain's surroundings.

Telencephalic dopaminergic nuclei, such as the nucleus accumbens and the caudate-putamen, have been conserved in their gross and microscopic structure throughout evolution from rodents (Bertler and Rosengren, 1959) to humans (Sano et al., 1959), whereas the structural organization of the mesotelencephalic dopaminergic circuits, most strictly involved in human pathologies such as depression and psychosis, shows significant differences between rodents and primates (Berger, 1992).

Such differences in primates include much larger terminal fields of innervation and a more detailed "mapping," different peptide expression, and much earlier prenatal development (Berger et al., 1991). Recent data show that the major development of the cerebral cortex in primates was accompanied (or produced?) by a similar expansion of the dopaminergic input to all cortical layers, with a specific and laminar redistribution of the dopaminergic terminals. Berger (1992) has speculated that cortical dopamine targets that developed most recently in phylogeny are of particular functional value and that the mesocorticolimbic dopaminergic system is involved in more complex integrative functions than previously assumed.

For several authors the mesolimbic and mesocortical dopamine circuits have long been misconceptualized (Le Moal and Simon, 1991) as simple reward or reinforcement systems (Wise, 1989). Instead, they motivate and coordinate the functions of higher brain areas that mediate planning and foresight, promote states of eagerness, and direct finalized movement in both animals and humans (Panksepp, 1998). These systems make animals intensely interested in exploring the world but by the same means make animals susceptible to environmental stimuli that have been sought and consumed. In mammals, especially primates, the dopaminergic system generates and sustains curiosity, and it efficiently facilitates learning. It is particularly effective when memorizing information about where resources are situated and the best way to obtain that which is needed for survival, including food, water, warmth, and sex (Panksepp, 1998).

MISMATCH THEORY AND DOPAMINERGIC SYSTEM

Large sets of data (Nesse and Williams, 1994) have allowed the definition of a field theory called "evolutionary mismatch," which derives largely from the fact that current environmental conditions are different from those in which the human central nervous system evolved. This mismatch between evolved traits and contemporary lifestyle, the lack of evolutionary trade-offs (e.g., selection of some traits over others), and historical constraints (e.g., how a trait has evolved) has resulted in the poor specialization of selected traits, as well as a particular susceptibility to mental disorders.

To explain the somatic correlates of such an evolutionary view of disease, it is assumed that pathogens that attack humans evolve faster than we do. If the ever-mutating environmental conditions (where change is mostly due to technology) could be assimilated to organic pathogens, their rapid rate of evolution and change would impose a pressure that is not paralleled by evolution of the brain structures that can analyze, process, and elaborate on such rapid variations. For example, a poor fit between strongly evolved traits (e.g., dependency) and the current urban social environment may explain the increased frequency of anxiety and depressive disorders (McGuire and Troisi, 1998).

However, current views on evolutionary mismatch theory lack a definition of which precise brain areas or neuronal circuits are involved in coding such evolved traits and to what extent neurobiology can be applied to the topographical localization of a specific psychopathology. We will attempt to demonstrate that some mismatched behaviors are deeply rooted in normal physiology and therefore in evolution of the dopaminergic system.

The appetitive and consummatory phases of behaviors triggered by environmental cues that are associated with survival properties (whether rewarding or aversive for the individual) are known to be mediated by sensory-specific dopaminergic neuronal circuits. Dopaminergic systems are involved in mechanisms that determine satiety to food (Ahn and Phillips, 1999), sex (Fiorino et al., 1997), and drugs of abuse (Fibiger, 1987). In all these conditions, the most important dopamine systems involved are those of the terminal fields of the prefrontal cortex (Cenci et al., 1992) and the nucleus accumbens (Phillips et al., 1993), both originating from neurons located in the ventral tegmental area of the midbrain.

Whether stimulation of these neurons mediates the incentive salience (Berridge and Robinson, 1998) or associative learning (Bassareo and Di Chiara, 1997) capacities of a reward is still intensely debated. According to the first hypothesis, rewarding (and thus also adverse) stimuli that have acquired motivational significance (salience) are part of a phenomenon that is neither unitary nor subjective; dopamine-related neural circuits mediate only a specific component of reward, i.e., attribution of incentive salience to an otherwise neutral event. In contrast, others have argued that mesolimbic dopaminergic pathways serve only to respond to specific stimuli that possess high motivational impact as a result of their novelty, unpredictability, specific sensory modalities, or occurrence under a deprivation state; in these conditions, dopamine neurons define the substrate for precise associative learning abilities. Attributing the first capacity to the mesocortical and the second to the mesolimbic dopaminergic system has recently been proposed (Bassareo and Di Chiara, 1997).

From an evolutionary perspective, the two mechanisms must be equally important in the attribution of an incentive to ethnologically relevant stimuli and must facilitate, by means of both incentive salience and associative learning, the selection and memory of appropriate behavioral responses. The conservation of such principles throughout evolution explains why pharmacological manipulations of the dopaminergic transmission can similarly modify basic behaviors in distant species such as lizards and rats (Fig. 1-2). Stimulation of the dopaminergic transmission will increase these behaviors, whereas blocking dopaminergic receptors or lesions of the dopaminergic pathways will decrease them. This confirms that dopamine is an important neurotransmitter coding for sensory-specific responses, in the sense that a perceived environmental cue is acted on cognitively either with an increase (through curiosity and reward) or a decrease (through fear and aversion) in exploration (Blackburn et al., 1992). Electrophysiological recordings have indicated key cortical and subcortical dopaminergic regions involved in these motivated behaviors. In primates, a particular role is given to the connections between the nucleus accumbens and the frontal cortex (Rolls, 1999), which we consider primary sites for the evolutionary mismatch between the dopaminergic system and the ability to process significant change-related information to guide coherent behavioral responses.

ROLE OF MONOAMINERGIC SYSTEM IN EVOLUTION OF VERTEBRATE NERVOUS SYSTEM

Animals with big brains are scarce because bigger neuronal structures cost more in terms of energy expenditure, development time, and anatomical complexity. It was always supposed that a better diet (i.e., caloric value) was the start for the development of a larger cerebral mass. Jacobs et al. (1996) described how a duplication of the gene coding for a retinal cone pigment in an ancestor of prosimians about 40 million years ago resulted in the development of trichromatic vision. This ability to see in color was instrumental in detecting ripe fruit and gave an immediate evolutionary advantage over green-leaf eaters. At about the same time the system for

- Establishing a "territory"
- Showing place preference
- Hunting
- Greeting
- Grouping socially
- Feeding and drinking
- Grooming
- Courting
- Mating
- Breeding
- Maternal behavior
- Playing (mammals only)

Mac Lean, 1985

FIG. 1-2. Special forms of basic behaviors. Manipulating dopaminergic transmission by drugs or lesions can modify basic behaviors present in distant species, demonstrating that physiology of the limbic system has not changed fundamental capacities for several thousands of years. Adapted from Mac Lean (1985).

color vision and emotional communication via facial expression expanded, the olfactory bulb is thought to have regressed in primates.

Recently this hypothesis was confirmed by showing that a highly predictable relationship exists between the relative size of the neocortex and the total brain (Finlay and Darlington, 1995). When the sizes of 10 measured brain divisions from 131 species are plotted as a function of total brain size, the two most expanded structures in all species are, in fact, the neocortex and striatum (caudate-putamen; nucleus accumbens and internal capsule), in contrast with that of the olfactory bulb. Thus two dopaminergic structures—one connected to taste-related reward and satiety and the other to olfactory satiety—seemed to be mutually exclusive in their development and to have conserved these complementary characteristics in modern humans (Rolls and Rolls, 1997). The neural mechanisms of sensory-specific satiety in primates are implemented in the orbitofrontal cortex, which has an important integrative function. Neurons in this region of the cortex were indeed found to respond to stimulation of the taste, olfactory, or visual systems. In addition, some neurons were found with bimodal responses, e.g., responding to both taste and olfactory or taste and visual stimuli. Because these multimodal neurons were found in close proximity to unimodal neurons and because the unimodal sensory neurons were intermingled, the orbitofrontal cortex may represent the first cortical area of convergence for these three modalities in primates (Rolls and Baylis, 1994).

EVOLUTION OF ENZYMES

The acquisition of the behaviors modulated by dopaminergic innervation has been so indispensable in survival that the enzymatic machinery needed to synthesize dopamine appeared early in phylogenesis. A rudimentary nervous system, that of the sea pansy *Renilla koellikeri (cnidaria)*, can synthesize dopamine; such synthesis is inhibited by alpha-methyl-*p*-tyrosine (Pani and Anctil, 1994). In this invertebrate, dopamine gives bioluminescence and produces muscular contractions, which are likely used to capture food or avoid danger. Dopamine is insufficient to result in such superior animal characteristics as the ability to feel pleasure and pain. The neurochemical basis of the effects of dopaminomimetic drugs in other distant organisms has not been fully elucidated, but the hyperkinesia induced by cocaine in *Planaria* specimens suggests that the selective site for presynaptic dopamine reuptake is already present in this flatworm (Palladini et al., 1996). Goldfish show place preference for water bowls where they have received amphetamine, a drug of abuse that selectively increases dopaminergic transmission (Lett and Grant., 1989). In the cephalochordate amphioxus, a group related to vertebrates, the presence of dopamine (but not norepinephrine) was assayed. In contrast, two distinct genes homologous to the jawed vertebrate dopamine D1 and β-adrenergic receptor genes were shown to be extant in representatives of the earliest craniates, lamprey and hagfish, paralleling a high dopamine and norepinephrine content throughout their brain (Vincent et al., 1998).

EVOLUTION OF RECEPTOR FAMILY

The evolving vertebrate nervous system was accompanied by major gene duplication events that generated novel organs along with a definite sympathetic system that could monitor and control them. Vertebrate neural pathways synthesizing monoamine neurotransmitters (mostly dopamine and norepinephrine) were subsequently recruited to process increased information demands by mediating psychomotor functions, such as selective attention/predictive reward and emotional drive, via activation of multiple catecholamine receptor subtypes linked to G-protein.

At least 1,000 million years ago, all classical transmitter ligand molecules evolved the ability to activate a wide range of ion channels, resulting in excitation, inhibition, and biphasic or multiphasic responses. In this respect the invertebrate receptors that have so far been cloned show striking homologies with mammalian receptors, indicating that many basic receptor subtypes evolved early, probably at least 800 million years ago (Walker et al., 1996).

The evolution of these receptor-mediated events was similarly driven by forces of gene duplication at the cephalochordate/vertebrate transition. In Amphioxus, one catecholamine receptor gene was found that, based on molecular phylogeny and functional analysis, formed a monophyletic group with both vertebrate dopamine D1 and β-adrenergic receptor classes (Vincent et al., 1998). These data suggest that a D1/β-receptor gene duplication was required for the elaboration of novel catecholamine psychomotor adaptive responses and that a noradrenergic system specifically emerged at the origin of vertebrate evolution. Recent data have confirmed that the dopamine D1A, D1B, and D1C receptors share molecular, pharmacological, and functional attributes that unambiguously allow for their evolutionary classification as distinct D1 receptor subtypes in the vertebrate phylum (Cardinaud et al., 1997).

These receptors conserve a fairly stable secondary structure, a moderate and reasonably steady rate of sequence change, and usually lack introns within their coding sequence. Several results indicate that the first event to occur within this gene superfamily was the divergence of the catecholamine receptors from the muscarinic acetylcholine receptors, which occurred before the divergence of the arthropod and vertebrate lineages. Subsequently the ability to activate specific second-messenger pathways diverged independently in both the muscarinic and the catecholamine receptors. This appears to have occurred after the divergence of the arthropod and vertebrate lineages but before the divergence of the avian and mammalian lineages. However, the second-messenger pathways activated by adrenergic and dopamine receptors did not diverge independently. Rather the ability of the catecholamine receptors to bind to specific ligands, such as epinephrine, norepinephrine, dopamine, or octopamine, was repeatedly modified in evolutionary history and in some cases was modified after the divergence of the second-messenger pathways (Fryxell, 1995).

When the distribution of the D1 and D2 dopaminergic receptors in the brain of a mouse, rat, or cat is compared with that of a monkey, similarities are found only in the basal ganglia; the highest density is in the caudate-putamen, nucleus accumbens, olfactory tubercle, and substantia nigra. Apart from these nuclei, and particularly in more recent structures such as the cerebellum and the frontal cortex, the absolute and relative values of the dopamine receptor subtypes are completely different in primates, suggesting that the transcriptional control of the gene encoding for the dopaminergic receptors has also undergone profound changes throughout evolution (Camps et al., 1990).

CONDITIONS THAT HAVE EVOLVED AND THAT INTERFERE WITH FUNCTION OF DOPAMINERGIC SYSTEM

Several conditions that have an important influence on the dopaminergic system physiology have profoundly changed during evolution (Fig. 1-3).

Drugs of Abuse

The ability to extract, purify, and synthesize psychoactive compounds has increased their availability to the general population in quantities and qualities never experienced in the history of humankind. In addition, the development of new routes of administration (e.g., hypodermic needles, smoking, organic solvents) has increased the penetration of drugs of abuse into the brain and have contributed to a change in the traditional relationship between the use of the natural source of the drug (e.g., chewing of coca leaves) to that of its active component (e.g., intravenous injection of cocaine hydrochloride).

Drugs of abuse offer a remarkable example of evolutionary mismatch at the level of the dopaminergic system and help to clarify its role in the general physiology of the central nervous system. If drugs of abuse that act on the dopaminergic system

- **Drugs of abuse**
- **Stress**
- **Chronic sleep deprivation**
- **Chronic emotional reactions**
- **Chronic antidepressants**
- **Withdrawal from various drugs**

FIG. 1-3. Conditions that have changed throughout evolution and that interfere with functions of dopaminergic system.

(i.e., all of them, directly or indirectly) were used solely for their hedonic and "reward producing" potential, then the pure ability to experience pleasure would be the only capacity to be mainly affected by chronic use. Instead, after a variable period of use, all drugs of abuse that determine dependence interfere with the global adaptation of an individual to its environment, producing not only an impairment of hedonic capacities but also a more disruptive effect on cognitive and emotional abilities that are necessary for effective interaction with the world (maladaptation).

The limbic portion of the dopaminergic system is essential for generation of the basic emotions that mediate various prosocial behaviors (such as maternal care, playfulness, and friendship) and have been learned and evolved to influence motivational states and, ultimately, to increase fitness. All these behaviors, along with the emotions related to them and their cognitive implications, are profoundly altered in a drug addict, perhaps much more than just the capacity to experience pleasure or avoid pain (whether physical or psychological). Drugs of abuse that convey a signal that falsely indicates the arrival of a huge fitness benefit (higher than food, water, sex, etc.) actively change behavioral hierarchies; as a consequence, seeking drugs increases in frequency to the point where it becomes the only dominant behavior, displacing all other adaptive traits (Nesse and Berridge, 1997).

Stress

Both acute and chronic stress have a detrimental impact on the normal function of the dopaminergic system (Pani et al., 2000). The response of the dopaminergic system to stress is neither homogenous nor generalized, and numerous results suggest that mesoprefrontal cortex dopaminergic projections are selectively activated by sudden changes in environmental conditions, regardless of whether they are expected (Kaneyuki et al., 1991).

The fine tuning of dopamine extracellular concentration in the medial prefrontal cortex seems to be essential for the decision-making protocols of the central nervous system, because excessive dopamine activity is detrimental to the spatial working memory functions of the medial prefrontal cortex in the rat and monkey (Murphy et al., 1996a). This supports the idea of a critical range of dopamine turnover for optimal prefrontal cortical cognitive functioning, with reduced or excessive dopamine turnover leading to cognitive impairment. Several data indicate ventral tegmental area projections (Murphy et al., 1996b), dopamine receptors (Steketee and Kalivas, 1991), and ventral tegmental area dopamine cells with a loss of inhibitory tone (Sorg and Steketee, 1992) as important regulatory sites for maintaining superior cognitive functions. The increased ability to remove dopamine in chronically stressed animals has also indicated that altered dopamine clearance may serve as an adaptive mechanism in the medial prefrontal cortex (Meiergerd et al., 1997). It has been further suggested that increased D1 receptor stimulation during stress may serve to take the medial prefrontal cortex "off-line" to allow posterior cortical and subcortical structures to regulate more "primitive" forms of behavior (Zahrt et al., 1997). Because dopaminergic innervation of the medial prefrontal cortex can regulate the activity of subcortical dopamine innervations, disruption of the medial prefrontal cortex dopamine fibers may result in the altered biochemical responsiveness of the dopamine subcortical innervations (Deutch et al., 1990).

In humans, the balance between cortical and subcortical dopaminergic activity may protect against psychotic decompensation from chronic endogenous or exogenous insult (Friedhoff et al., 1995). However, failure of this coping mechanism may well contribute to the vulnerability of the medial prefrontal cortex in many neuropsychiatric disorders related to the stress response (Finlay and Zigmond, 1997).

Stimuli that increase the release of dopamine in the medial prefrontal cortex or nucleus accumbens, whether natural (water, food, and sex) or artificial (drugs of abuse), can be heavily affected by stress. The exposure to acute inescapable shock interferes with the capacity to consume a highly palatable diet. The magnitude and duration of the response vary across different strains of mice (Griffiths et al., 1992), suggesting that a genetic component is important for encoding this reaction modality of the brain dopamine system. Sexual behavior of male rats is also impaired by long-term stress, which leads to decreased activity of dopamine neurons (Sato and Kumamoto, 1992). Prenatally stressed male rats do not exhibit copulation during sexual behavior tests, and no significant changes in dopamine release are seen during exposure to estrous females, suggesting a deficit in dopamine neurotransmission in the nucleus accumbens (Wang et al., 1995), which can be reversed acutely by apomorphine or by L-dopa plus carbidopa, a dopa decarboxylase inhibitor (Sugiura et al., 1997).

Chronic Emotional Reactions

Emotional responses can be difficult to differentiate from generic reactions to stress in laboratory animals and humans. In addition, emotions such as empathy seem to be uniquely human and are therefore impossible to mimic in animal models. In contrast, several animal behaviors such as freezing, self-grooming, exploration, and defecation have been considered valid somatic correlates to human emotional responses in which the dopaminergic system is involved. In all the models, the chronic nature of the stimulus is essential to produce a stable change in the physiology of the dopaminergic system. This can be due to generic stress such as sleep disruption, time shifts, poor physical activity, increased physical constraints, and unnatural social rules. In diseases in which dopamine function is compromised, humans exhibit a constellation of emotional symptoms, suggesting that the dopamine system is important in the integration of several functions. A dorsal tier of dopamine neurons receives input from the ventral (limbic-related) striatum and from the amygdala and projects widely throughout the cortex. Through these projections, the limbic system has an enormous influence on dopamine output and can therefore affect the emotional and motivational ''coloring'' of a wide range of behaviors (Haber and Fudge, 1997).

The lateral-basolateral amygdala receives sensory input from environmental stimuli and, along with the central amygdala, mediates conditional fear. Through its projections to forebrain, midbrain, and hindbrain, the central amygdala governs behavioral, autonomic, and endocrine responses that characterize a central fear state (Davis, 1992). Revelations about the amygdala-based fear system have led to considerable progress in delineating the neural connections and cellular mechanisms that underlie aversive emotionality. Recent results provide electrophysiological evidence of neural discharge in the central amygdala as a consequence of repeated low-current, high-frequency electrical stimulation of the ventral tegmental area (Gelowitz and Kokkinidis, 1999).

The introduction of Roman high-avoidance (RHA) and Roman low-avoidance (RLA) rats, two selectively bred lines that differ in their level of emotionality, into an unfamiliar environment, the application of a high-intensity loud noise, or immobilization are associated with increased extracellular cortical DOPAC levels in the RHA but not the RLA line, suggesting that the differently evoked emotional reactions may produce a common activation of cognitive processes (Bertolucci-D'Angio et al., 1990). This difference in reaction to a stressful stimulus according to the genetic makeup of an individual is an essential function of the mesencephalic dopaminergic neurons and of their role in the organization of behavioral responses that are the reflection of a heightened attention of the animal to cope with the stressor (D'Angio et al., 1988). They seem to facilitate the functions of the integrative structures they innervate and to have a coordinated functioning, regulating the information transfer between these structures (Louilot et al., 1989).

The study of fear and the role of the dopaminergic system in rodents has produced inconsistent results. Although some results suggest an important relationship between social reactivity and motor activity, as well as an important, albeit strain-dependent, role for D1 receptors in mediating specific emotional behaviors (Gendreau et al., 1997), others demonstrate that long-term administration of low, presynaptic doses of the D2 antagonist *l*-sulpiride is highly effective in an animal model of anticipatory anxiety/panic behavior (Cavazzuti et al., 1999). However, recent findings suggest that quinpirole (a D2 agonist) decreases fear by blocking the retrieval of a learned association between a conditioned and an unconditioned stimulus (Nader and LeDoux, 1999).

Chronic Sleep Deprivation

Humans have conserved mechanisms, like those that exist in other animals, that detect changes in day length and make corresponding adjustments in the duration of nocturnal periods. Several studies from Wehr et al. (1995) have suggested that modern use of artificial light after dark and artificial darkness during the daytime suppresses responses in men (Wehr, 1998) to seasonal changes in the duration of the natural scoto- and photoperiod that might otherwise occur at a given latitude, producing a chronic disturbance in the sleep pattern and decreasing, overall, the total amount of sleep. It is difficult to conceive that chronic sleep deprivation in humans could be obtained and maintained without any activation in the stress axis. Acute and chronic sleep deprivation per se is to be considered a cause of stress in humans.

Sleep deprivation in rats has been extensively studied in our laboratory as a possible animal model of mania. After sleep deprivation (approximately 72 hr), the rat does not fall asleep as soon as it is returned to its home cage but shows wakefulness for about 30 min, during which the animal presents a cohort of symptoms that appear to mimic those present in idiopathic mania. In particular, the animal displays a high degree of hyperactivity, irritability, aggressiveness, hypersexuality, and stereotypy. The model not only confirmed that sleep loss often precedes, and may trigger, a manic episode (Gessa et al., 1995), but it also allowed the discovery of an active role of the limbic dopamine and opioid system in the generation of arousal and insomnia related to sleep deprivation-induced stress (Fadda et al., 1993).

CONCLUSIONS

The brain of *Homo sapiens sapiens* developed on the African plains in populations of 100,000–200,000 individuals; today there are 6 billion of us worldwide. Can the structural organization and the neuronal plasticity of the human brain still control the evolution of the environment humans have created? Some influential neurobiologists have expressed strong doubts (Changeux, 1983) (Fig. 1-4). Is the functional uncoupling of the associative learning capacities of the prefrontal cortex the site of the dopaminergic evolutionary mismatch?

Environmentally induced changes in the activity of the dopaminergic system, either by conventional (food, water, sex, etc.) or nonconventional (drugs of abuse, chronic stress, emotional reactions, etc.) stimuli are thought to code for reward-aversion, sensory-motor, incentive-salience mechanisms that are needed to associate the learned outcome of that stimuli with a definite emotional state of the individual. The dopaminergic innervation to the prefrontal cortex is essential for processing and elab-

- **1550 Screwdriver**
- **1690 Steam engine**
- **1770 Electric battery**
- **1853 Hyperdermic needle**
- **1876 Telephone**
- **1885 Automobile engine**
- **1886 Coca-cola**
- **1903 Airplane**
- **1920 Radio broadcast**
- **1926 Television**
- **1948 Transistors**
- **1962 Minicomputer**
- **1969 Moonlanding**
- **1972 Videogames**
- **1978 Test tube baby**
- **1988 Patented animal life**
- **1992 Global internet**
- **2000 Human genome sequence**

FIG. 1-4. Significant inventions and technological advancement. During the last 500 years, and particularly during the last century, the human brain has produced and experienced a grade of technological advancement unknown in its entire history.

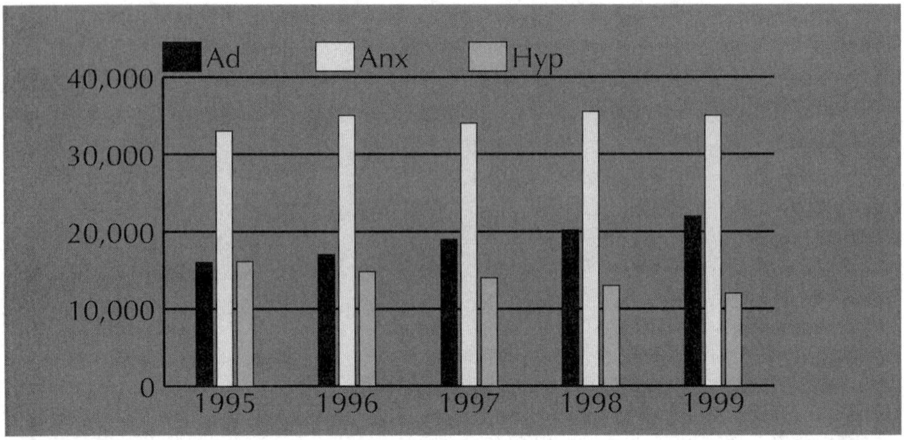

FIG. 1-5. Italian market for antidepressants (Ad), anxiolytics (Anx), and hypnotics (Hyp) from 1995 to 1999. Number of psychotropic prescriptions, especially antidepressants, sold in Italy constantly increases, and in 1998 and 1999 sales surpassed 20 million. Italy's population is about 57 million. The experience of other industrialized countries is similar.

orating on the "expectancy" of the events and in the working memory related to them, in both rats and monkeys (Murphy et al., 1996a). The dorsolateral portion of the prefrontal cortex is important in monitoring the context of the situation in relation to how and what reward is given (Watanabe, 1996). Patients with prefrontal lesions are poor in assessing how actions relate to goals. Results suggest that prefrontal cortical lesions provoke a selective impairment in managerial knowledge that may contribute to difficulties in the formulation and execution of plans (Sirigu et al., 1995).

Neurons that are critical for the computation of sensory-specific satiety in the monkey are located in the orbitofrontal cortex, and in humans decision-making processes depend on signals arising in the prefrontal cortex in association with peripheral somatovisceral signals that can introduce biases in the reasoning processes (Damasio, 1996). When normal subjects experience situations that they associate with the possibility of negative consequences, they sense a peripheral reaction (mainly an adrenergic response) and learn to make decisions accordingly. Damage to the orbitofrontal cortex in adulthood as well as in early life (Anderson et al., 1999) disrupts the capacity to make these physiological responses and impairs this ability to make crucial social decisions.

It is tempting to speculate that evolution did not select and shape the dopaminergic system solely to convey pleasure but instead utilized the "pleasure principle" to gain better survival chances and effective reproduction rates in an ever-changing environment. The radical changes between the conditions in which the human brain evolved (Wilson, 1993) and the conditions in which it now lives might contribute to explaining why clinicians more frequently treat issues concerning a growing sense of despair and anhedonia (Fig. 1-5).

References

Ahn S, Phillips AG (1999). Dopaminergic correlates of sensory-specific satiety in the medial prefrontal cortex and nucleus accumbens of the rat. *J Neurosci* 19,RC29.

Anderson SW, Bechara A, Damasio H, et al. (1999). Impairment of social and moral behavior related to early damage in human prefrontal cortex. *Nature Neurosci* 11,1032–1037.

Bassareo V, Di Chiara G (1997). Differential influence of associative and nonassociative learning mechanisms on the responsiveness of prefrontal and accumbal dopamine transmission to food stimuli in rats fed ad libitum. *J Neurosci* 17,851–861.

Berger B (1992). Dopaminergic innervation of the frontal cerebral cortex. Evolutionary trends and functional implications. In: *Advances in Neurology*, Chauvel P, Delgado-Escueta G, et al., eds. New York: Raven, vol. 57, pp. 525–544.

Berger B, Gaspar P, Verney C (1991). Dopaminergic innervation of the cerebral cortex: unexpected differences between rodents and primates. *Trends Neurosci* 14,21–27 [erratum (1991) 14,119].

Berridge KC, Robinson TE (1998). What is the role of dopamine in reward: hedonic impact, reward learning, or incentive salience? *Brain Res Rev* 28,309–369.

Bertler A, Rosengren E (1959). Occurrence and distribution of catecholamine in brain. *Acta Physiol Scand* 47,350–361.

Bertolucci-D'Angio M, Serrano A, Scatton B (1990). Mesocorticolimbic dopaminergic systems and emotional states. *J Neurosci Meth* 34,135–142

Blackburn JR, Pfaus JG, Phillips AG (1992). Dopamine functions in appetitive and defensive behaviors. *Progr Neurobiol* 39, 247–279.

Camps M, Kelly PH, Palacios JM (1990). Autoradiographic localization of dopamine D1 and D2 receptors in the brain of several mammalian species. *J Neural Transm Gent Sect* 80,105–127.

Cardinaud B, Sugamori KS, Coudouel S, et al. (1997). Early emergence of three dopamine D1 receptor subtypes in vertebrates. Molecular phylogenetic, pharmacological, and functional criteria defining D1A, D1B, and D1C receptors in European eel *Anguilla anguilla. J Biol Chem* 272,2778–2787.

Cavazzuti E, Bertolini A, Vergoni AV, et al. (1999). l-Sulpiride, at a low, non-neuroleptic dose, prevents conditioned fear stress-induced freezing behavior in rats. *Psychopharmacology (Berl)* 143,20–23.

Cenci MA, Kalén P, Mandel RJ, et al. (1992). Regional differences in the regulation of dopamine and noradrenaline release in medial frontal cortex, nucleus accumbens and caudate-putamen: a microdialysis study in the rat. *Brain Res* 581,217–228.

Changeux JP (1983). *L'Homme Neuronal.* Paris: Fayard.

Damasio AR (1996). The somatic marker hypothesis and the possible functions of the prefrontal cortex. *Philos Trans R Soc Lond B Biol Sci* 351,1413–1420.

D'Angio M, Serrano A, Driscoll P, et al. (1988). Stressful environmental stimuli increase extracellular DOPAC levels in the prefrontal cortex of hypoemotional (Roman high-avoidance) but not hyperemotional (Roman low-avoidance) rats. An in vivo voltametric study. *Brain Res* 451,237–247.

Darwin C (1859). *The Origin of Species by Means of Natural Selection.* London: John Murray, p. 488.

Davis M (1992). The role of the amygdala in conditioned fear. In: *The Amygdala: Neurobiological Aspects of Emotion, Memory, and Mental Dysfunction*, Aggleton JP, ed. New York: Wiley, pp. 255–305.

Deutch AY, Clark WA, Roth RH (1990). Prefrontal cortical dopamine depletion enhances the responsiveness of mesolimbic dopamine neurons to stress. *Brain Res* 521,311–315.

Divac I (1995). Monotremunculi and brain evolution. *Trends Neurosi* 18,2–4.

Fadda P, Martellotta MC, Gessa GL, et al. (1993). Dopamine and opioid interactions in sleep deprivation. *Progr Neuropsychopharmacol Biol Psychiatry* 17,269–278.

Fibiger HC (1987). Role of catecholamine transmitters in reward systems: implications for the neurobiology of affect. In: *Brain Reward Systems and Abuse*, Oreland E, ed. New York: New York Press, pp. 61–74.

Finlay BL, Darlington RB (1995). Linked regularities in the development and evolution of mammalian brains. *Science* 268,1578–1584.

Finlay JM, Zigmond MJ (1997). The effect of stress on central dopaminergic neurons: possible clinical implications. *Neurochem Res* 22,1387–1394.

Fiorino DF, Coury A, Phillips AG (1997). Dynamic changes in nucleus accumbens dopamine efflux during the Coolidge effect in male rats. *J Neurosci* 17,4849–4855.

Friedhoff AJ, Carr KD, Uysal S, et al. (1995). Repeated inescapable stress produces a neuroleptic-like effect on the conditioned avoidance response. *Neuropsychopharmacology* 13,129–138.

Fryxell KJ (1995). The evolutionary divergence of neurotransmitter receptors and second-messenger pathways. *J Mol Evol* 41,85–97.

Gelowitz DL, Kokkinidis L (1999). Enhanced amygdala kindling after electrical stimulation of the ventral

tegmental area: implications for fear and anxiety. *J Neurosci* 19,RC41.
Gendreau PL, Gariépy JL, Petitto JM, et al. (1997). D1 dopamine receptor mediation of social and nonsocial emotional reactivity in mice: effects of housing and strain difference in motor activity. *Behav Neurosci* 111,424–434.
Gessa GL, Pani L, Fadda P, et al. (1995). Sleep deprivation in the rat: an animal model of mania. *Eur J Neuropsychopharmacol Suppl* 5,89–93.
Greenfield PM (1994). Language tools and brain: the ontogeny and phylogeny of hierarchically organized sequential behavior. *Behav Brain Sci* 17,357–365 (commentary).
Griffiths J, Shanks N, Anisman H (1992). Strain-specific alterations in consumption of a palatable diet following repeated stressor exposure. *Pharmacol Biochem Behav* 42,219–227.
Haber SN, Fudge JL (1997) The interface between dopamine neurons and the amygdala: implications for schizophrenia. *Schizophr Bull* 23,471–482.
Jacobs GH, Neitz M, Deegan JF, et al. (1996). Trichromatic colour vision in New World monkeys. *Nature* 382,156–158.
Kaneyuki H, Yokoo H, Tsuda A, et al. (1991). Psychological stress increases dopamine turnover selectively in mesoprefrontal dopamine neurons of rats: reversal by diazepam. *Brain Res* 557,154–161.
Le Moal M, Simon H (1991). Mesocorticolimbic dopaminergic network: functional and regulatory roles. *Physiol Rev* 71,155–234.
Lett BT, Grant VL (1989). The hedonic effects of amphetamine and pentobarbital in goldfish. *Pharmacol Biochem Behav* 32,355–356.
Louilot A, Taghzouti K, Simon H, et al. (1989). Limbic system, basal ganglia, and dopaminergic neurons. Executive and regulatory neurons and their role in the organization of behavior. *Brain Behav Evol* 33,157–161.
Mac Lean PD (1985). Brain evolution relating to family, play and the separation call. *Arch Gen Psychiatry* 42,405–417.
McGuire MT, Troisi A (1998). *Darwinian Psychiatry*. New York: Oxford University Press.
Meiergerd SM, Schenk JO, Sorg BA (1997). Repeated cocaine and stress increase dopamine clearance in the rat medial prefrontal cortex. *Brain Res* 773,203–207.
Murphy BL, Arnsten AF, Goldman Rakic PS, et al. (1996a). Increased dopamine turnover in the prefrontal cortex impairs spatial working memory performance in rats and monkeys. *Proc Natl Acad Sci USA* 93,1325–1329.
Murphy BL, Arnsten AF, Jentsch JD, et al. (1996b). Dopamine and spatial working memory in rats and monkeys: pharmacological reversal of stress-induced impairment. *J Neurosci* 16,7768–7775.
Nader K, LeDoux J (1999). The dopaminergic modulation of fear: quinpirole impairs the recall of emotional memories in rats. *Behav Neurosci* 113,152–165.
Nesse RM, Berridge KC (1997). Psychoactive drugs in evolutionary perspective. *Science* 278,63–66.
Nesse RM, Williams GC (1994). *Why We Get Sick*. New York: Random House.
Palladini G, Ruggeri S, Stocchi F, et al. (1996). A pharmacological study of cocaine activity in planaria. *Comp Biochem Physiol C Pharmacol Toxicol Endocrinol* 115,41–45.
Pani AK, Anctil M. (1994). Evidence for biosynthesis and catabolism of monoamines in the sea pansy *Renilla koellikeri (cnidaria). Neurochem Int* 25,465–474.
Pani L, Porcella A., Gessa GL (2000). The role of stress in the pathophysiology of the dopaminergic system. *Mol Psychol* 5,14–21.
Panksepp J (1998). *Affective Neuroscience: the Foundations of Human and Animal Emotions*. New York: Oxford University Press, pp. 53–55.
Phillips AG, Atkinson LJ, Blackburn JR, et al. (1993). Increased extracellular dopamine in the nucleus accumbens of the rat elicited by a conditioned stimulus for food: an electrochemical study. *Can J Physiol Pharmacol* 71,387–393.
Povinelli DJ, Preuss TM (1995). Theory of mind: evolutionary history of a cognitive specialization. *Trends Neurosci* 18,418–424.
Rolls ET (1999). *The Brain and Emotions*. New York: Oxford University Press.
Rolls ET, Baylis LL (1994). Gustatory, olfactory, and visual convergence within the primate orbitofrontal cortex. *J Neurosci* 14,5437–5452.
Rolls ET, Rolls JH (1997). Olfactory sensory-specific satiety in humans. *Physiol Behav* 3,461–473.
Sano I, Gamo T, Kakimoto Y, et al. (1959). Distribution of catechol compounds in human brain. *Biochem Biophys Acta* 32,586–588.
Sato Y, Kumamoto Y (1992). Psychological stress and sexual behavior in male rats. II. Effect of psychological stress on dopamine and its metabolites in the critical brain areas mediating sexual behavior. *Nippon Hinyokika Gakkai Zasshi* 83,212–219.

Sirigu A, Zalla T, Pillon B, et al. (1995). Selective impairments in managerial knowledge following pre-frontal cortex damage. *Cortex* 31,301–316.

Sorg BA, Steketee JD (1992). Mechanisms of cocaine-induced sensitization. *Progr Neuropsychopharmacol Biol Psychiatry* 16,1003–1012.

Steketee JD, Kalivas PW (1991). Sensitization to psychostimulants and stress after injection of pertussis toxin into the A10 dopamine region. *J Pharmacol Exp Ther* 259,916–924.

Sugiura K, Yoshimura H, Yokoyama M (1997). An animal model of copulatory disorder induced by social stress in male mice: effects of apomorphine and L-dopa. *Psychopharmacol Berl* 133,249–255.

Vincent JD, Cardinaud B, Vernier P (1998). Evolution of monoamine receptors and the origin of motivational and emotional systems in vertebrates. *Bull Acad Natl Med* 182,1505–1514.

Walker RJ, Brooks HL, Holden-Dye L (1996). Evolution and overview of classical transmitter molecules and their receptors. *Parasitol Suppl* 113,3–33.

Wang CT, Huang RL, Tai MY, et al. (1995). Dopamine release in the nucleus accumbens during sexual behavior in prenatally stressed adult male rats. *Neurosci Lett* 200,29–32.

Watanabe M (1996). Reward expectancy in primate prefrontal neurons. *Nature* 382,629–632.

Wehr TA (1998). Effect of seasonal changes in daylength on human neuroendocrine function. *Horm Res* 49,118–124.

Wehr TA, Giesen HA, Moul DE, et al. (1995). Suppression of men's responses to seasonal changes in day length by modern artificial lighting. *Am J Physiol* 269,173–178.

Wilson DR (1993). Evolutionary epidemiology. Darwinian theory in the service of medicine and psychiatry. *Acta Biotheor* 41,205–218.

Wise RA (1989). The brain and reward. In: *The Neuropharmacological Basis of Reward*, Liebman J, Cooper SJ, eds. Oxford: Oxford University Press, pp. 248–262.

Zahrt J, Taylor JR, Mathew RG, et al. (1997). Supranormal stimulation of D1 dopamine receptors in the rodent prefrontal cortex impairs spatial working memory performance. *J Neurosci* 17,8528–8535.

2.

Neurobiological Features of Dopamine D2 Receptor Knockout Mice

Carole Mathis, Shiro Aoyama, Minoru Kobayashi, and Emiliana Borrelli

Dysfunctions of the dopaminergic system are involved in several human brain disorders. Neuropathologies such as Parkinson's disease and schizophrenia share alterations of dopaminergic transmission.

In Parkinson's disease the content of dopamine, norepinephrine, and serotonin is lower than normal (Hornykiewicz, 1966). However, dopamine is the most drastically reduced; this was the first finding to show an association between dopamine levels and a brain disease. Alteration of this neurotransmitter in other brain disorders, including depression, schizophrenia, and dementia, has been subsequently documented.

Dopamine is synthesized by mesencephalic neurons in the substantia nigra and ventral tegmental area (Graybiel, 1990). The substantia nigra and ventral tegmental area belong to the complex neural network that constitutes the basal ganglia. Three pathways arise from these locations: the nigrostriatal, mesocorticolimbic, and tuberoinfundibular. In this way dopamine affects various functions that range from the control of movements and hormone secretion to motivated and emotional behaviors (Jackson and Westlind-Daniesson, 1994).

The nigrostriatal pathway is involved in the control of movement and sensorimotor coordination. Indeed degeneration of these neurons leads to Parkinson's disease (Hornykiewicz, 1966; Seeman and Niznik, 1990), which is characterized by akinesia, bradykinesia, and resting tremors. The mesocorticolimbic pathway has influence on learning, memory, and motivated behaviors. This pathway is also involved in the establishment of the rewarding properties of drugs of abuse. It is well-established that drug intake leads to an increased release of dopamine in areas of the limbic system. The tuberoinfundibular pathway participates in control of the synthesis and release of pituitary hormones.

The dopaminergic transmission is transduced by membrane receptors of the seven transmembrane domain G-protein coupled family, whose activation leads to the stimulation or inhibition of intracellular second messengers. Two subclasses of dopamine receptors have been defined: 1) D1-like receptors comprising D1 (Dearry et al., 1990; Zhou et al., 1990) and D5 (Grandy et al., 1991; Sunahara et al., 1991) and 2) D2-like receptors comprising D2 (Bunzow et al., 1988; Dal Toso et al., 1989), D3 (Sokoloff et al., 1990), and D4 (Van Tol et al., 1991). D2-like receptors, in addition to inhibiting cAMP levels, might also couple to other cellular effectors (Picetti et al., 1997).

D1 and D2 are the most widely expressed, whereas D3, D4, and D5 receptors present a restricted pattern. D1 and D2 receptors are strongly expressed in the striatum by medium spiny neurons. Inside this structure, D1 and D2 receptors have been reported to be expressed in different subsets of neurons (Gerfen, 1992; Hersch et al., 1995; Yung et al., 1995). The presence of both receptors in the same neurons has been reported (Aizman et al., 2000; Ariano et al., 1997; Meador-Woodruff et al., 1991; Surmeier et al. 1996). Two efferent pathways arise from the striatum that project back to the substantia nigra: the striatonigral or direct pathway and the striatopallidal or indirect pathway. Striatonigral neurons contain D1 receptors, whereas striatopallidal neurons express D2 receptors.

Targeted mutagenesis of different components of the dopaminergic system has been used to finely elucidate the importance of each component in vivo (Accili et al., 1996; Baik et al., 1995; Drago et al., 1994; Giros et al., 1996; Xu et al., 1994a; Zhou and Palmiter, 1995). These studies have had and will have much impact on our knowledge about the importance of each gene composing the dopaminergic system.

DOPAMINE D2 RECEPTORS

D2S is the first dopamine D2 receptor cDNA isolated (Bunzow et al., 1988). This cDNA encodes for a protein of 415 amino acids containing seven stretches of hydrophobic amino acids, a classical feature of seven transmembrane domain G-protein coupled receptors. Transfected into mammalian cells, this cDNA displayed pharmacological features typical of the native striatal dopamine D2 receptor. Afterward, this cDNA was isolated from many other species including human. The human homologue is 96% identical to the rat receptor, with one amino acid deletion (Dal Toso et al., 1989). In situ hybridization analysis showed that the D2 receptor is highly expressed in the caudate putamen, nucleus accumbens, and olfactory tubercules. D2 receptor mRNAs are also highly expressed in the dopaminergic cell bodies of neurons within the substantia nigra pars compacta and ventral tegmental area, which suggests an autoreceptor role for the D2 receptor.

Later a novel cDNA was isolated—D2L. D2L is identical to D2S except that it contains an additional 29 amino acid in the putative third intracellular loop. D2L and D2S are generated from the same gene by alternative splicing (Dal Toso et al., 1989; Giros et al., 1989). D2L has a length of 444 amino acids in rat (Chio et al., 1990; Monsma et al., 1989) and mouse (Montmayeur et al., 1991) and 443 in human (Dal Toso et al., 1989; Giros et al., 1989; Grandy et al., 1989). Both isoforms have similar localization and pharmacological profile (Dal Toso et al., 1989; Giros et al., 1989; Monsma et al., 1990; Montmayeur et al., 1991). D2L is the most abundantly expressed, although the ratio of the two isoforms has been found inverted in the mesencephalon (Montmayeur et al., 1991). This underlies the possibility that the shorter isoform, D2S, might perform autoreceptor functions in vivo.

The 29-amino acid insert confers on D2L a G-protein coupling specificity different from D2S. We have shown that D2L and D2S inhibit adenylyl cyclase differently when transfected in cells that do not contain the α_2-subunit of the inhibitory G-protein (Montmayeur and Borrelli, 1991). Specifically D2L requires the presence of α_2-subunit of the inhibitory G-protein to inhibit adenylate cyclase more potently (Montmayeur et al., 1993). This indicates that the insert is involved in specifying the interaction of D2L with the α_2-subunit of the inhibitory G-protein; however, even in its absence this receptor can interact, although less efficiently, with other G-proteins.

Site-directed mutagenesis in the D2L insert was performed to identify the residues conferring the α_2-subunit of the inhibitory G-protein coupling specificity (Guiramand et al. 1995). The conversion of aspartate-249 into valine resulted in a mutated receptor that is not more dependent on the α_2-subunit of the inhibitory G-protein to efficiently inhibit adenylyl cyclase. This demonstrates a key role of the 29-amino acid insertion in the selection of the G-protein with which D2 receptor isoforms interact. These data suggest that the differential G-protein coupling characteristics between the two isoforms underlie functional differences and distinct regulations of the signaling pathways activated by D2L and D2S in vivo.

The cloned D2 receptor on ligand binding leads to inhibition of adenylyl cyclase as reported (Cote et al., 1983). However, this receptor has also been shown to be negatively coupled to phosphoinositide hydrolysis and Ca^{2+} mobilization (Picetti et al., 1997). Inhibition of phosphoinositide hydrolysis could explain the decrease of Ca^{2+} levels observed in pituitary cells after dopamine administration (Vallar and Meldolesi, 1989).

A promoter with characteristics of a housekeeping gene controls transcription of the D2 receptor gene. Nonetheless the D2 gene has a specific and restricted pattern of expression that underlies a strict regulation by cell-specific transcription factors. We have identified a functional retinoic acid responsive element in the D2 receptor promoter (Samad et al., 1997). Retinoic acid regulates transcription through the activation of nuclear receptor proteins that bind DNA.

Analysis of retinoid acid receptor-null mice supports our finding and shows that in these animals D2 receptor expression is reduced with a concomitant impairment of locomotor functions (Krezel et al., 1998). This finding assigns retinoic acid a central role in the control of gene expression in the central nervous system.

KNOCKOUT MICE AS MODEL SYSTEMS TO STUDY NEUROTRANSMITTER FUNCTIONS IN VIVO

The gene targeting technique has made defined alterations to genes possible in vivo (Bradley, 1987). Mutated genes are introduced into mouse embryonic stem cells that can be maintained indefinitely in culture in an undifferentiated state. However, upon return to the environment of the early embryo, these cells might contribute to the formation of the resulting chimeric animals. This way, any genetic alteration introduced in these cells can be transferred to recipient animals, and lines of mice bearing these mutations can be established. By using this approach, dopamine receptors in mutant mice have been generated (Accili et al., 1996; Baik et al., 1995; Drago et al., 1994; Xu et al., 1994b, 1997). These animals represent a great tool to discriminate the function of each receptor in vivo. In addition, the bias created by the use of other model systems in which either chemical or mechanical lesions are induced can be overcome, which, although useful, can be nonselective. Similarly the use of ligands to test the function of receptors in vivo presents the bias of drugs acting at multiple receptors with the consequent lack of specificity.

D2 RECEPTOR-DEFICIENT MICE

The generation of mice lacking the expression of dopamine D2 receptors (Baik et al., 1995) results in motor behavior impairment of mutant mice. Slower movements and abnormal gait with sprawled hind legs are characteristic. The motor behavior of D2 receptor mutants was analyzed and quantified using several behavioral tests, such as the open field ring test and rotarod test. In all tests D2 receptor mutants failed to behave as their wild-type littermates, thus indicating that loss of D2 receptor function greatly impairs locomotion (Baik et al. 1995).

D2 receptor-deficient mice show a slight reduction of their body weight resulting from a 10–15% reduction in water and food intake, which shows an involvement of D2 receptor in the control of feeding behavior. Absence of D2 receptors cannot be compensated by other members of the dopamine receptor's family, as established by studies at the mRNA and protein levels. In the striatum of D2 receptor mutant mice a strong elevation of the enkephalin levels was observed. This was paralleled by a slight decrease of substance P expression, whereas the level of expression of dynorphin seemed to be unaltered (Baik et al., 1995). These striking findings are reminiscent of the modifications observed in the striatum of 6-hydroxydopamine lesioned animals (Gerfen et al., 1990). Thus reduction of dopamine obtained in these lesioned animals seems to preferentially affect D2 receptor-mediated functions.

The search for compensatory changes in the expression level of components of systems related to the dopaminergic showed an increase of expression, at the cortical level, of glutamic acid decarboxylase (GAD). This enzyme is the limiting enzyme in GABA synthesis. Accordingly, D2 receptor antagonist-induced catalepsy is mainly mediated via activation of the striatopallidal GABA pathways (Ogren and Fuxe, 1988); in addition, chronic administration of the D2 receptor antagonists induces an increase in striatal GAD mRNA levels (Laprade and Soghomonian, 1995). We suggest that increased GAD expression in the cortex of D2 receptor-deficient mice might represent a compensatory mechanism to overcome the increased stimulation of the striatopallidal pathway. However, this hypothesis must be confirmed by appropriate experiments.

D2 RECEPTOR IS THE DOPAMINERGIC AUTORECEPTOR

Among the D2-like family the D2 receptor is the most abundantly expressed in the substantia nigra and ventral tegmental area. D3 receptors share a common presynaptic localization in dopaminergic neurons with D2 receptors (Levesque et al., 1992). However, D2 are the most abundant receptors in these cells. Therefore to establish whether the presynaptic function of D2 receptors could be compensated by D3 receptors we recorded the firing of dopaminergic neurons in the ventral tegmental area and substantia nigra pars compacta from D2 receptor-deficient mice and compared it with recordings from wild-type littermates.

In contrast to recordings from wild-type animals, dopamine (10–100 mM) and quinpirole (1–3 mM) applied on dopaminergic cells recorded from D2 receptor-deficient mice sections caused neither a hyperpolarization nor an inhibition of the spontaneous firing (Mercuri et al., 1997). Preliminary results, obtained by microdialysis and voltammetry on D2 receptor mutants, agree with electrophysiological studies on a clear autoreceptor role for D2 receptors. Thus despite the presence of D2 and D3 receptors in substantia nigra and ventral tegmental area a total loss of dopaminergic inhibition was observed in sections from D2 receptor-deficient mice. This shows that D2 is the receptor mediating this function in the substantia nigra and ventral tegmental area. However, an effect of D3 receptors on a restricted number of neurons cannot be excluded.

Reduced fertility was observed in the breeding of homozygous D2 receptor-deficient mice, indicating alterations of the hypothalamic-pituitary-gonadal axis. We have more recently assessed that D2 receptor-deficient mice have high levels of circulating prolactin, which may be the cause of fertility problems (Saiardi et al., 1997). In addition, large hyperplasias are found in pituitaries of D2 receptor-deficient mice. These findings suggest a role for D2 receptors not only in the regulation of prolactin synthesis and release but also in the control of pituitary cell proliferation.

The phenotypic changes observed in D2 receptor-deficient animals support an essential role for these receptors in the dopaminergic control of physiological function connected to movement and regulation of hormone secretion.

ANIMAL MODELS OF NEUROPATHOLOGIES

The diagnosis of Parkinson's disease is classically confirmed by the degeneration of dopaminergic neurons in the substantia nigra. Destruction of the nigrostriatal pathway and the consequent decrease in striatal dopamine are the most distinctive biochemical characteristics. The activities of tyrosine hydroxylase and DOPA decarboxylase, both involved in dopamine synthesis, are decreased in the substantia nigra and striatum (Agid et al., 1989).

A reduction of DAT binding sites in parkinsonian postmortem brains has also been reported (Niznik et al., 1991). However, the dopaminergic neural system does not degenerate as a whole; the nigrostriatal pathway, for example, is more severely affected than the mesocortical or the mesolimbic systems. Within the striatum, the putamen is most severely affected; given the role of the striatum in the control of motor function, this explains the observed movement disorders.

Normal movements result from a coordinated balance of cortical and thalamic excitation of the striatonigral and striatopallidal pathways that regulate the tonic activity of the substantia nigra pars reticulata neurons. Although neural control of movement also involves other neural circuits, when the dopaminergic system is deregulated the control of coordinated movement is lost. Genetic ablation of D2 receptor results in parkinsonian-like locomotor phenotype. We are aware that the mechanisms underlying Parkinson's and D2 receptor-deficient mice symptoms are not identical; however, the similitude of the locomotor phenotype is intriguing. It suggests that lack of dopamine in Parkinson's disease might particularly affect D2 receptor function in the basal ganglia circuitry and that the D2 receptor is key in motor skills control. Indeed, observations that D2 receptor-deficient mice have impaired locomotion are consistent not only with akinesia in Parkinson's disease but also with hypoactivity resulting from antagonist blockade of dopamine receptors.

Recall that D1 receptor knockout mice display either normal (Drago et al., 1994) or mild hyperactivity (Xu et al., 1994a) in contrast to D2 receptor-deficient mice (Baik et al., 1995). Moreover in dopamine-deficient mice a significant improvement of locomotion and stereotypes was obtained when they were treated with low doses of D2 receptor agonist, indicating that D1 receptor stimulation is not required for D2 receptor-mediated behaviors. Thus we believe that a fine characterization of D2 receptor-deficient mice will help understand the basal mechanisms responsible for the movement disorders of Parkinson's disease. These mice might be used to test alternative drugs that can rescue the locomotor phenotype. In addition, a novel specific D2 receptor agonist may provide a more efficient therapeutic strategy to relieve parkinsonian movement disorders.

We have recently shown that a novel adenosine A2A selective antagonist, KW-6002, can rescue the phenotype of D2 receptor-deficient mice. Results strongly support A2A antagonists as potential alternative therapy for dopamine deficiencies. Blockade of A2A receptors in D2 receptor-null mice reestablishes their locomotor activity and coordination of movements (Aoyama et al., 2000). In addition, blockade lowers enkephalin levels to normal. This means that A2A receptors can regulate, in the absence of D2 receptors, locomotor activity, coordination of movement, and gene expression. These results encourage the possibility of A2A antagonists for treatment of Parkinson's disease as a potential nondopaminergic approach either alone or as an adjunct to levodopa or dopamine agonist therapy.

The generation of knockout mice has added novel tools to study the function of different proteins in vivo. Each mutant represents a great tool to analyze the involvement of proteins in the control of different physiological functions and, as is the case for dopamine receptors, to test novel pharmacological therapies in vivo.

REFERENCES

Accili D, Fishburn CS, Drago J, et al. (1996). A targeted mutation of the D3 dopamine receptor gene is associated with hyperactivity in mice. *Proc Natl Acad Sci USA* 93,1945–1949.

Agid Y, Cervera P, Hirsch E, et al. (1989). Biochemistry of Parkinson's disease 28 years later: a critical review *Mov Disord* 4,S126–S144.

Aizman O, Brismar H, Uhlen P, et al. (2000). Anatomical and physiological evidence for D1 and D2 dopamine receptor colocalization in neostriatal neurons. *Nature Neurosci* 3,226–230.

Aoyama S, Kase H, Borrelli E (2000). Rescue of locomotor impairment in dopamine D2 receptor deficient mice by an adenosine A2A receptor antagonist. *J Neurosci* 20,5848–5852.

Ariano MA, Larson ER, Noblett KL, et al. (1997). Coexpression of striatal dopamine receptor subtypes and excitatory amino acid subunits. *Synapse* 26,400–414.

Baik J-H, Picetti R, Saiardi A, et al. (1995). Parkinsonian-like locomotor impairment in mice lacking dopamine D2 receptors. *Nature* 377,424–428.

Bradley A (1987). In: *Teratocarcinomas and Embryonic Stem Cells: a Practical Approach*, Robertson EJ, ed. Oxford: IRL Press, pp. 113–151.

Bunzow JR, Van Tol HHM, Grandy DK, et al. (1988). Cloning and expression of a rat D2 dopamine receptor. *Nature* 336,783–787.

Chio CL, Hess GF, Graham RS, et al. (1990). A second molecular form of D2 dopamine receptor in rat and bovine caudate nucleus. *Nature* 343,266–269.

Cote TE, Frey EA, Grewe CW, et al. (1983). Evidence that the D2 dopamine receptor in the intermediate lobe of the rat pituitary gland is associated with an inhibitory guanyl nucleotide component. *J Neurol Trans Suppl* 18,139–147.

Dal Toso R, Sommer B, Ewert M, et al. (1989). The dopamine D2 receptor: two molecular forms generated by alternative splicing. *EMBO J* 8,4025–4034.

Dearry A, Gingrich JA, Falardeau P, et al. (1990). Molecular cloning and expression of the gene for a human D1 dopamine receptor. *Nature* 347,72–75.

Drago J, Gerfen CR, Lachowicz JE, et al. (1994). Altered striatal function in a mutant mouse lacking D1A dopamine receptor. *Proc Natl Acad Sci USA* 91,12564–12568.

Gerfen CR (1992). The neostriatal mosaic: multiple levels of compartmental organization. *Trends Neurosci* 15,133–139.

Gerfen CR, Engber TM, Mahan LC, et al. (1990). D1 and D2 dopamine receptor-regulated gene expression of striatonigral and striatopallidal neurons. *Science* 250,1429–1432.

Giros B, Jaber M, Jones SR, et al. (1996). Hyperlocomotion and indifference to cocaine and amphetamine in mice lacking the dopamine transporter. *Nature* 379,606–612.

Giros B, Sokoloff P, Martres MP, et al. (1989). Alternative splicing directs the expression of two D2 dopamine receptor isoforms. *Nature* 342,923–926.

Grandy DK, Marchionni MA, Makam H, et al. (1989). Cloning of the cDNA and gene for a human D2 dopamine receptor. *Proc Natl Acad Sci USA* 86,9762–9766.

Grandy DK, Zhang YA, Bouvier C, et al. (1991). Multiple human D5 dopamine receptor genes: a functional receptor and two pseudogenes. *Proc Natl Acad Sci USA* 88,9175–9179.

Graybiel AM (1990). Neurotransmitters and neuromodulators in the basal ganglia. *Trends Neurosci* 13,244–254.

Guiramand J, Montmayeur J-P, Ceraline J, et al. (1995). Alternative splicing of the dopamine D2 receptor directs specificity of coupling to G-proteins. *J Biol Chem* 270,7354–7358.

Hersch SM, Ciliax BJ, Gutekunst CA, et al. (1995). Electron microscopic analysis of D1 and D2 dopamine receptor proteins in the dorsal striatum and their synaptic relationships with motor corticostriatal afferents. *J Neurosci* 15,5222–5237.

Hornykiewicz O (1966). Dopamine and brain function. *Pharmacol Rev* 18,925–964.

Jackson DJ, Westlind-Daniesson A (1994). Dopamine receptors: molecular biology, biochemistry and behavioural aspects. *Pharmacol Ther* 64,291–369.

Krezel W, Ghyselinck N, Samad AT, et al. (1998). Impaired locomotion and dopamine signaling in retinoid receptor mutant mice. *Science* 279,863–867.

Laprade N, Soghomonian JJ (1995). Differential regulation of mRNA levels encoding for the two isoforms of glutamate decarboxylase (GAD65 and GAD67) by dopamine receptors in the rat striatum. *Brain Res Mol Brain Res* 34,65–74.

Levesque D, Diaz J, Pilon C, et al. (1992). Identification, characterization, and localization of the dopamine D3 receptor in rat brain using 7-[^{3}H]hydroxy-N,N-di-n-propyl-2-aminotetralin. *Proc Natl Acad Sci USA* 89,8155–8159.

Meador-Woodruff JH, Mansour A, Healy DJ, et al. (1991). Comparison of the distributions of D1 and D2 dopamine receptor mRNAs in rat brain. *Neuropsychopharmacology* 5,231–242.

Mercuri NB, Saiardi A, Bonci A, et al. (1997). Loss of autoreceptor function in dopaminergic neurons from dopamine D2 receptor deficient mice. *Neuroscience* 79,323–327.

Monsma FJ, Mahan LC, McVittie LD, et al. (1990). Molecular cloning and expression of a D1 dopamine receptor linked to adenylate cyclase activation. *Proc Natl Acad Sci USA* 87,6723–6727.

Montmayeur JP, Bausero P, Amlaiky N, et al. (1991). Differential expression of the mouse D2 dopamine receptor isoforms. *FEBS Lett* 278,239–243.

Montmayeur J-P, Borrelli E (1991). Transcription mediated by a cAMP-responsive promoter element is reduced upon activation of dopamine D2 receptors. *Proc Natl Acad Sci USA* 88,3135–3139.

Montmayeur J-P, Guiramand J, Borrelli E (1993). Preferential coupling between dopamine D2 receptors and G-proteins. *Mol Endocrinol* 7,161–170.
Niznik HB, Fogel EF, Fassos FF, et al. (1991). The dopamine transporter is absent in parkinsonian putamen and reduced in the caudate nucleus. *J Neurochem* 56,192–198.
Ogren SO, Fuxe K (1988). D1 and D2 receptor antagonists induce catalepsy via different efferent striatal pathways. *Neurosci Lett* 85,333–338.
Picetti R, Saiardi A, Abdel Samad T, et al. (1997). Dopamine D2 receptors in signal transduction and behavior. *Crit Rev Neurobiol* 11,121–142.
Saiardi A, Bozzi Y, Baik J-H, et al. (1997). Antiproliferative role of dopamine: loss of D2 receptors causes hormonal dysfunction and pituitary hyperplasia. *Neuron* 19,115–126.
Samad AT, Krezel W, Chambon P, et al. (1997). Regulation of dopaminergic pathways by retinoid activation of the D2 receptor promoter by members of the retinoic acid receptor-retinoid X receptor family. *Proc Natl Acad USA* 94,14349–14354.
Seeman P, Niznik HB (1990). Dopamine receptors and transporters in Parkinson's disease and schizophrenia. *FASEB J* 4,2737–2744.
Sokoloff P, Giros B, Martres MP, et al. (1990). Molecular cloning and characterization of a novel dopamine receptor (D3) as a target for neuroleptics. *Nature* 347,146–151.
Sunahara RK, Guan HC, O'Dowd BF, et al. (1991). Cloning of the gene for a human dopamine D5 receptor with higher affinity for dopamine than D1. *Nature* 350,614–619.
Surmeier DJ, W.J., S., Yan Z (1996). Coordinated expression of dopamine receptors in neostriatal medium spiny neurons. *J Neurosci* 16,6579–6591.
Vallar L, Meldolesi J (1989). Mechanisms of signal transduction at the dopamine D2 receptor. *Trends Pharmacol Sci* 10,74–77.
Van Tol HH, Bunzow JR, Guan H-C, et al. (1991). Cloning of the gene for a human dopamine D4 receptor with high affinity for the antipsychotic clozapine. *Nature* 350,610–614.
Xu M, Hu XT, Cooper DC, et al. (1994a). Dopamine D1 receptor mutant mice are deficient in striatal expression of dynorphin and in dopamine-mediated behavioral responses. *Cell* 79,945–955.
Xu M, Koeltzow TE, Santiago GT, et al. (1997). Dopamine D3 receptor mutant mice exhibit increased behavioral sensitivity to concurrent stimulation of D1 and D2 receptors. *Neuron* 19,837–848.
Xu M, Moratalla R, Gold LH, et al. (1994b). Elimination of cocaine-induced hyperactivity and dopamine-mediated neurophysiological effects in dopamine D1 receptor mutant mice. *Cell* 79,729–742.
Yung KK, Bolam JP, Smith AD, et al. (1995). Immunocytochemical localization of D1 and D2 dopamine receptors in the basal ganglia of the rat: light and electron microscopy. *Neuroscience* 65,709–730.
Zhou Q-Y, Grandy DK, Thambi L, et al. (1990). Cloning and expression of human and rat D1 dopamine receptors. *Nature* 347,76–80.
Zhou Q-Y, Palmiter RD (1995). Dopamine-deficient mice are severely hypoactive, adipsic, and aphagic. *Cell* 83,1197–1209.

3.

Differential Effects of Typical and Atypical Antipsychotics on Neurotransmitter Receptor Expression and Function

Robert E. Smith, Daniel J. Healy, and James H. Meador-Woodruff

ABSTRACT

Despite 40 years of investigation, the mechanisms of action of antipsychotic medications are not well-known. The initial characterization of antipsychotics revealed modulatory effects on dopaminergic pathways, but recent work has indicated effects on multiple neurotransmitter systems. The discovery of atypical antipsychotics highlights the putative role of nondopaminergic receptors in the pathophysiology of schizophrenia. However, disagreement remains over what differentiates typical and atypical antipsychotics. In this review, we focus on the distinct patterns of neuroanatomical adaptations of dopamine, serotonin, glutamate, γ-aminobutyric acid, and cholinergic receptors induced by typical and atypical antipsychotics. We critically review reported pharmacological differences between typical and atypical antipsychotics and their effects on the region- or circuit-specific expression of certain receptor subtypes. Where relevant, molecular signaling processes are linked to both therapeutic and adverse effects of antipsychotic medications. Finally, we discuss prevailing hypotheses regarding the etiology of the clinical efficacy and adverse effects of antipsychotic medications at the molecular level.

INTRODUCTION

Dysfunctional dopaminergic neurotransmission has been a favored etiology for the pathogenesis of schizophrenia and other psychotic syndromes for more than 25 years, based in part on the observations that dopaminergic agonists can induce psychotic symptoms and that dopamine receptor antagonists are often clinically efficacious for psychosis (Davis et al., 1991). Specifically, antipsychotic clinical potency has been positively correlated with dopamine D2-like receptor affinity. Antipsychotic-mediated dopamine receptor blockade is almost immediate, however, whereas clinical improvement often takes weeks to months, suggesting the hyperdopaminergic hypothesis of schizophrenia is overly simplistic. In addition, antipsychotic-mediated dopamine receptor blockade frequently results in only mild to moderate clinical improvement. Consequently, the view of antipsychotics as exclusively dopamine receptor antagonists has been modified to include putative effects on other neurotransmitter receptor systems.

The recent introduction of newer "atypical" antipsychotics has stimulated a reconsideration of antipsychotic mechanisms of action. These new antipsychotics are considered atypical because of their favorable motor side effect profile and efficacy against negative (deficit) and positive psychotic symptoms compared with older, "typical" antipsychotics (Kinon and Lieberman, 1996). Atypicals have significantly higher ratios of serotonin 5-hydroxytryptamine $(HT)_2$/dopamine D2 or dopamine D4/dopamine D2 receptor affinities compared with typicals, perhaps providing a pharmacologic basis for observed clinical differences (Kinon and Lieberman, 1996).

These pharmacological differences reflect the varying effects on receptor expression and function after treatment with atypical versus typical antipsychotics. However, receptor function and expression are not determined by anatomic location or pharmacologic regulation. Different types of neurotransmitter receptors are found throughout the brain on neurons grouped in distinct circuits, and, for a given receptor, functional coupling to cellular processes may be highly variable (O'Donnell and Grace, 1998). Disparate regulation of neurotransmitter receptors is not limited to a comparison of typicals and atypicals. Differential regulation of receptor subtypes from the same receptor class has been demonstrated after antipsychotic treatment, illustrating the complexity of antipsychotic effects on the brain.

Variation in experimental design confounds comparison of many studies that demonstrate anatomic differences in antipsychotic-induced receptor expression. There is significant discordance among studies owing to differences in dose, route, frequency, and duration of antipsychotic treatment. For example, some studies have used depot forms of haloperidol, whereas others have employed daily injections or oral dosing, resulting in steady state versus peak and trough blood levels, respectively. In addition, discordance between studies is also due to variation in the assay utilized. For example, some investigators utilize in situ hybridization, receptor autoradiography, and/or Western blots, whereas others employ Northern blots and/or reverse transcriptase-polymerase chain reaction (RT-PCR), yielding results that may vary owing to technical considerations. Nevertheless, data from rigorous application of multiple techniques allow comparisons of receptor expression at multiple levels of gene organization, supporting the contention that antipsychotics affect the expression and function of neuroreceptors at multiple levels, including mRNA expression, mRNA processing, translation, intracellular signaling, and/or receptor localization. Despite these variables, it is clear that antipsychotics induce unique, region-specific patterns of receptor expression. Studies of neurochemical anatomy may facilitate the elucidation of the clinical, pharmacological, and anatomical properties of antipsychotics by measuring receptor expression in motor, limbic, and other circuits.

In this review, we focus on the distinct patterns of neuroanatomical adaptations of dopamine, serotonin, glutamate, γ-aminobutyric acid (GABA), and cholinergic receptors induced by typical and atypical antipsychotics. Rodent experiments with similar dose, route, and treatment duration will be highlighted. Studies that utilize anatomically specific methods, such as in situ hybridization and receptor autoradiography, will be emphasized. We critically review reported pharmacological differences between typical and atypical antipsychotics and their effects on the region- or circuit-specific expression of certain receptor subtypes. Finally, we discuss prevailing hypotheses regarding the etiology of the clinical efficacy and adverse effects of antipsychotic medications at the molecular level.

DOPAMINE RECEPTORS

The dopamine hypothesis of antipsychotic efficacy arose from the observation that clinical potency was positively correlated with dopamine D2-like receptor affinity (Davis et al., 1991). Therefore modulation of dopamine receptor expression has been a topic of intense study. Two families of dopamine receptors have been identified: 1) D1-like family, consisting of the positively adenylyl cyclase-coupled D1 and D5 receptors, and 2) D2-like family, consisting of the negatively adenylyl cyclase-coupled D2, D3, and D4 receptors. D3 and D4 receptors are distributed predominantly in limbic regions of the rodent brain, whereas D1 and D2 receptors are broadly distributed in both motor and limbic regions. Low levels of D5 receptor mRNA are located in the rat hippocampus (HPC), but the D5 receptor is notably absent from motor structures and most limbic regions in rodent brain.

D1 Receptors

Both typical and atypical antipsychotics regulate D1 receptor expression. D1 receptor mRNA was up-regulated 21–35% after 14 days of haloperidol (2.0 mg/kg/d) in the nucleus accumbens (ACB), caudate-putamen (CPU), HPC, and cingulate cortex (Cg) (Damask et al., 1996; Ritter and Meador-Woodruff, 1997). In contrast, D1 receptor mRNA was down-regulated 19% in the ACB by 14 days of clozapine (20 mg/kg/d), but up to 3 weeks of haloperidol (1–4 mg/kg/d) did not affect D1 receptor mRNA in the ACB or CPU (Damask et al., 1996, Fox et al., 1994, Jaber et al., 1994). For this review, limbic areas are broadly defined as the HPC, frontal cortex (FC)/Cg, ACB, and ventral tegmental area, whereas motor areas include the CPU and substantia nigra (primary motor regions of cortex are rarely included in these types of studies).

In similar experiments, D1 receptor binding in the CPU was unaffected by 3–4 weeks of haloperidol (0.4–2.0 mg/kg/d) (Huang et al., 1997; Laruelle et al., 1992; O'Dell et al., 1990; See et al., 1990; Shapiro et al., 1995; Tarazi et al., 1997; Wan et al., 1996). Conversely, 4–8 months of haloperidol decanoate decreased D1 receptor binding by 20% in the CPU (Laruelle et al., 1992; Sasaki et al., 1998). These alterations in receptor binding were not replicated in two other studies where haloperidol was administered orally (1.5 mg/kg/d) (Florijn et al., 1997; See et al., 1990).

Reports of the effects of clozapine have been similarly inconsistent. Three weeks of clozapine (15–30 mg/kg/d) increased D1 receptor binding by 23–43% in the CPU and by 12–43% in the ACB (Huang et al., 1997; O'Dell et al., 1990; See et al., 1990). However, several other studies did not demonstrate changes in D1 receptor binding in the CPU or ACB despite similar treatment conditions (20–25 mg/kg/d for 3 weeks) (Tarazi et al., 1997; Wan et al., 1996). Part of the observed discrepancy between these similar studies may be due to the lack of control for serotonin receptor affinity. Binding of the ligand ^{3}H-SCH23390 may reflect changes in serotonin rather than D1 receptor expression (O'Dell et al., 1990; Sasaki et al., 1998; See et al., 1990; Wan et al., 1996). In a related study, 8 months of oral clozapine (25–29.2 mg/kg/d) did not alter D1 receptor binding in the CPU, substantia nigra, or ACB (Florijn et al., 1997; See et al., 1990). The preponderance of these results suggests that neither acute nor chronic clozapine administration affects D1 receptor binding in the CPU.

D2 Receptors

One consistent effect of typical antipsychotic treatment is the up-regulation of D2 receptor binding in the CPU (Damask et al., 1996). However, although some studies have found concomitant changes in D2 receptor mRNA levels after typical antipsychotic treatment, most studies have found minimal or no change (Damask et al., 1996). Likewise, there is discordance regarding the effects of haloperidol on the D2 receptor mRNA isoforms D2L and D2S. These isoforms, which differ by the presence or absence of an 87 base pair exon, were both increased in the CPU in three separate studies after up to 16 days of haloperidol (2–4 mg/kg/d), whereas three other studies found no change in CPU isoform expression after up to 35 days of haloperidol (1–5 mg/kg/d) (Fishburn et al., 1994; Martres et al., 1992; Matsunaga et al., 1991; Rogue et al., 1991; Sora et al., 1992; Srvastava et al., 1990). None of these studies detected a shift in the ratio of D2L or D2S receptor splice variant to total D2 receptor mRNA levels in the CPU, suggesting that haloperidol does not alter mRNA processing for this receptor in this region. In contrast, D2 mRNA processing in FC and Cg was altered by 15 days of haloperidol (4 mg/kg/d), with a significant increase in the D2L:D2S ratio (Martres et al., 1992). These studies suggest that haloperidol may regulate dopamine receptor isoform expression at the level of mRNA processing in the limbic cortex but not the striatum.

Effects of atypical antipsychotics on striatal D2 expression and function have not been as rigorously evaluated. However, clozapine treatment appears to decrease D2 receptor mRNA in ACB and CPU, whereas there is no change in D2 mRNA after clozapine (25 mg/kg/day for 3 weeks) (Damask et al., 1996; See et al., 1996). Further study is necessary to confirm the disparate effects of typical versus atypical antipsychotics on striatal D2 receptor expression.

Several studies have examined extrastriatal D2 receptor mRNA expression. After 2 weeks of clozapine (20 mg/kg/d) the level of D2 receptor mRNA was increased in HPC by approximately 100%, whereas the level of D2 receptor mRNA in the HPC was decreased 39% after haloperidol (2.0 mg/kg/d) (Ritter and Meador-Woodruff, 1997). These opposing effects were also observed in the FC and Cg (Damask et al., 1996). However, changes in cortical expression of D2 mRNA were not observed after up to 15 days of haloperidol (4 mg/kg/d) in two other studies (Fox et al., 1994; Martres et al., 1992). These findings highlight the differential, region-specific effects of both typical and atypical antipsychotics on D2 receptor expression (Table 3-1).

D3 Receptors

In most reports, changes in D3 receptor mRNA expression were not detected in the ACB or HPC after 1–2 weeks of clozapine (20 mg/kg/d) or haloperidol (0.5–5.0 mg/kg/d) (Damask et al., 1996; Fox et al., 1994; Ritter and Meador-Woodruff, 1997; Wang et al., 1996). One study demonstrated increased D3 mRNA in whole brain after haloperidol (3 mg/kg/d for 32 days) or clozapine (30 mg/kg/d for 4 days), whereas a more anatomically specific study found increased D3 mRNA in the CPU after clozapine (Buckland et al., 1992a, 1993; Hurley et al., 1996). The increase in the CPU was not associated with increased D3 receptor binding in the same animals (Hurley et al., 1996) nor have any other groups demonstrated changes in D3 receptor binding in CPU or ACB after up to 8 months of treatment with typical or atypical antipsychotics (Florijn et al., 1997; Tarazi et al., 1997). These results, in contrast to the strong evidence indicating that haloperidol increases D2 receptor binding in the CPU, provide a molecular basis for the notion that the clinical efficacy of haloperidol is associated with differing molecular effects on members of the D2-like receptor family (Table 3-1).

TABLE 3-1. Comparison of D_2 and D_3 receptor mRNA and binding studies

Drug	Receptor	Effect	Location	No. of studies	Time	Dose (mg/kg/d)
Haloperidol	D_2 binding	↑	CPU	many	variable	variable
Haloperidol	D_2 mRNA	-	CPU	many	variable	variable
Haloperidol	D_{2S} & D_{2L} mRNA	↑	CPU	3	15–16 days	2–4
Haloperidol	D_{2S} & D_{2L} mRNA	-	CPU	3	7–35 days	1–5
Haloperidol	D_{2S}/D_{2L} ratio	-	CPU	6	7–35 days	1–5
Clozapine	D_2 mRNA	↓	CPU/ACB	2	14–21 days	20–33.8
Haloperidol	D_3 mRNA	-	ACB/HPC	4	7–14 days	0.5-5
Haloperidol	D_3 mRNA	-	CPU	1	21 days	5
Haloperidol	D_3 binding	-	CPU/ACB	2	1–8 months	1.5
Clozapine	D_3 mRNA	-	ACB/HPC	4	7–14 days	20
Clozapine	D_3 mRNA	↑	CPU	1	21 days	20
Clozapine	D_3 binding	-	CPU/ACB	3	3–32 weeks	20–25

↑ increase; ↓ decrease; - no change.

D4 Receptors

The high affinity of D4 receptors for clozapine has made this receptor the source of much interest, because typical antipsychotics have greater affinity for the D2 receptor. Several mRNA studies have yielded disparate results. D4 receptor mRNA in the HPC was decreased by 33% after 2 weeks of treatment with haloperidol (2.0 mg/kg/d), but no effect was detected after clozapine (20 mg/kg/d) (Ritter and Meador-Woodruff, 1997). In contrast, a 2-fold increase in D4 mRNA was detected by RT-PCR in the CPU 28 days after one injection (25 mg/kg) of haloperidol decanoate (Schoots et al., 1995). However, the RT-PCR experiments were conducted without a D4-specific internal control, such as a known amount of a mutant D4 receptor, which would be amplified by the same primers as the native D4 receptor. Thus, detection of even a 2-fold increase of D4 mRNA by PCR may at best only reflect a change in mRNA levels before amplification of < 3%, assuming that control and experimental samples were reverse transcribed and amplified with similar efficiency.

Until recently, the lack of selective D4 ligands has made it difficult to directly examine D4 receptor regulation at the posttranscriptional level. However, based on an indirect subtraction determination of D4 receptor binding, both clozapine (25 mg/kg/d for 1 month) and haloperidol (1.5 mg/kg/d for 28 days) increased ^{3}H-nemonapride binding in the CPU, in the presence of nonradioactive raclopride, a D2 and D3 receptor selective ligand. This effect persisted after 8 months of treatment with either drug (Schoots et al., 1995; Tarazi et al., 1997a,b).

However, there is doubt whether this method accurately measures D4 receptor binding. First, there are low levels of D4 receptor mRNA expressed in the CPU or in regions that project to the CPU in the rat (Damask et al., 1996; Schoots et al., 1995). Second, recent studies demonstrated that nemonapride also labels serotonin and sigma receptors, which are likely present in the CPU and, unless subtracted out, may confound detection of the D4 receptor (Noda-Saita et al., 1999; Tang et al., 1997). Although current evidence does not support a differential effect of typical versus atypical antipsychotics on D4 receptor mRNA expression, the preferential D4 versus D2 binding attributed to clozapine is tantalizing owing to the unique clinical efficacy of clozapine and other atypical antipsychotics.

D5 Receptors

D5 receptor mRNA levels in the HPC were unchanged by 14 days of either haloperidol (2.0 mg/kg/d) or clozapine (20 mg/kg/d) treatment (Ritter and Meador-Woodruff, 1997). Further, whole brain D5 mRNA was not altered by haloperidol treatment (3 mg/kg/d for 32 days) (Buckland et al., 1992b).

Dopaminergic Signal Transduction

Several studies have evaluated the effects of treatment with typical and atypical antipsychotics on various signal transduction pathways. Protein kinase C and phospholipase C activity and isoform expression were differentially regulated in various areas of the rat brain by acute (one dose) and chronic (3 weeks) treatment with typical or atypical antipsychotics (Dwivedi and Pandey, 1999), whereas both inositol triphosphate and cAMP were significantly increased in CPU of rats challenged with 5 mg/kg haloperidol (Kaneko et al., 1992) (Table 3-2).

TABLE 3-2. Effects of typical and atypical antipsychotics on signaling pathways

Antipsychotic	Effect on signaling	Localization	Duration	Dose/day (mg/kg)
Acute dosing				
Haloperidol	↑ IP-3, ↑ cAMP	CPU	One dose	5
Haloperidol	↑ AC	HEK cells	–	In vitro
Haloperidol	↓ $G_i\alpha$, $G_s\alpha$, β	CPU	2 weeks	3
Haloperidol	↑PKC in membrane ↓PKC in cytosol	Cortex, HPC, STR	One dose	1
Haloperidol	↑AC activity (21%) ↓ $G_i\alpha$ protein	Fr, STR	2 weeks	6
Clozapine	↑ $G_i\alpha$, $G_s\alpha$, β	CPU	2 weeks	20
Clozapine	No effect on PKC or PtdIns-PLC	Cortex, HPC, STR	One dose	20
Clozapine	↓ AC activity (20 and 31%)	Fr, STR	2 weeks	20
Chronic dosing				
Haloperidol	No effect on multiple G protein isoforms	STR, SN, PFC, HPC	22 days	0.5
Haloperidol	↓ PKC in membrane ↓PKC in cytosol No effect on PtdIns-PLC	Cortex, HPC, STR	3 weeks	1
Haloperidol	No effect on AC or PKC	CPU	4 weeks	1
Haloperidol	No effect on inositol	CPU	52 weeks	1
Clozapine	No effect on multiple G protein isoforms	STR, SN, PFC, HPC	20 days	20
Clozapine	↓ PKC in membrane ↓PKC in cytosol No effect on PtdIns-PLC	Cortex, HPC, STR	3 weeks	20
Clozapine	No effect on AC or PKC	CPU	4 weeks	20
Clozapine	No effect on inositol monophosphate	CPU	52 weeks	25

Although these well-executed studies are informative regarding the broad effects of antipsychotics, they do not indicate which receptors, if any, are linked to various components of signaling pathways. Other reports have implicated linkage of both adenylyl cyclase and phosphoinositide second messenger pathways to D1-like receptors (Pizzi et al., 1988; Simmonds and Strange, 1985; Vallar and Meldolesi 1989). Various reports have implicated linkage of both adenylyl cyclase and phosphoinositide second messenger pathways to the D2-like receptors (Pizzi et al., 1988; Simmonds and Strange 1985; Vallar and Meldolesi 1989). Haloperidol reversed quinpirole-mediated inhibition of adenylyl cyclase activity in HEK cells transfected with the D2-like receptors (McAllister et al., 1995). In this study, binding of agonist to D2 and D4 receptors was attenuated by pretreatment of the HEK membranes with a GTP analogue. Occupation of the intracellular G-protein site by the GTP analogue presumably causes an allosterically mediated alteration in the dopamine binding site, resulting in the decreased agonist binding observed for the D2 and D4 transfectants. Agonist binding to the D3 transfectant was not significantly altered by the GTP analogue, indicating a potential difference in the functional coupling of G-protein second messengers. HEK cells and neurons likely have dissimilar expression of G-protein isoforms, which may explain the observed difference. Alternatively, this difference in second messenger coupling may be an integral property of the D3 receptor (McAllister et al., 1995).

In another study of D2-like receptors, effects mediated via D4 receptor activation (inhibition of calcium current) were independent of adenylate cyclase inhibition (Mei et al., 1995). In a related study, clozapine blocked D4 receptor-mediated inhibition of cAMP accumulation and NaH-1 dependent extracellular acidification (Chio et al., 1994). cAMP accumulation required protein kinase C, whereas acidification did not, suggesting involvement of other signaling pathways. Regardless of the mechanism, variation in the second messenger coupling of D2-like receptors could explain the disparate clinical effects of these drugs. Supporting this contention, differences in D2-like receptor linked G-protein isoform expression were detected in the CPU of rat brains harvested from animals pretreated for 14 days with either 3 mg/kg haloperidol or 20 mg/kg clozapine (Gupta and Mishra, 1992). In the same animals, Western blot analysis of tissue homogenates demonstrated decreased $G_{i\alpha}$, $G_{s\alpha}$, and β-subunits after treatment with haloperidol. In contrast, the $G_{i\alpha}$, $G_{s\alpha}$, and β-subunits were increased with clozapine (Gupta and Mishra, 1992). Consistent with these findings, antipsychotic treatment had significant effects on GTPγS-mediated adenylyl cyclase activity in the frontal cortex and striatum of rats. After 14 days of haloperidol (6 mg/kg per day), adenylyl cyclase activity was increased 21% in the frontal cortex, whereas olanzapine (20 mg/kg per day) significantly decreased adenylyl cyclase activity in the frontal cortex (20%) and striatum (31%) (Kaplan et al., 1999). Haloperidol resulted in a decreased immunoreactivity for $G_{i\alpha}$ subunits in the cortex but not the striatum, a finding similar to that of previous studies. These studies hint at the potential complexity of the dopamine receptor linkage to second messenger pathways.

Results from some studies employing chronic (>2 weeks) dosing regimens are not consistent with the reported effects on signaling pathways after acute (up to 14 days) administration of antipsychotics. Clozapine or haloperidol for 4–52 weeks did not affect CPU inositol monophosphate or adenylyl cyclase response to D2 agonist nor binding levels of adenylyl cyclase or protein kinase C (Rubinstein et al., 1989; Wan et al., 1996). In addition, no differences in various G-protein isoforms were detected by Western blot analysis in the striatum, substantia nigra, prefrontal cortex, or HPC of rats treated for 22 days with 0.5 mg/kg/day subcutaneous haloperidol or 20 mg/kg/d clozapine (Meller and Bohmaker 1996). Although variation in dose, route, and strain of animal may explain some observed differences, analysis of transcript or protein expression levels may be insufficient to detect functional differences in signaling. Alternatively, chronic antipsychotic administration may sensitize signaling pathways, such that differences in second messengers are not detected.

Although many studies investigating antipsychotic effects have focused on individual components of signaling pathways, others have utilized functional endpoints such as proliferation assays or expression of specific genes. The agonist quinpirole stimulated proliferation of NG 108-15 cells transfected with the D3 receptor, an effect potentiated by coadministration of forskolin, a compound that increases cAMP production. However, in related experiments utilizing the same transfectant, quinpirole attenuated forskolin-mediated cAMP production. The inhibitory effect of quinpirole was antagonized by haloperidol. The "opposite and synergistic" effects of cAMP are consistent with data indicating that cAMP signaling is not required for, but may potentiate, mitogenesis (Griffon et al., 1997; Kavanaugh et al., 1988; Schwartz et al., 1998; van Corven et al., 1989). D3 receptor-mediated mitogenesis is dependent on specific G-protein isoform coupling (Pilon et al., 1994; Seabrook et al., 1994; Sokoloff and Schwartz, 1995). Thus, haloperidol may exert a wide range of seemingly contradictory effects, which depend on the subtype, concentration, and second messenger coupling of specific dopamine receptors.

Mitogenesis may be a useful endpoint for demonstrating intact and functional coupling to signaling pathways in vitro, but analysis of such pathways in vivo is impractical, because mitogenesis is not a typical neuronal response to a stimulus. Recent work has utilized gene expression as an end-point in the evaluation of D1 and D3 receptor signaling in the rat brain. For example, c-fos and substance P mRNA levels were measured via in situ hybridization analysis of the islands of Calleja. Results indicate that granule cells in this region express D1 and D3, but not D2, receptors (Diaz et al., 1995; Schwartz et al., 1998).

Costimulation of the D1 and D3 receptors with specific agonists and/or antagonists yielded interesting results. c-fos expression was attenuated by the D3 agonist and increased by the D1 agonist, a result predicted by the previously described effects on cAMP production. This result is supported by several studies that demonstrated increased c-fos levels after treatment with D3 antagonists (Merchant et al., 1996; Shafer and Levant 1998; Vahid-Ansari et al., 1996). The presence of such opposing pathways in the same cell suggests a form of tonic regulation allowing precise control of intracellular signaling mediated via the dopamine neurotransmitter system. In contrast, in the ACB, D1 and D3 receptor coactivation was not antagonistic. In this area, treatment with D1 and D3 agonists resulted in synergistic upregulation of substance P mRNA expression, suggesting linkage to, and activation of, parallel signaling mechanisms such as the mitogen-activated protein kinase pathway. These results indicate that antipsychotics may exert different effects on signaling pathways in adjacent neurons.

Studies that investigate the effects of antipsychotics on gene expression represent an important step in the process of determining the relationship between biological mechanisms and function. However, few studies with a functional endpoint, which may translate to humans, have evaluated antipsychotic effects on signaling pathways. One well-designed study evaluated the effects of haloperidol in the striatum of wild-type and protein kinase A regulatory subunit-knockout mice. In the wild type animals, treatment with haloperidol led to increased levels of c-fos and neurotensin mRNA in the striatum and induced a cataleptic response, effects blocked in the knockout mice (Adams et al., 1997). This study directly links haloperidol-mediated regulation of signaling pathways with a functional endpoint that correlates with the motor side effects of haloperidol in humans.

Other work has begun to evaluate the proximate effects on intracellular signaling after treatment with antipsychotics. DARPP-32, a small phosphoprotein found in medium-sized spiny neurons of the neostriatum, is a potent inhibitor of protein phosphatase-1 (Fienberg et al., 1998; Nishi et al., 1997). Protein phosphatase-1 regulates the phosphorylation status of many neuronal phosphoproteins, including the NR1 subunit of the NMDA glutamate receptor (Fienberg et al., 1998). These findings demonstrate that dopamine agonists and dopamine antagonists differentially regulate phosphorylation of DARPP-32, indicating a central role for this protein when considering the molecular effects of antipsychotics on signaling pathways.

In summary, although there is not good consensus on the patterns of dopamine receptor expression that result from typical and atypical antipsychotic treatment, the observed differences in second messenger coupling between the dopamine receptors have broad implications for understanding the effects of antipsychotic medications. For example, haloperidol may directly modulate striatal protein kinase activity, altering gene expression, possibly resulting in motor side effects (Adams et al., 1997). Effects of antipsychotics may not be limited to the receptor level. Trifluoperazine directly bound calcium binding proteins and inhibited various protein kinases at micromolar concentrations (Agopyan and Krnjevic, 1993; Levin and Weiss, 1978). In addition, the discovery and characterization of PSD-95/DIg/ZO-1 (PDZ) domain-containing proteins have generated multiple new candidates genes, which if abnormally expressed or disrupted may lead to aberrant dopaminergic neurotransmission. Spinophillin, which contains one PDZ domain, has been shown to interact with the D2 dopamine receptor, F-actin, and protein phosphatase-1, presumably to localize specific components of a signaling complex (Smith et al., 1999). Such proteins, which putatively link signaling machinery to intracellular receptor domains, have not been investigated from the point of view of antipsychotic regulation. Nevertheless the rich and diverse nature of second messenger coupling taken with the varying affinities of drugs such as haloperidol and clozapine for the dopamine receptors provides a theoretical basis for understanding the therapeutic and adverse effects of antipsychotic drugs at a molecular level.

SEROTONIN RECEPTORS

The high affinity of serotonin 5-HT_2-like receptors for atypical antipsychotics may underlie some of the unique clinical therapeutic profile of these drugs (Kinon and Lieberman, 1996). However, few studies have examined antipsychotic regulation of serotonin receptor expression.

5-HT_{2A} Receptors

After 2 weeks of clozapine (25 mg/kg/d), 5-HT_{2A} receptor mRNA in the Cg was decreased 28%, and 5-HT_{2A} receptor binding in the FC and Cg was decreased 66% (Burnet et al., 1996a). This is consistent with several other studies that demonstrated decreases in cortical 5-HT_2 receptor binding after clozapine treatment and suggests that expression of the 5-HT_{2A} receptor may be regulated at the level of transcription (Burnet et al., 1996a; Kuoppamaki et al., 1995; Lee and Tang, 1984; O'Dell et al., 1990; Reynolds et al., 1983; Wilmot and Szczepanik, 1989). Unlike the FC and Cg, 5-HT_{2A} receptor mRNA and binding were unchanged in piriform cortex, suggesting that these effects are region specific (Burnet et al., 1996a). In contrast to the studies with clozapine, treatment with up to 3 weeks of either haloperidol (1.0–2.0 mg/kg/d) or haloperidol decanoate (25 mg/kg) did not affect 5-HT_{2A} receptor binding or mRNA levels in the FC or Cg (Andree et al., 1986; Burnet et al., 1996a,b; Kuoppamaki et al., 1995; O'Dell et al., 1990; Wilmot and Szczepanik, 1989). These findings highlight the apparent differences in the regulation of receptor expression between typical and atypical antipsychotics.

5-HT_{2C} Receptors

Haloperidol (1.0–2.0 mg/kg/d) or clozapine (25 mg/kg/d) for 2 weeks had no effect on 5-HT_{2C} receptor mRNA or binding in the ACB (Burnet et al., 1996a). Further, fluphenthixol treatment (0.2 mg/kg/d for 10 weeks) did not alter 5-HT_{2C} receptor mRNA in whole brain extracts (De La Concha et al., 1991).

5-HT_6 Receptors

5-HT_6 receptor mRNA was decreased after 2 weeks of clozapine (20 mg/kg/d) in the HPC but not in the FC, ACB, or CPU (Frederick and Meador-Woodruff, 1999). Similar to 5-HT2 receptor data, haloperidol (2.0 mg/kg/d) did not affect 5-HT_6 receptor mRNA levels (Frederick and Meador-Woodruff, 1999).

Consistent with their pharmacology, atypical antipsychotics may be more likely to induce alterations in serotonin receptor expression compared with typicals. These effects are limited to certain subtypes of serotonin receptors in selected limbic regions. Nevertheless such a difference in receptor regulation may explain observed differences in clinical efficacy between typical and atypical antipsychotics.

GLUTAMATE RECEPTORS

Converging lines of evidence implicate glutamate receptors in schizophrenia (Javitt and Zukin, 1991). Glutamate receptors are divided into four families: NMDA, AMPA, kainate, and metabotropic, which are activated by glutamate but modulated by other ligands acting at unique binding sites (Hollmann and Heinemann, 1994). NMDA, AMPA, and kainate receptors are multimeric associations of specific subunits that form ligand-gated ion channels. Metabotropic receptors are seven transmembrane domain G-protein coupled receptors encoded by eight separate genes: mgluR1–mgluR8. The NMDA receptor subunits are encoded by five genes: NR1 and NR2A–NR2D (Hollmann and Heinemann, 1994). NR1 is expressed as one of eight isoforms owing to the alternative splicing of exons 5, 21, and 22 (Durand et al., 1993; Hollmann and Heinemann, 1994). AMPA receptor subunits are derived from a family of four genes termed gluR1–gluR4, each of which can be processed into a flip or flop isoform by alternative splicing. Kainate receptor subunits are derived from genes for the low affinity gluR5–gluR7 and high affinity KA1–KA2 subunits.

The NMDA subtype, the best characterized of the ionotropic glutamate receptors, contains a unique glycine binding site that must be occupied before glutamate-mediated channel activation (Hollmann and Heinemann, 1994). In addition, there are unique sites that bind noncompetitive antagonists and polyamines. Assembled AMPA receptors also contain several binding sites: one for glutamate, one at which competitive antagonists such as CNQX bind, and one where desensitization modulators exert their influence (Bleakman and Lodge, 1998). Kainate receptors contain a glutamate binding site, but other binding sites have not been well characterized. Because expression of binding sites is influenced by the subunit composition of the final assembled ionotropic receptor, the pharmacological regulation of ionotropic glutamate receptors depends in part on the unique combination of subunits.

Once such phenotypic variant generated in the laboratory, the NR1 homomer, forms nonfunctional receptors that bind only glycine (Boeckman and Aizenman, 1994; Grimwood et al., 1995). NR2 subunits must coassemble with NR1 for formation of functional ligand-gated ion channels (Lynch et al., 1994; Monyer et al., 1992). This structure-function relationship extends to specific subunits. The NR2A variant is linked with competitive antagonists of the glutamate binding site, like CGP39653, and the NR2B variant with the polyamine binding site (Gallagher et al., 1996; Lynch et al., 1994; Varney et al., 1996). Finally, NMDA receptors with NR2A or NR2B subunits bind MK-801, a phencyclidine site agonist, more avidly than those containing NR2C or NR2D receptors (Lynch et al., 1994).

Although less is known about the association between AMPA or kainate receptor subunits and binding site properties, subunit composition affects AMPA receptor calcium conductance and the sensitivity of kainate receptors to glutamate (Geiger et al., 1995; Sommer et al., 1992; Swanson et al., 1997). There are no studies demonstrating differential binding site properties of metabotropic receptor subtypes mgluR1–mgluR8, although there are pharmacological differences between the subtypes (Conn and Pin, 1997).

Taken together, these studies demonstrate the importance of subunit composition in determining functional properties of ionotropic glutamate receptors. Further, there may be multiple populations of each receptor subtype mediating glutamatergic neurotransmission.

Although the NMDA receptor subtype is most often implicated in schizophrenia, there is mounting evidence that AMPA, kainate, and metabotropic receptors affect NMDA receptor activity. Specifically, activation of presynaptic kainate receptors facilitates glutamate release and/or decreases GABAergic activity, creating a functional interface with postsynaptic NMDA and AMPA receptors (Chittajalu et al., 1996, 1999; Clarke et al., 1997; Cunha et al., 1997; Frerking et al., 1998; Lodge and Bleakman, 1997; Rodriguez-Moreno et al., 1997). Presynaptic metabotropic glutamate receptors also appear to affect glutamate release, and metabotropic modulators affect NMDA receptor function (Alagarsamy et al., 1998; Kishi et al., 1998; Moghaddam and Adams, 1998). Further, the NMDA receptor ion channel is blocked at physiological concentrations of magnesium (Hollmann and Heinemann, 1994). This blockade is voltage-dependent, such that partial depolarization of the cell

TABLE 3-3. Comparison of NR1 receptor mRNA studies

Drug	Receptor	Effect	Location	No. of studies	Time	Dose (mg/kg/d)
Haloperidol	NR1 mRNA	↑	CPU	2	21–30 days	1–1.8
Haloperidol	NR1 mRNA	–	CPU	2	14–28 days	0.5–2
Haloperidol	NR1 mRNA	–	ACB	2	14–21 days	1–2
Haloperidol	NR1 mRNA	–	CPU/ACB	1	26 weeks	1
Haloperidol decanoate	NR1 mRNA	–	CPU/ACB	1	16 weeks	25 mg/kg/wk
Clozapine	NR1 mRNA	↓	ACB	1	21 days	30
Clozapine	NR1 mRNA	↑	CPU	1	28 days	30
Clozapine	NR1 mRNA	–	CPU	4	3–26 days	30–35
Clozapine	NR1 mRNA	–	ACB	2	3–26 weeks	35
Clozapine	NR1 exon 5 mRNA	↑	CPU	1	28 days	30
Haloperidol	NR1 exon 5 mRNA	↑	CPU	1	28 days	0.5
Haloperidol decanoate	NR1 exon 22 mRNA	↑	CPU	1	4 months	1

↑ increase; ↓ decrease; – no change.

membrane is required to extrude magnesium and allow ion flow though the NMDA receptor channel. Activation of postsynaptic AMPA or metabotropic receptors likely provides this permissive function, because these receptors are extensively colocalized with NMDA receptors at glutamatergic terminals (Bekkers and Stevens, 1989; He et al., 1998).

Finally, there is evidence for both postsynaptic kainate receptors and presynaptic AMPA and NMDA receptors (Berreta and Jones, 1996; Breukel et al., 1998; Castillo et al., 1997; Chittajalu et al., 1996; DiBiasi et al., 1996; Patel and Croucher, 1997; Vignes and Collingridge, 1997), suggesting further complexity for the interaction of glutamate receptors. Therefore receptor composition and anatomical localization of binding sites are vital components of glutamatergic neurotransmission; examination of glutamate receptor expression must explain these complexities.

NMDA Receptors

NR2 subunits appear to be differentially regulated by antipsychotics, although few studies have been published. NR2C mRNA levels were decreased 19–28% in the FC and ACB after 3 weeks of clozapine (30 mg/kg/d) (Riva et al., 1997, 1999). In these studies, no alterations in NR2 subunit mRNA levels were detected in the CPU or HPC. In contrast, one study detected an increase in NR2B, but not NR2A, mRNA in the CPU after 4 weeks of clozapine (30 mg/kg/d) (Meshul et al., 1996). Assessment of NR2 subunits after haloperidol is similarly contradictory. NR2A–NR2C mRNAs were increased in the CPU by 20–47% after treatment for 3 weeks with haloperidol (1.0 mg/kg/d), whereas no changes were detected in the HPC, ACB, or FC (Riva et al., 1997). However, in a similar study, NR2A or NR2B mRNA levels in CPU were unchanged after haloperidol (0.5 mg/kg/d) for 4 weeks (Meshul et al., 1996). Such disparate results may be due to differences in duration and dose of antipsychotic, illustrating the need for coordination of study conditions.

Other studies have focused on antipsychotic regulation of NR1 subunit mRNA expression and processing (Table 3-3). After 3 weeks of clozapine (30 mg/kg/d), NR1 mRNA levels were decreased in the ACB by 32%, although no changes were detected in the CPU, HPC, or FC (Riva et al., 1997). In contrast, after 3 weeks of haloperidol (1.0 mg/kg/d), NR1 mRNA in the CPU was increased by 20%, although no effect was detected in the HPC, ACB, or FC (Riva et al., 1997). Consistent with this finding, total NR1 immunoreactivity was increased in the CPU after haloperidol for 1 month (Fitzgerald et al., 1995). These results were not replicated in a similar study.

Total NR1 mRNA levels in the CPU were increased after 4 weeks of clozapine (30 mg/kg/d) but not haloperidol (0.5 mg/kg/d) (Meshul et al., 1996). In addition, treatment with neither clozapine (35 mg/kg/d for 21 days) nor haloperidol (1.8–2.0 mg/kg/d for 14–21 days) affected total NR1 mRNA levels in the CPU or ACB, whereas NR1 immunoreactivity was not altered after 25 days of clozapine (35 mg/kg/d) (Brene et al., 1998; Eastwood et al., 1994, Fitzgerald et al., 1995). Finally, chronic treatment with haloperidol decanoate (25 mg/kg/3 weeks for 16 weeks), haloperidol (1.0 mg/kg/d for 26 weeks), or clozapine (35 mg/kg/d for 26 weeks) did not lead to persistent changes in total NR1 mRNA in FC, CPU, or ACB (Brene et al., 1998; Eastwood et al., 1996). Such region-, dose- and duration-dependent differences in receptor expression suggest that the physiological responses to antipsychotic treatment are dynamic, indicating the need for additional timepoints when evaluating the effects of antipsychotic treatment.

Several studies have demonstrated that antipsychotics may affect mRNA processing (Table 3-3). Expression of NR1 exon 5-containing mRNA in the CPU was increased after either clozapine (30 mg/kg/d) or haloperidol (0.5 mg/kg/d) for 4 weeks (Meshul et al., 1996). In addition, exon 22-NR1 immunoreactive dendritic spines were increased in the CPU of rats treated for 4 months with haloperidol decanoate (1.0 mg/kg/d), suggesting that NR1 mRNA processing changes may persist beyond the acute response to antipsychotic treatment. These results indicate that analysis of total mRNA levels, versus evaluation of the expression of specific exon-containing isoforms, may be insufficient to detect antipsychotic-mediated changes in gene expression occurring via mRNA processing. Studies that examine expression of both specific exon-containing isoforms and protein levels in the same animals would be useful to resolve this inconsistency.

The difficulty in interpreting NMDA receptor subunit mRNA level data extends to binding studies. This is not unexpected considering that, in part, subunit expression determines binding site expression. ^{3}H-MK-801 binding was reduced by 17–30% in the FC after clozapine (25–30 mg/kg/d) or haloperidol (1.5 mg/kg/d) for 3–4 weeks (Giardino et al., 1997; Tarazi et al., 1996). In addition, a reduction in ^{3}H-MK-801 binding was detected in the CPU for up to 8 months after either clozapine (25 mg/kg/d) or haloperidol (1.5 mg/kg/d) for 4 weeks (Tarazi et al., 1996). In other studies, these effects were not observed with lower doses of clozapine (20 mg/kg/d for 3 weeks) or haloperidol (0.5 mg/kg/d for 3 weeks) nor were there significant changes in ^{3}H-MK-801 binding in the FC after 3–8 months of either drug (Johnson et al., 1994; McCoy and Richfield, 1996; Meshul et al., 1996; Ossowska et al., 1996, 1999; Tarazi et al., 1996). However, binding of a competitive antagonist to the glutamate binding site was increased in rats treated for 3 months with clozapine (30 mg/kg/d) or haloperidol (1.0 mg/kg/d), perhaps suggesting a time-dependent shift in binding site regulation by antipsychotics (Ossowska et al., 1999).

Discrepancies in the studies of the effects of haloperidol may be explained by differences in the percentage of rodents that develop vacuous chewing movements. Rats that did not develop vacuous chewing movements after 36 weeks of haloperidol (28.5 mg/kg/3 weeks) had significantly decreased ^{3}H-MK-801 binding in the CPU, whereas those rats that developed vacuous chewing movements did not downregulate ^{3}H-MK-801 binding in the CPU (Hamid et al., 1998). These results suggest that there are subpopulations of animals with differential sensitivities to antipsychotics. Thus, studies that do not account for such phenotypic variations may yield contradictory results.

AMPA Receptors

Several studies have demonstrated that clozapine and haloperidol have differential effects on AMPA receptor subunit expression. Treatment with haloperidol (2.0 mg/kg/d) for 2 weeks resulted in a 15–50% decrease in gluR2 and gluR4 mRNA levels in FC, CPU, and ACB. Treatment with clozapine for 2 weeks (20 mg/kg/d) led to a 15–30% decrease in gluR3 mRNA expression in the FC, CPU, and ACB and a similar decrease in gluR4 mRNA levels in CPU and ACB (Healy and Meador-Woodruff, 1997). Clozapine and haloperidol had similar effects on hippocampal AMPA receptor expression. gluR1 was increased, and gluR2, gluR3, and gluR4 mRNA levels were decreased in the HPC by 18–51% after 2 weeks of haloperidol (2.0 mg/kg/d). In contrast, 2 weeks of clozapine (20 mg/kg/d) led to increased gluR1 mRNA and decreased gluR3 and gluR4 mRNA levels in the HPC by 29–45% (Meador-Woodruff et al., 1996). Tascedda et al. (1999) found relatively little change in AMPA receptor subunit mRNA levels; gluR1, gluR2, and gluR3 mRNA levels in the ACB, CPU, or HPC were not altered after haloperidol (1.0 mg/kg/d) for 3 weeks, whereas decreased gluR3 mRNA expression in the ACB was the only alteration in subunit mRNA detected after clozapine (30 mg/kg/d).

Similar to studies of total subunit mRNA levels, AMPA receptor mRNA processing is also regulated by antipsychotics. Clozapine (30 mg/kg/d for 21 days), but not haloperidol (1.0 mg/kg/d for 21 days), led to a 28% decrease in the gluR2 flip splice variant in the ACB, whereas a similar study did not detect any effect with lower doses of clozapine (20 mg/kg/d) or haloperidol (0.5 mg/kg/d) (McCoy et al., 1998; Tascedda et al., 1999). Supporting the notion of an effect on mRNA processing, an increase in the gluR2 flip:flop ratio was detected in the CPU and HPC after 2 weeks of haloperidol (2.0 mg/kg/d) (Eastwood et al., 1996). In this study, there was no significant change in total gluR2 mRNA levels, indicating an alteration in gluR2 mRNA processing. Increases in the gluR2 flip:flop ratio persisted after 16–26 weeks of haloperidol (1.8 mg/kg/d) or haloperidol decanoate (25 mg/kg/3 weeks) but not clozapine (35 mg/kg/d) (Brene et al., 1998; Eastwood et al., 1996).

AMPA receptor subunit protein levels are also regulated by haloperidol and clozapine. Fitzgerald et al. (1995) found increases in gluR1 immunoreactivity in rat CPU and FC after haloperidol (1.8 mg/kg/d for 30 days) or clozapine (35 mg/kg/d for 25 days), whereas gluR2 immunoreactivity was increased in the FC, ACB, and HPC after clozapine. These studies differ from subunit mRNA studies, suggesting that there may be dissociation between the regulation of AMPA receptor subunit mRNA and protein expression or turnover.

Antipsychotic treatment differentially affected agonist binding. ^{3}H-AMPA in the FC, HPC, ACB, and CPU was increased 30–45% after 3 weeks of haloperidol (0.5 mg/kg/d) but not clozapine (20 mg/kg/d) (McCoy et al., 1996). However, ^{3}H-AMPA binding was unchanged after 6 months of fluphenazine decanoate (30 mg/kg/month) (Johnson et al., 1994). Further, binding of the antagonist ^{3}H-CNQX was unaffected by 1–8 months of treatment with haloperidol or clozapine (McCoy et al., 1996;

Tarazi et al., 1996). Thus antipsychotics may only transiently regulate selected AMPA receptor binding sites.

Kainate Receptors

Few studies have examined antipsychotic regulation of kainate receptor expression. After clozapine (20 mg/kg/d for 14 days), increased gluR5–gluR7 and KA2 mRNA levels were detected in the HPC, and increased gluR7 mRNA was detected in the FC, Cg, and CPU (Healy and Meador-Woodruff, 1997; Meador-Woodruff et al., 1996). After haloperidol, modest increases were observed in KA2 mRNA in the CPU and gluR5 mRNA in the HPC (Healy and Meador-Woodruff, 1996; Meador-Woodruff et al., 1997). In addition, the KA2 subunit was up-regulated in the HPC and FC, but not the CPU, after 4 months of haloperidol decanoate (25 mg/kg/3 weeks), suggesting that the changes observed after a brief dosing regimen may persist (Eastwood et al., 1996).

Neither relatively short term (28 days) nor long term (8 months) clozapine (25 mg/kg/d) or haloperidol (1.5 mg/kg/d) affected ^{3}H-kainate binding in the CPU, ACB, FC, Cg, HPC, ventral tegmental area, or substantia nigra (Tarazi et al., 1996).

The multiple levels of gene organization of ionotropic glutamate receptor expression make it difficult to generalize about patterns of glutamate receptor expression associated with typical or atypical antipsychotic treatments. Nevertheless changes in glutamate receptor expression observed after treatment with antipsychotic medications sufficiently establish glutamate neurotransmitter pathways as a target for future investigation.

Metabotropic Receptors

To date, no studies have directly examined the regulation of metabotropic glutamate receptor expression by antipsychotics.

GABA RECEPTOR EXPRESSION

GABAergic dysfunction has previously been implicated in the pathophysiology of schizophrenia, and several studies have demonstrated selective effects of antipsychotics on GABA receptor expression (Benes, 1998). There are three GABA receptor families: $GABA_A$, $GABA_B$, and $GABA_C$. Although $GABA_A$ and $GABA_B$ receptors are abundantly expressed in limbic and motor regions, most studies on antipsychotic regulation of GABA receptor expression have focused on the $GABA_A$ family. Similar to ionotropic glutamate receptors, $GABA_A$ receptors are ligand gated ion channels formed from the assembly of variably spliced α-, β-, γ-, [gd]-, [ge]-, [gp]-, [gq]-, or [gr]-subunits, all encoded by separate genes (Sieghart et al., 1999). $GABA_A$ receptor subunits form multiple receptor binding sites, including a GABA agonist site, a benzodiazepine modulatory site, an ion channel site, a barbiturate site, and a steroid modulatory site. Binding sites are also associated with the presence of selected subunits in the assembled receptor. For example, the benzodiazepine site is associated with the presence of the γ_2- subunit in the final receptor.

After 4 weeks of clozapine or olanzapine (0.1–1.0 mg/kg/d), the GABA agonist site binding of ^{3}H-muscimol in the HPC was decreased by 50%, whereas binding after haloperidol (0.01–0.1 mg/kg/d) was attenuated only 15% (Farnbach-Pralong et al., 1998). In the CPU, ^{3}H-muscimol binding was modestly, but significantly, decreased (7%) after 24 weeks of fluphenazine decanoate (30 mg/kg/month) (Johnson et al., 1994). In addition, binding to the steroid site with ^{3}H-TBPS was increased by 12% after 21 weeks of haloperidol decanoate (30 mg/kg/3 weeks) (Sasaki et al., 1997). In contrast, other studies found no change in agonist or benzodiazepine site binding in the CPU after 8–12 months of haloperidol (1.4–1.6 mg/kg/d) (Rupniak et al., 1987; See et al., 1990).

One proposed link between the clinical effects of antipsychotics involves the relationship of vacuous chewing movements in the rat, suggested by some to model tardive dyskinesia, and changes in GABA receptor binding. Rats that developed significant vacuous chewing movements after being treated with 21 weeks of haloperidol decanoate (30 mg/kg/3 weeks) had greater increases in ^{3}H-TBPS binding in the CPU compared with rats without these movements, suggesting that $GABA_A$ receptor binding changes may be related the motor side effects of typical antipsychotics (Sasaki et al., 1997). Consistent with this interpretation is the demonstration by multiple groups that agonist site binding is increased in the substantia nigra after 1–8 months of haloperidol (Frey et al., 1987; Gale, 1980; Huffman and Ticku, 1983; See et al., 1990). This effect is specific for the GABA agonist site, because benzodiazepine binding is unaffected in animals treated similarly (See et al., 1990). Further, clozapine did not affect binding to either the GABA agonist or benzodiazepine site, supporting the idea that alterations in $GABA_A$ receptor binding may be associated with some motor side effects of typical antipsychotics. Neither $GABA_A$ subunit expression nor $GABA_B$ receptor expression have been examined in studies of antipsychotic regulation, which may clarify these previous reports.

CHOLINERGIC RECEPTORS

Muscarinic cholinergic receptors have clinically significant affinities for some antipsychotics, which regulate expression of these receptors. Muscarinic receptor density in the CPU was decreased by 17% after 12 weeks of oral fluphenazine (0.005% w/v in drinking water), whereas after 12 weeks of clozapine (0.075% w/w in the diet), muscarinic receptor density was increased by 20% in the CPU, FC, and HPC (Friedman et al., 1983). Muscarinic receptor expression was unchanged after up to 6 weeks of either typical or atypical antipsychotics (Akiyama et al., 1987; Boyson et al., 1988; Friedman et al., 1983; Kajiyama and Nomura, 1981). Further, the effects noted after 12 weeks of typical antipsychotic treatment in CPU may be transient, because muscarinic receptor densities were not changed after 8 months of oral haloperidol (1.57 mg/kg/d) or oral clozapine (29.2 mg/kg/d) (See et al., 1990). Discrepancies in the above studies may be due to shifts in the expression of specific muscarinic receptor subtypes, because the studies were performed before the muscarinic receptor subtypes were cloned and reflect the total population of these receptors. Consistent with this notion, a recent study demonstrated that m2 protein levels in the CPU were increased after one injection of fluphenazine decanoate (12.5 mg/kg) but not after 2 weeks of clozapine (20 mg/kg/d) (Cawley et al., 1993).

Finally, typical and atypical antipsychotics have modest effects on second messenger systems associated with muscarinic receptors. Six weeks of haloperidol (1.5 mg/kg/d) attenuated carbachol-stimulated inositol monophosphate accumulation by 33% in the CPU, HPC, and FC (Li et al., 1992). This effect was not detected in the CPU or HPC after 4 weeks of haloperidol (5 mg/kg/d) or in the CPU after 52 weeks of haloperidol or clozapine (Akiyama et al., 1987; Rubinstein et al., 1989).

These studies suggest that there may be differences between the effects of typical and atypical antipsychotics on muscarinic receptor expression, and future studies focusing on selective labeling of the muscarinic subtypes may prove fruitful. There are no studies examining the effects of antipsychotics on nicotinic cholinergic receptor expression.

CONCLUSIONS

Several patterns emerge from an examination of the effects of typical and atypical antipsychotics on dopamine, serotonin, glutamate, GABA, and cholinergic receptor expression in specific brain areas. These effects differ for various neurotransmitter receptors, particularly for receptor subtypes within a neurotransmitter receptor family. For example, D2, but not D3, receptor binding is increased in the CPU and ACB after haloperidol but not clozapine (Table 3-1). This effect was limited to D2 binding, because D2 mRNA levels in the CPU were unchanged. These results illustrate the varying effects on receptor expression after treatment with atypical versus typical antipsychotics. However, receptor function is not solely determined by anatomic location or pharmacologic regulation. For a given receptor, functional coupling to cellular processes may be highly variable. For example, D1 and D3 receptor activation led to up-regulation of gene expression in the ACB but inhibited it in the islands of Calleja. These results indicate that a specific receptor may have opposing, seemingly contradictory, effects on adjacent neurons.

Comparisons between many of the studies we reviewed are limited by differences in drugs, dosing, and routes of administration. For example, comparison of two separate studies that evaluated NR2A expression after treatment with haloperidol were inconsistent: one detected an increase in NR2A and the other no change. Although the studies used a similar duration of treatment, one used 1.0 mg/kg of haloperidol and the other 0.5 mg/kg. Such differences in experimental design make comparisons of results difficult and diminish potential contributions to the field. Future studies on the effects of typical and atypical antipsychotics on receptor expression should try to minimize such differences by utilizing a study design approximating analogous studies.

Examination of receptor expression at multiple levels of gene organization using neuroanatomical techniques has revealed exciting new targets for investigation of the effects of antipsychotics. For example, the alterations in NR1 splice variants detected after antipsychotic treatment suggest that the effects of antipsychotics extend to mRNA processing. The association of changes in the expression of specific exons with the expression and regulation of other genes, such as receptor anchoring proteins, is a direction future studies should pursue.

Despite numerous studies designed to elucidate the effects of antipsychotics on the rat brain, only a few firm conclusions may be postulated. Antipsychotic effects on receptor expression are highly variable and depend on the functional coupling of specific receptors to intracellular signaling pathways. Thus identical receptors found on adjacent neurons may display disparate responses to the same antipsychotic. Such responses may be specific to typical versus atypical antipsychotics on the basis of well delineated pharmacologic differences.

Future studies have great potential to improve our understanding of antipsychotic effects. Such studies will be most useful if they 1) simultaneously examine multiple neurotransmitter systems in the same sets of animals treated with typical and atypical antipsychotics; 2) examine multiple receptor subtypes of the same neurotransmitter system; 3) measure receptor expression in multiple, interconnected regions that comprise limbic and motor circuits; and 4) measure receptor expression at multiple levels of gene organization. Comprehensive studies of this kind will facilitate the interpretation of these data, because dose, duration, and route of administration will be held constant; these confounds are currently major limitations when comparing studies of this kind.

REFERENCES

Adams MR, Brandon EP, Chartoff EH, et al. (1997). Loss of haloperidol induced gene expression and catalepsy in protein kinase A-deficient mice. *Proc Natl Acad Sci USA* 94,12157–12161.

Agopyan N, Krnjevic K (1993). Effects of trifluoperazine on synaptically evoked potentials and membrane properties of CA1 pyramidal neurons of rat hippocampus in situ and in vitro. *Synapse* 13,10–19.

Akiyama K, Sato M, Yamada N, et al. (1987). Effect of chronic administration of haloperidol (intermittently) and haloperidol-decanoate (continuously) on D2 dopamine and muscarinic cholinergic receptors and on carbachol-stimulated phosphoinositide hydrolysis in the rat striatum. *Jpn J Psychiatry Neurol* 41,311–320.

Alagarsamy S, Marino MJ, Rouse ST, et al. (1998). Activation of NMDA receptors reverses desensitization of mGluR5 in native and recombinant systems. *Nature Neurosci* 2,234–240.

Andree TH, Mikuni M, Tong CY, et al. (1986). Differential effect of subchronic treatment with various neuroleptic agents on serotonin-2 receptors in rat cerebral cortex. *J Neurochem* 46,191–197.

Bekkers JM, Stevens CF (1989). NMDA and non-NMDA receptors are co-localized at individual excitatory synapses in cultured rat hippocampus. *Nature* 341,230–233.

Benes F (1998). Model generation and testing to probe neural circuitry in the cingulate cortex of postmortem schizophrenic brain. *Schizophr Bull* 24,219–230.

Bleakman D, Lodge D (1998). Neuropharmacology of AMPA and kainate receptors. *Neuropharmacology* 37,1187–1204.

Boeckman FA, Aizenman E (1994). Stable transfection of the NMDAR1 subunit in Chinese hamster ovary cells fails to produce a functional N-methyl-D-aspartate receptor. *Neurosci Lett* 173,189–192.

Boyson SJ, McGonigle P, Luthin GR, et al. (1988). Effects of chronic administration of neuroleptic and anticholinergic agents on densities of D2 dopamine and muscarinic cholinergic receptors in rat stria-

tum. *J Pharmacol Exp Ther* 244,987–993.
Brene S, Messer C, Nestler EJ (1998). Expression of messenger RNAs encoding ionotropic glutamate receptors in rat brain: regulation by haloperidol. *Neuroscience* 84,813–823.
Breukel AIM, Besselen E, Lopes da Silva FH, et al. (1998). A presynaptic N-methyl-D-aspartate autoreceptor in rat hippocampus modulating amino acid release from a cytoplasmic pool. *Eur J Neurosci* 10,106–114.
Buckland PR, O'Donovan MC, McGuffin P (1992a). Changes in dopamine D1, D2, and D3 receptor mRNA levels in rat brain following antipsychotic treatment. *Psychopharmacology* 106,479–483.
Buckland PR, O'Donovan MC, McGuffin P (1992b). Lack of effect of chronic antipsychotic treatment on dopamine D5 receptor mRNA level. *Eur J Neuropsychopharmacol* 2,405–409.
Buckland PR, O'Donovan MC, McGuffin P (1993). Clozapine and sulpiride up-regulate dopamine D3 receptor mRNA levels. *Neuropharmacology* 32,901–907.
Burnet PWJ, Chen CPL-H, McGowan S, et al. (1996a). The effects of clozapine and haloperidol on serotonin-1A, -2A and -2C receptor gene expression and serotonin metabolism in the rat forebrain. *Neuroscience* 73,531–540.
Burnet PWJ, Eastwood SL, Harrison PJ (1996b). 5-HT1A and 5-HT_{2A} receptor mRNAs and binding site densities are differentially altered in schizophrenia. *Neuropsychopharmacology* 15,442–455.
Castillo PE, Malenka RC, Nicoll RA (1997). Kainate receptors mediate a slow postsynaptic current in hippocampal CA3 neurons. *Nature* 388,182–186.
Cawley Jr TA, Shickley TJ, Ruggieri MR, et al. (1993). Effect of chronic neuroleptic treatment on central and peripheral muscarinic receptors. *J Pharmacol Exp Ther* 267,134–139.
Chio CL, Drong RF, Riley DT, et al. (1994). D4 dopamine receptor-mediated signaling events determined in transfected Chinese hamster ovary cells. *J Biol Chem* 269,1813–11819.
Chittajallu R, Braithwaite SP, Clarke VRJ, et al. (1999). Kainate receptors: subunits, synaptic localization and function. *Trends Pharmacol Sci* 20,26–35.
Chittajallu R, Vignes M, Dev KK, et al. (1996). Regulation of glutamate release by presynaptic kainate receptors in the hippocampus. *Nature* 379,78–81.
Clarke VRJ, Ballyk BA, Hoo KH, et al. (1997). A hippocampal gluR5 kainate receptor regulating inhibitor synaptic transmission. *Nature* 389,599–603.
Conn PJ, Pin J-P (1997). Pharmacology and functions of metabotropic glutamate receptors. *Ann Rev Pharmacol Toxicol* 37,205–237.
Cunha RA, Constantino MD, Ribeiro JA (1997). Inhibition of [^{3}H]-γ-aminobutyric acid release by kainate receptor activation in rat hippocampal synaptosomes. *Eur J Pharmacol* 323,167–172.
Damask SP, Bovenkirk KA, de le Pena G, et al. (1996). Differential effects of clozapine and haloperidol on dopamine receptor mRNA expression in rat striatum and cortex. *Mol Brain Res* 41,241–249.
Davis KL, Kahn RS, Ko G, et al. (1991). Dopamine in schizophrenia: a review and reconceptualization. *Am J Psychiatry* 148,1474–1486.
De La Concha A, McKie J, Hodgkinson S, et al. (1991). Stereospecific effect of flupenthixol on neuroreceptor gene expression. *Mol Brain Res* 10,123–127.
DeBiasi S, Minelli A, Melone M, et al. (1996). Presynaptic NMDA receptors in the neocortex are both auto- and heteroreceptors. *Neuroreport* 7,2773–2776.
Diaz J, Leívesque D, Lammers CH, et al. (1995). Phenotypical characterization of neurons expressing the dopamine D3 receptor. *Neuroscience* 65,731–745.
Durand GM, Bennett MVL, Zukin RS (1993). Splice variants of the N-methyl-D-aspartate receptor NR1 identify domains involved in regulation by polyamines and protein kinase C. *Proc Natl Acad Sci USA* 90,6731–6735.
Dwivedi Y, Pandey GN (1999). Effects of treatment with haloperidol, chlorpromazine, and clozapine on protein kinase C (PKC) and phosphoinositide-specific phospholipase C (PI-PLC) activity and on mRNA and protein expression of PKC and PLC isozymes in rat brain. *J Pharmacol Exp Ther* 291,688–704.
Eastwood SL, Porter RHP, Harrison PJ (1996). The effect of chronic haloperidol on glutamate receptor subunit (gluR1, gluR2, KA1, KA2, NR1). mRNAs and glutamate binding protein mRNA in rat forebrain. *Neurosci Lett* 212,163–166.
Eastwood SL, Story P, Burnet PWJ, et al. (1994). Differential changes in glutamate receptor subunit messenger RNAs in rat brain after haloperidol treatment. *J Psychopharmacol* 8,196–203.
Farbach-Pralong D, Bradbury R, Copolov D, et al. (1998). Clozapine and olanzapine treatment decreases rat cortical and limbic $GABA_A$ receptors. *Eur J Pharmacol* 349,R7–R8.
Fienberg AA, Hiroi N, Mermelstein PG, et al. (1998). DARPP-32: regulator of the efficacy of dopaminergic neurotransmission. *Science* 281,838–842.

Fishburn CS, David C, Carmon S, et al. (1994). The effect of haloperidol on D2 dopamine receptor subtype mRNA levels in the brain. *FEBS Lett* 339,63–66.
Fitzgerald LW, Deutch AY, Gasic G, et al. (1995). Regulation of cortical and subcortical glutamate receptor subunit expression by antipsychotic drugs. *J Neurosci* 15,2453–2461.
Florijn WJ, Tarazi FI, Creese I (1997). Dopamine receptor subtypes: differential regulation after 8 months treatment with antipsychotic drugs. *J Pharmacol Exp Ther* 280,561–569.
Fox CA, Mansour A, Watson Jr SJ (1994). The effects of haloperidol on dopamine receptor gene expression. *Exp Neurol* 130,288–303.
Frederick JA, Meador-Woodruff JH (1999). Effects of clozapine and haloperidol on 5-HT_6 receptor mRNA levels in rat brain. *Schizophr Res* 38,7–12.
Frerking M, Malenka RC, Nicoll RA (1998). Synaptic activation of kainate receptors on hippocampal interneurons. *Nature Neurosci* 1,479–486.
Frey JM, Ticku MJ, Huffman RD (1987). GABAergic supersensitivity within the pars reticulata of the rat substantia nigra following chronic haloperidol administration. *Brain Res* 425,73–84.
Friedman E, Gianutsos G, Kuster J (1983). Chronic fluphenazine and clozapine elicit opposite changes in brain muscarinic receptor binding: implications for understanding tardive dyskinesia. *J Pharmacol Exp Ther* 226,7–11.
Gale K (1980). Chronic blockade of dopamine receptors by anti-schizophrenic drugs enhances GABA binding in substantia nigra. *Nature* 283,569–570.
Gallagher MJ, Huang H, Pritchett DB, et al. (1996). Interactions between ifenprodil and the NR2B subunit of the *N*-methyl-D-aspartate receptor. *J Biol Chem* 271,9603–9611.
Geiger JRP, Melcher T, Koh D-S, et al. (1995). Relative abundance of subunit mRNAs determines gating and Ca_{2+} permeability of AMPA receptors in principal neurons and interneurons in rat CNS. *Neuron* 15,193–204.
Giardino L, Bortolotti F, Orazzo C, et al. (1997). Effect of chronic clozapine administration on [^{3}H]MK801-binding sites in the rat brain: a side-preference action in cortical areas. *Brain Res* 762,216–218.
Griffon N, Pilon C, Sautel F, et al. (1997). Two intracellular pathways for the dopamine D3 receptor: opposite and synergistic interactions with cyclic AMP. *J Neurochem* 67,1–9.
Grimwood S, LeBourdelles B, Whiting PJ (1995). Recombinant human NMDA homomeric NMDAR1 receptors expressed in mammalian cells form a high-affinity glycine antagonist binding site. *J Neurochem* 64,525–530.
Gupta SK, Mishra RK (1992). Effects of chronic treatment of haloperidol and clozapine on levels of G-protein subunits in rat striatum. *J Mol Neurosci* 3,197–201.
Hamid EH, Hyde TM, Baca SM, et al. (1998). Failure to down regulate NMDA receptors in the striatum and nucleus accumbens associated with neuroleptic-induced dyskinesia. *Brain Res* 796,291–295.
He Y, Janssen WGM, Morrison JH (1998). Synaptic coexistence of AMPA and NMDA receptors in the rat hippocampus: a postembedding immunogold study. *J Neurosci Res* 54,444–449.
Healy DJ, King RE, Bovenkerk KA, et al. (1997). Clozapine and haloperidol differentially regulate AMPA and kainate receptor subunit mRNA levels in rat cortex and striatum. *Mol Brain Res* 47,331–338.
Hollmann M, Heinemann S (1994). Cloned glutamate receptors. *Annu Rev Neurosci* 17,31–108.
Huang N, Ase AR, Hebert C, et al. (1997). Effects of chronic neuroleptic treatments on dopamine D1 and D2 receptors: homogenate binding and autoradiographic studies. *Neurochem Int* 30,277–290.
Huffman RD, Ticku MJ (1983). The effects of chronic haloperidol administration on GABA receptor binding. *Pharmacol Biochem Behav* 19,199–204.
Hurley MJ, Stubbs CM, Jenner P, et al. (1996). Effect of chronic treatment with typical and atypical neuroleptics on the expression of dopamine D2 and D3 receptors in rat brain. *Psychopharmacology* 128,362–370.
Jaber M, Tison F, Fournier MC, et al. (1994). Differential influence of haloperidol and sulpiride on dopamine receptors and peptide mRNA levels in the rat striatum and pituitary. *Mol Brain Res* 23,14–20.
Javitt DC, Zukin SR (1991). Recent advances in the phencyclidine model of schizophrenia. *Am J Psychiatry* 148,1301–1308.
Johnson AE, Liminga U, Liden A, et al. (1994). Chronic treatment with a classical neuroleptic alters excitatory amino acid and GABAergic neurotransmission in specific regions of the rat brain. *Neuroscience* 63,1003–1020.
Kajiyama H, Nomura Y (1981). Alteration in dopaminergic and muscarinic cholinergic receptors after subchronic treatment with haloperidol in the developing rat brain. *J Pharm Dyn* 4,85–90.

Kaneko M, Sato K, Horikoshi R, et al. (1992). Effect of haloperidol on cyclic AMP and inositol triphosphate in rat striatum in vivo. *Prostagl Leukotr Essential Fatty Acids* 46,53–57.

Kaplan GB, Leite-Morris KA, Keith DJ (1999). Differential effects of treatment with typical and atypical antipsychotic drugs on adenylyl cyclase and G proteins. *Neurosci Lett* 273,147–150.

Kavanaugh WM, Lewis LT, Ives HE, et al. (1988). Serotonin-induced deoxyribonucleic acid synthesis in vascular smooth muscle cells involved in a novel, pertussis toxin-sensitive pathway. *Mol Endocrinol* 2,599–605.

Kinon BJ, Lieberman JA (1996). Mechanisms of action of atypical antipsychotic drugs: a critical analysis. *Psychopharmacology* 124,2–34.

Kishi A, Ohno M, Watanabe S (1998). Spermidine, a polyamine site agonist, attenuates working memory deficits caused by blockade of hippocampal muscarinic receptors and mGluRs in rats. *Brain Res* 793,311–314.

Kuoppamaki M, Palvimaki E-P, Hietala J, et al. (1996). Differential regulation of rat 5-HR_{2A} and 5-HT_{2C} receptors after chronic treatment with clozapine, chlorpromazine and three putative atypical antipsychotic drugs. *Neuropsychopharmacology* 13,139–150.

Laruelle M, Jaskiw GE, Lipska BK, et al. (1992). D1 and D2 receptor modulation in rat striatum and nucleus accumbens after subchronic and chronic haloperidol treatment. *Brain Res* 575,47–56.

Lee T, Tang SW (1984). Loxapine and clozapine decrease serotonin (S2), but do not elevate dopamine (D2), receptor numbers in the rat brain. *Psychiatr Res* 12,277–285.

Levin RM, Weiss B (1978). Specificity of the binding of trifluoperazine to the calcium-dependent activator of phosphodiesterase and to a series of other calcium-binding proteins. *Biochim Biophys Acta* 540,197–204.

Li R, Wing LL, Kirch DG, et al. (1992). Effects of chronic nicotine and haloperidol administration on muscarinic receptor-mediated phosphoinositide turnover in rat brain slices. *Psychopharmacology* 109,248–250.

Lodge D, Bleakman D (1997). A hippocampal gluR5 kainate receptor regulating inhibitory synaptic transmission. *Nature* 389,599–603.

Lynch DR, Anegawa NJ, Verdoorn T, et al. (1994). N-methyl-D-aspartate receptors: different subunit requirements for binding of glutamate antagonists, glycine antagonists, and channel-blocking agents. *Mol Pharmacol* 45,540–545.

Martres MP, Sokoloff P, Giros B, et al. (1992). Effects of dopaminergic transmission interruption on the D2 receptor isoforms in various cerebral tissues. *J Neurochem* 58,673–679.

Matsunaga T, Ohara K, Natsukari N, et al. (1991). Dopamine D2-receptor mRNA level in rat striatum after chronic haloperidol treatment. *Neurosci Res* 12,440–445.

McAllister G, Knowles MR, Ward-Booth SM, et al. (1995). Functional coupling of human D2, D3, and D4 dopamine receptors in HEK293 cells. *J Recept Sign Trans Res* 15,267–281.

McCoy L, Cox C, Richfield EK (1998). Antipsychotic drug regulation of AMPA receptor affinity states and GluR1, GluR2 splice variant expression. *Synapse* 28,195–207.

McCoy L, Cox C, Richfield EK (1996). Chronic treatment with typical and atypical antipsychotics increases the AMPA-preferring form of AMPA receptor in rat brain. *Eur J Pharmacol* 318,41–45.

McCoy L, Richfield EK (1996). Chronic antipsychotic treatment alters glycine-stimulated NMDA receptor binding in rat brain. *Neurosci Lett* 213,137–141.

Meador-Woodruff JH, King RE, Damask SP, et al. (1996). Differential regulation of hippocampal AMPA and kainate receptor subunit expression by haloperidol and clozapine. *Mol Psychiatry* 1,41–53.

Mei YA, Griffon N, Buquet C, et al. (1995). Activation of dopamine D4 receptor inhibits an L-type calcium current in cerebellar granule cells. *Neuroscience* 68,107–116.

Meller E, Bohmaker K (1996). Chronic treatment with antipsychotic drugs does not alter G protein alpha or beta subunit levels in rat brain. *Neuropharmacology* 35,1785–1791.

Merchant KM, Figur LM, Evans DL (1996). Induction of c-fos mRNA in rat medial prefrontal cortex by antipsychotic drugs: role of dopamine D2 and D3 receptors. *Cereb Cortex* 6,561–570.

Meshul CK, Bunker GL, Mason JN, et al. (1996). Effects of subchronic clozapine and haloperidol on striatal glutamatergic synapses. *J Neurochem* 67,1965–1973.

Moghaddam B, Adams BW (1998). Reversal of phencyclidine effects by a group II metabotropic glutamate receptor agonist in rats. *Science* 281,1349–1352.

Monyer H, Sprengel R, Schoepfer R, et al. (1992). Heteromeric NMDA receptors: molecular and functional distinction of subtypes. *Science* 256,1217–1220.

Nishi, A, Snyder GL, Greengard P (1997). Bidirectional regulation of DARPP-32 phosphorylation by dopamine. *J Neurosci* 17,8147–8155.

Noda-Saita K, Matsumoto M, Hidaka K, et al. (1999). Dopamine D4-like binding sites labeled by

[^{3}H]nemonapride include substantial serotonin 5-HT_{2A} receptors in primate cerebral cortex. *Biochem Biophys Res Commun* 255,367–370.

O'Dell SJ, La Hoste GJ, Widmark CB, et al. (1990). Chronic treatment with clozapine or haloperidol differentially regulates dopamine and serotonin receptors in rat brain. *Synapse* 6,146–153.

O'Donnell P, Grace AA (1998). Dysfunctions in multiple interrelated systems as the neurobiological bases of schizophrenic symptom clusters. *Schizophr Bull* 24,267–283.

Ossowska K, Pietraszek M, Wardas J (1996). Further evidence for the subsensitivity of striatal AMPA receptors induced by chronic haloperidol administration: an autoradiographic study. *Naunyn-Schmiedeberg's Arch Pharmacol* 353,384–388.

Ossowska K, Pietraszek M, Wardas J, et al. (1999). Chronic haloperidol and clozapine administration increase the number of cortical NMDA receptors in rats. *Naunyn-Schmiedeberg's Arch Pharmacol* 359,280–287.

Patel DR, Croucher MJ (1997). Evidence for a role of presynaptic AMPA receptors in the control of neuronal glutamate release in the rat forebrain. *Eur J Pharmacol* 332,143–151.

Pilon C, Levesque D, Dimitriadou V, et al. (1994). Functional coupling of the human dopamine D3 receptor in a transfected NG 108-15 neuroblastoma-glioma hybrid cell line. *Eur J Pharmacol* 268,129–139.

Pizzi M, DaPrada M, Valerio A, et al. (1988). Dopamine D2 receptor stimulation inhibits inositol phosphate generating system in rat striatal slices. *Brain Res* 456,235–240.

Reynolds GP, Garrett NJ, Rupniak N, et al. (1983). Chronic clozapine treatment of rats down-regulates cortical 5-HT2 receptors. *Eur J Pharmacol* 89,325–326.

Ritter LM, Meador-Woodruff JH (1997). Antipsychotic regulation of hippocampal dopamine receptor messenger RNA expression. *Biol Psychiatry* 42,155–164.

Riva MA, Tascedda F, Lovati E, et al. (1997). Regulation of NMDA receptor subunit messenger RNA levels in the rat brain following acute and chronic exposure to antipsychotic drugs. *Mol Brain Res* 50,136–142.

Rodriguez-Moreno A, Herreras O, Lerma J (1997). Kainate receptors presynaptically downregulate GABAergic inhibition in the rat hippocampus. *Neuron* 19,893–901.

Rogue P, Hanauer A, Zwiller J, et al. (1991). Up-regulation of dopamine D2 receptor mRNA in rat striatum by chronic neuroleptic treatment. *Eur J Pharmacol* 207,165–168.

Rubinstein JE, Hitzemann RJ, Ashby CR, et al. (1989). Long term treatment with antipsychotics does not alter the phosphoinositide response to muscarinic or D2 dopaminergic agonists in rat striatum. *Brain Res* 496,385–388.

Rupniak NMJ, Prestwich SA, Horton RW, et al. (1987). Alterations in cerebral glutamic acid decarboxylase and [^{3}H]-flunitrazepam binding during continuous treatment of rats for up to one year with haloperidol, sulpiride, or clozapine. *J Neural Transm* 68,113–125.

Sasaki T, Kennedy JL, Nobrega JN (1997). Localized changes in GABA receptor-gated chloride channel in rat brain after long-term haloperidol: relation to vacuous chewing movements. *Synapse* 25,73–79.

Sasaki T, Kennedy JL, Nobrega JN (1998). Regional brain changes in [^{3}H]SCH 23390 binding to dopamine D1 receptors after long-term haloperidol treatment: lack of correspondence with the development of vacuous chewing movements. *Behav Brain Res* 90,125–132.

Schoots O, Seeman P, Guan H-C, et al. (1995). Long-term haloperidol elevates dopamine D4 receptors by 2-fold in rats. *Eur J Pharmacol* 289,67–72.

Schwartz JC, Diaz J, Bordet R, et al. (1998). Functional implications of multiple dopamine receptor subtypes: the D1/D3 receptor coexistence. *Brain Res Rev* 26,236–242.

Seabrook GR, Kemp JA, Freedman SB, et al. (1994). Functional expression of human D3 dopamine receptors in differentiated neuroblastoma x glioma NG108-15 cells. *Br J Pharmacol* 111,391–393.

See RE, Lynch AM, Sorg BA (1996). Subchronic administration of clozapine, but not haloperidol or metaclopromide, decreases dopamine D2 receptor messenger RNA levels in the nucleus accumbens and caudate-putamen in rats. *Neuroscience* 72,99–104.

See RE, Toga AW, Ellison G (1990). Autoradiographic analysis of regional alterations in brain receptors following chronic administration and withdrawal of typical and atypical neuroleptics in rats. *J Neural Transm* 82,93–109.

Shafer RA, Levant B (1998). The D3 dopamine receptor in cellular and organismal function. *Psychopharmacology (Berl)* 135,1–16.

Shapiro LA, Offord SJ, Ordway GA (1995). The effect of chronic treatment with a novel aryl-piperazine antipsychotic on monoamine receptors in rat brain. *Brain Res* 677,250–256.

Sieghart W, Fuchs K, Tretter V, et al. (1999). Structure and subunit composition of $GABA_A$ receptors.

Neurochem Int 34,379–385.
Simmons SH, Strange PG (1985). Inhibition of phospholipid breakdown by D2 dopamine receptors in dissociated bovine anterior pituitary cells. *Neurosci Lett* 60,267–272.
Smith FD, Oxford GS, Milgram SL (1999). Association of the D2 dopamine receptor third cytoplasmic loop with spinophilin, a protein phosphatase-1-interacting protein. *J Biol Chem* 274,19894–19900.
Sokoloff P, Schwartz JC (1995). Novel dopamine receptors half a decade later [see comments]. *Trends Pharmacol Sci* 16,270–275.
Sommer B, Burnashev N, Verdoorn TA, et al. (1992). A glutamate receptor channel with high affinity for domoate and kainate. *EMBO J* 11,1651–1656.
Sora I, Fujiwara Y, Tomita H, et al. (1992). Lack of effect of haloperidol or methamphetamine treatment on the mRNA levels of two dopamine D2 receptor isoforms in rat brain. *Jpn J Psychiatry Neurol* 46,967–973.
Swanson GT, Kamboj SK, Cull-Candy SG (1997). Single-channel properties of recombinant AMPA receptors depend on RNA editing, splice variation, and subunit composition. *J Neurosci* 17,58–69.
Tang SW, Helmeste DM, Fang H, et al. (1997). Differential labeling of dopamine and sigma sites by [^{3}H]nemonapride and [^{3}H]raclopride in postmortem human brains. *Brain Res* 765,7–12.
Tarazi FI, Florijn WJ, Creese I (1996). Regulation of ionotropic glutamate receptors following subchronic and chronic treatment with typical and atypical antipsychotics. *Psychopharmacology* 128,371–379.
Tarazi FI, Florijn WJ, Creese I (1997). Differential regulation of dopamine receptors after chronic typical and atypical antipsychotic drug treatment. *Neuroscience* 78,985–996.
Tascedda F, Lovati E, Blom JMC, et al. (1999). Regulation of ionotropic glutamate receptors in the rat brain in response to the atypical antipsychotic Seroquel (quetiapine fumarate). *Neuropsychopharmacology* 21,211–217.
Vahid-Ansari F, Nakabeppu Y, Robertson GS (1996). Contrasting effects of chronic clozapine, Seroquel(TM) (ICI 204,636) and haloperidol administration of deltaFosB-like immunoreactivity in the rodent forebrain. *Eur J Neurosci* 8,927–936.
Vallar L, Meldolesi L (1989). Mechanism of signal transduction at the dopamine D2 receptor. *Trends Pharmacol Sci* 10,74–77.
van Corven EJ, Groenink A, Jalink K, et al. (1989). Lysophosphatidate-induced cell proliferation: identification and dissection of signaling pathways mediated by G proteins. *Cell* 59,45–54.
Varney MA, Jachec C, Deal C, et al. (1996). Stable expression and characterization of recombinant human heteromeric N-methyl-D-aspartate receptor subtypes NMDAR1A/2A and NMDAR1A/2B in mammalian cells. *J Pharmacol Exp Ther* 279,367–378.
Vignes M, Collingridge GL (1997). The synaptic activation of kainate receptors. *Nature* 388,179–182.
Wan DC, Dean B, Pavey G, et al. (1996). Treatment with haloperidol or clozapine causes changes in dopamine receptors but not adenylate cyclase or protein kinase C in the rat forebrain. *Life Sci* 59,2001–2008.
Wang W, Hahn K-H, Bishop JF, et al. (1996). Up-regulation of D3 dopamine receptor mRNA by neuroleptics. *Synapse* 23,232–235.
Wilmot CA, Szczepanik AM (1989). Effects of acute and chronic treatments with clozapine and haloperidol on serotonin (5-HT2) and dopamine (D2) receptors in rat brain. *Brain Res* 487,288–298.

4.

Dopamine-Glutamate Interactions

Werner J. Schmidt

ABSTRACT

A transmitter system does not work in isolation—it interacts with other transmitters. A critical balance exists between dopamine and glutamate in the basal ganglia. Dopamine and glutamate, via the NMDA receptor, seem to exert opposite effects on animal behavior. This has implications for understanding the role of dopamine in various diseases and for developing therapies designed to restore normal balance between dopamine and glutamate. In Parkinson's disease dopamine activity is reduced, and there is an overweight of glutamate activity in several structures of the basal ganglia. Thus pharmacologically reducing abnormal glutamate activities may be a strategy to treat parkinsonian symptoms and perhaps to reduce glutamatergic excitotoxicity. A deficient glutamatergic activity, possibly of the corticofugal projection to the basal ganglia, may underlie schizophrenia. In the development of addictive behavior and after withdrawal from addictive drugs, changes occur in the dopaminergic system. There is evidence that for these processes of neuroplasticity glutamate is crucial. Elucidation of these mechanisms may lead to new anticraving therapies or perhaps even to a cure from addictive behavior.

INTRODUCTION

The brain dopamine system originates in the midbrain. Most dopaminergic neurons project to the striatum/nucleus accumbens complex and to other basal ganglia nuclei as well as to the prefrontal cortex, amygdala, and hippocampus. Glutamatergic input to the basal ganglia originates in the neocortex, amygdala, and hippocampus. This review will focus on the basal ganglia because dopamine-glutamate interactions are most intricate there.

Although much has been researched, the functions of the basal ganglia are still enigmatic. The fact that basal ganglia do not project directly on the spinal motor output makes research difficult. Originally basal ganglia were considered to represent primitive motor nuclei, subserving postural and supportive control. Later the basal ganglia were considered to be involved in the generation of motor programs (Kornhuber, 1974), which the cortex cannot generate on its own. Neither assumption need be abandoned in the light of more recent findings, but today the basal ganglia are considered crucial in more aspects of behavioral control. They are involved in procedural and incentive learning and even have cognitive capabilities; e.g., they are involved in switching from one behavioral activity to another (Cools et al., 1984; Schmidt, 1984) as well as in decision-making according to internal representations and goals (Knowlton et al., 1996; Schultz et al., 1997).

FUNCTIONAL ANATOMY OF BASAL GANGLIA

In phylogenetically old vertebrates (e.g., fish), the basal ganglia represent the origin of a descending system. With the transition of animals to a terrestrial habitat, the development of the neocortex and, because of its close interconnections, an increase in thalamic volume and capacity happens. At this evolutionary stage, the output of basal ganglia is no longer directed solely to lower brain structures; loops are formed from basal ganglia to the thalamus and back to the basal ganglia and in higher species from basal ganglia via the thalamus additionally to the neocortex and back to the basal ganglia (Fig. 4-1). The main input structure of the basal ganglia is the striatum. The cortical input to the striatum terminates predominantly on spiny output neurons: the thalamic input to the striatum terminates on cholinergic interneurons that impinge on those spiny output neurons that project to the external segment of globus pallidus. This is the origin of the "indirect pathway" that projects from the striatum via the external segment of the globus pallidus, subthalamic

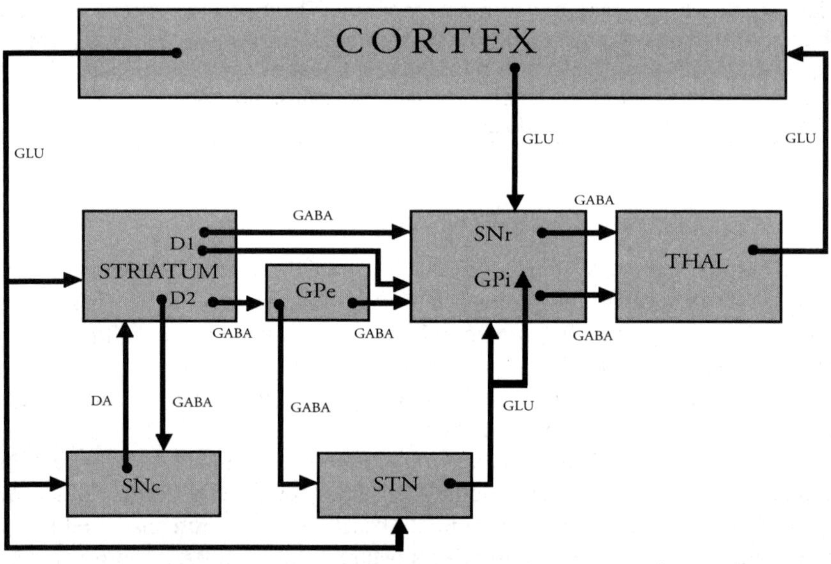

FIG. 4-1. Circuitry and neurotransmitters of basal ganglia. GLU, L-glutamic ACID; GABA, γ-aminobutyric acid; D1, dopamine D1 receptor; D2, dopamine D2 receptor; SNr, substantia nigra pars reticulata; Gpe, globus pallidus external segment; GPi, globus pallidus internal or medial segment; THAL, thalamus; DA, dopamine; SNc, substantia nigra pars compacta; STN, subthalamic nucleus.

nucleus (STN), and internal segment of globus pallidus to the thalamus. The projection from the striatum via the substantia nigra pars reticulata to the thalamus constitutes the direct pathway.

On the basis of these anatomical and functional findings, the following consideration has been advanced: a cortical input to the striatum results in activation of the striatal neurons, giving rise to direct and indirect pathways (Fig. 4-2). Because of the different numbers of neurons between the striatum and thalamus, this results in disinhibition (by the direct pathway) and inhibition (by the indirect pathway) of the thalamus. It has been hypothesized that by way of this dual influence, the basal ganglia can facilitate "wanted" behavior and inhibit "unwanted" behavior (Graybiel, 1993; Schmidt, 1994; Schmidt and Kretschmer, 1997). Although we cannot know what is wanted or unwanted in a certain context, this hypothesis has some attractive features because it explains some so far unexplained observations (e.g., both facilitatory and inhibitory behavioral effects of basal ganglia electrostimulation have been reported).

Within the striatum, dopamine inhibits the neurons of the indirect loop via D2 receptors and stimulates neurons of the direct loop via D1 receptors. Enhanced dopamine activity results in disinhibition of the thalamus, in increased thalamocortical signal, and behaviorally in psychomotor activation. Reduced dopamine activity results in inhibition of the thalamus and behaviorally in akinesia and rigidity (parkinsonism) (Fig. 4-3). Besides this presumably tonic dopamine activity, there also appears to exist a phasic dopamine signal deriving from phasic activation of

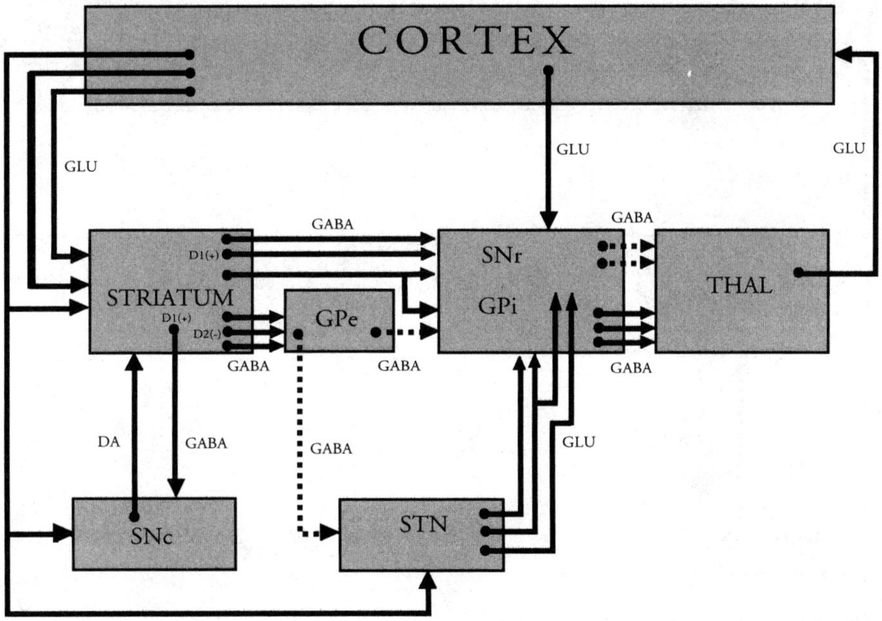

FIG. 4-2. Enhanced activity of GLUergic corticostriatal neurons. *Solid lines*, increased activity; *broken lines*, reduced activity. See Fig. 4-1 for abbreviations.

dopamine neurons. This dopamine signal may be involved in a process of evaluation, contributing to the decision of what is "wanted" and of what is "unwanted."

PARKINSON'S DISEASE

Degeneration of mesencephalic dopaminergic neurons underlies Parkinson's disease. The dopamine deficit in the projection areas leads, via the two basal ganglia pathways, to an increased GABAergic inhibition of thalamic nuclei (Fig. 4-3). This and the resulting decrease of thalamocortical activity are considered the cause of akinesia. A tonically active cortical glutamatergic innervation of the striatum/accumbens is prerequisite for the expression of akinesia and rigidity because lesions of the prefrontal cortex or blockade of NMDA receptors in the striatum counteract akinesia and rigidity in the rat (Schmidt and Kretschmer, 1997). The loss of dopaminergic inhibition, and in turn the relative overactivity in the striatum, result in increased activity of the striatopallidal GABAergic neurons. Findings of reduced GABA/benzodiazepine receptor density in the globus pallidus external segment of postmortem parkinsonian patients or MPTP-treated monkeys are in accordance with this view (Crossman, 1990). Although there is a relative glutamate overactivity in the striatum/accumbens, STN, and substantia nigra pars compacta, there is absolute glutamate overactivity in the substantia nigra pars reticulata and the globus pallidus internal segment (Fig. 4-3). Thus Parkinson's disease can be con-

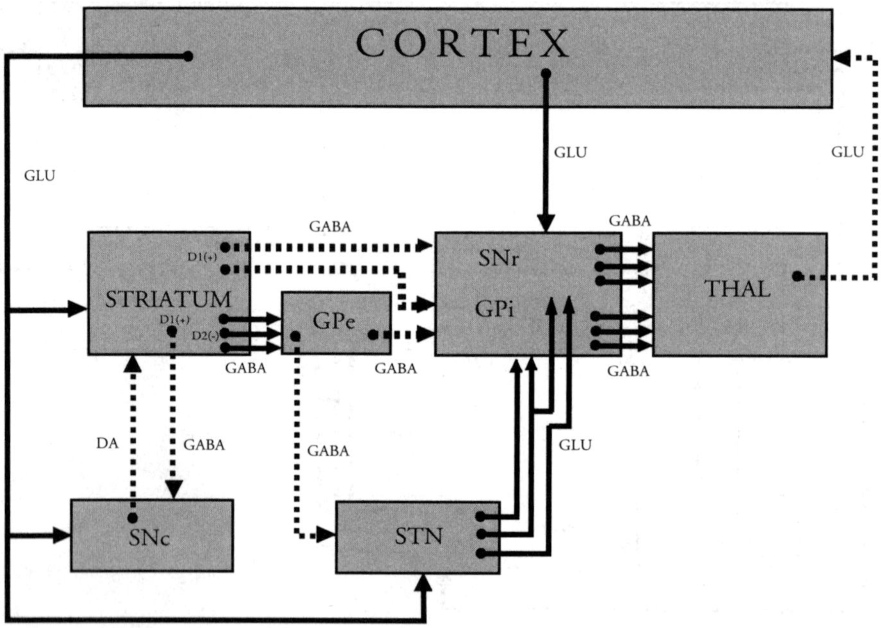

FIG. 4-3. Reduced activity of dopaminergic neurons originating in SNc. *Solid lines*, increased activity; *broken lines*, reduced activity. See Fig. 4-1 for abbreviations.

sidered a primary dopamine deficiency syndrome and a secondary glutamate overactivity syndrome.

Glutamate Receptor Antagonists as Antiparkinsonian Drugs?

The uncompetitive NMDA receptor antagonist dizocilpine (MK-801) could antagonize haloperidol-induced parkinsonism in the rat (Schmidt and Bubser, 1989) as well as movement initiation deficits (Hauber and Schmidt, 1990). Competitive NMDA receptor antagonists and antagonists at the glycine binding site of the NMDA receptor have qualitatively similar actions, but their locomotion-inducing effects are much weaker. All these NMDA receptor antagonists synergize with classical antiparkinsonian drugs such as L-dopa, bromocriptine, or scopolamine.

Although, the antiparkinsonian effects of amantadine, memantine, and budipine are partly due to their NMDA receptor antagonism, no NMDA receptor antagonist has so far been introduced as a new antiparkinsonian drug. The reasons are the strong side effects (e.g., psychotomimesis) and cognitive (mainly learning and memory) disturbances.

However, the NMDA receptor blockers may prove beneficial in reversing side effects of chronic L-dopa treatments. Some recent clinical studies report parkinsonian patients suffering from L-dopa-induced dyskinesias. When these individuals received adjuvant treatment with an NMDA receptor antagonist (e.g., dextromethorphan, dextrorphan, or amantadine) dyskinesia scores were substantially lowered while parkinsonian scores remained unchanged (Blanchet et al., 1997; Verhagen-Metman et al., 1998). A process of decreased efficacy of chronic L-dopa treatment that is reminiscent of the wearing-off fluctuations occurring in Parkinson's disease has also been observed in parkinsonian rats and monkeys. In these cases, one dose of dizocilpine could reduce the loss of efficacy of L-dopa (Blanchet et al., 1997). Several attempts have been made to explain these provocative findings. Our recent research suggests that these effects may be explained by adopting a state dependency interpretation. This means that the side effects of chronic L-dopa treatment that have developed in the absence of an NMDA receptor antagonist cannot be expressed in the presence of an NMDA receptor blocker (Schmidt et al., 1999; Tzschentke and Schmidt, 1998, 1999).

AMPA receptor antagonists have no antiparkinsonian activity; they even reduce the antiparkinsonian effects of NMDA receptor antagonists or L-dopa (Zadow and Schmidt, 1994). Little is known about the effects of ligands of metabotropic glutamate receptors (Kronthaler and Schmidt, 1998).

Neurodegeneration and Neuroprotection

Parkinson's disease is an active disease process in which nigral cell death is accelerated. The primary cause for the cell death is still unknown, but free radicals, metabolic stress, and excitotoxicity may contribute. Considering the role of excitotoxicity it can be seen from Fig. 4-3 that the decreased dopamine in turn causes increased glutamate tone in several basal ganglia nuclei. The midbrain dopamine cell groups receive two main glutamatergic inputs: one from the prefrontal cortex and one from the STN, which may contribute to nigral neurodegeneration in Parkinson's disease. In the 6-OH dopamine model, lesioning of the STN protects the nigral dopamine neurons (Rodriguez et al., 1998). This finding supports the view that excitotoxicity contributes to cell death in midbrain dopamine neurons.

Cell degeneration in Parkinson's disease is not confined to the midbrain because other structures also degenerate. This extranigral pathology comprises several limbic structures, mainly the amygdala and related structures (Braak et al. 1996) and those structures in the basal ganglia circuitry in which a relative (striatum/accumbens) or an absolute glutamate hyperactivity exists (STN, globus pallidus internal segment, substantia nigra pars reticulata) (Fig. 4-3). Our recent experiments provide evidence for a chronic cellular stress (c-fos, c-Jun expression) in these structures (Pedersen and Schmidt, 2000). Thus a loss of dopamine transforms the basal ganglia circuitry in a "destructive network." From these findings it may be concluded that an early dopamine substitution therapy slows neurodegeneration in Parkinson's disease. Indeed in several recent studies this has been shown. As an animal model of Parkinson's disease, degeneration of substantia nigra pars compacta was induced by bilateral injection of 6-OH dopamine into the striata, which caused a retrograde degeneration of the midbrain dopamine cell groups. In this model, the ergot-like alkaloids cabergoline or lisuride reduced the loss of dopaminergic cells. Furthermore, lisuride normalized presynaptic striatal DA metabolism of the remaining axon terminals (Pedersen et al., 1998).

Preliminary results from clinical studies indicate that newly developed dopamine receptor agonists (e.g., ropinirol, pramipexol, or pergolid) have some neuroprotective properties besides their symptomatic effects. From these data, two possibilities for neuroprotective therapies emerge: 1) blocking glutamatergic neurotoxicity by reducing glutamate activity and 2) replacement of dopamine in early stages of Parkinson's disease to restore normal transmitter balance in the basal ganglia loops.

SCHIZOPHRENIA

For a long time, the dopamine hypothesis has dominated speculation and discussion about the pathophysiology of schizophrenia, and dopamine agonist-induced behavioral stimulation in animals and humans has been considered to model the disease. However, in accordance with the basal ganglia circuitry just depicted, it has been found that glutamate antagonists can also induce behavioral "psychomotor" stimulation. A psychomotor stimulant effect of an NMDA receptor antagonist was described in 1986: local infusions of AP-5 into the striatum elicited stereotyped sniffing and, to a lesser extent, horizontal locomotion. Infusions into the nucleus accumbens elicited mainly locomotion and sniffing to a lesser extent. These psychomotor stimulant effects of NMDA receptor antagonists were specifically antagonized by the atypical antipsychotic drug clozapine. The classical neuroleptics (e.g., haloperidol) were much weaker in this respect (Schmidt, 1986). This is of special interest because it is well-known that clozapine does not antagonize stereotypies elicited by dopamine agonists; on the contrary, clozapine even enhances dopamine agonist-induced sniffing. Uncompetitive NMDA receptor antagonists that can be administered peripherally (e.g., phencyclidine or dizocilpine) even have stronger psychomotor stimulant effects.

The symptoms shown in Table 4-1 may suggest that NMDA receptor antagonist-induced behavior represents a better animal model of schizophrenia than dopamine agonist-induced behavior, especially because PCP-induced disturbances of social behavior in rats may be used to screen neuroleptics with some potency against negative symptoms (Sams-Dodd, 1995). PCP-induced symptoms often resemble schizophrenic symptoms in humans (Kornhuber and Weller, 1997; Steinpreis, 1996; Tamminga et al., 1995).

ADDICTION

Drugs of addiction use the brain reward system to mediate their hedonic/euphoric effects. Within the course of behaviors leading to reward, dopamine seems to be involved in the appetitive phase that is associated with approach. Robinson and Berridge (1993) suggest that dopamine attributes incentive salience to previously neutral stimuli. Opiates seem to be involved in the consummatory phase of the reward process (Di Chiara and North, 1992).

Glutamate is an essential transmitter in the brain reward system (especially the glutamatergic neurons from the prefrontal cortex to the ventral tegmental area), and disruption of these neurons interferes with the effects of various addictive drugs (Tzschentke and Schmidt, 1999). Brain glutamate is also involved in the process of sensitization and possibly in withdrawal states.

Sensitization

When repeated administration of a drug causes progressive augmentation of a behavioral response, this phenomenon is called behavioral sensitization (the oppo-

TABLE 4-1. Effects of dizocilpine (MK-801) or phencyclidne on animal behavior

Enhancement of
Horizontal locomotion
Sniffing
Repetitive head movements
Reduction of
Exploration
Dicrimination
Disturbances of
Prepulse inhibition in acoustic startle response
Cognition
Learning
Social behavior

site of tolerance). In animals, many drugs of addiction, especially psychostimulants, induce sensitization of locomotor behavior. If sensitization has developed in an individual, it is stable. Therefore it is believed to provide a useful animal model for the intensification of drug-seeking behavior that characterizes addiction in humans and promotes relapse (Wolf, 1998).

It has been shown that sensitization of locomotor behavior is accompanied by a progressive increase in the activity of neurons of the ventral tegmental area and in turn by a progressive increase of dopamine release in the nucleus accumbens (Wolf, 1998).

Because sensitization represents a process of neural plasticity and because we know that many forms of neural plasticity depend on glutamatergic mechanisms, it was reasonable to investigate whether glutamatergic processes are involved in behavioral sensitization and, if so, whether these could be blocked by glutamate receptor antagonists. Indeed it has been shown that expression of sensitized behavior could be blocked if animals receive a joint treatment of the sensitizing drug with an NMDA receptor antagonist during the sensitizing period. This was also the case if the NMDA receptor antagonist was infused directly into the ventral tegmental area (Wolf, 1998).

However, close examination of these experiments showed that, at least in some cases, the daily increase (during the sensitizing period) in the locomotor response was not blocked by NMDA receptor antagonists (only the sensitized response to the sensitizing drug after the period of sensitization). Actually debate is ongoing regarding to what extent NMDA receptor antagonists block development of sensitization or whether sensitization is not expressed because of a state dependency effect brought about by the NMDA receptor antagonists (Tzschentke and Schmidt, 1998, 1999). It is well-known that NMDA receptor antagonists produce a strong internal cue and can make retrieval of learned behavior state dependent (Jackson et al., 1992; Schmidt et al., 1999). Applying this to explain the sensitization experiments would mean that behavior (i.e., sensitization of locomotion) that is learned under the influence of an NMDA receptor antagonist cannot be expressed in the absence of an NMDA receptor antagonist.

Withdrawal

During chronic drug intake, several compensatory changes occur in the brain. After cessation of alcohol consumption, the activity of the glutamatergic system may increase. If the anticraving drug acamprosate mediates its effects by its NMDA receptor-blocking effects, than this would strongly support the hypothesis of a glutamate hyperactivity after withdrawal and possibly as one source for craving. Recently it has been shown that acamprosate also counteracts aversive effects after morphine withdrawal (Kratzer and Schmidt, 1998). Glutamate activity is also crucial in reinstatement of cocaine-seeking behavior. It was found that AMPA agonists induced reinstatement of cocaine-seeking behavior in rats (Kalivas and Cornish, 1999).

REFERENCES

Blanchet PJ, Papa SM, Verhagen Merman L, et al. (1997). Modulation of levodopa-induced motor response complications by NMDA-antagonists in Parkinson's disease. *Neurosci Biobehav Rev* 21,447–453.

Braak H, Braak E, Yilmazer D, et al. (1996). Pattern of brain destruction in Parkinson's and Alzheimer's diseases. *J Neural Transm* 103,455–490.

Cools AR, Jaspers R, Schwarz M, et al. (1984). Basal ganglia and switching motor programs. In: *Basal Ganglia: Structure and Function*, McKenzie JS, Kemm RE, Wilcock LN, eds. New York: Plenum, pp. 513–544.

Crossman AR (1990). A hypothesis on the pathophysiological mechanisms that underlie levodopa- or dopamine agonist-induced dyskinesia in Parkinson's disease: implications for future strategies in treatment. *Movement Disorders* 5:100–108.

Di Chiara G, North RA (1992). Neurobiology of opiate abuse.*Trends Pharmacol Sci* 13,185–193.

Graybiel AM (1993). Functions of the nigrostriatal system. *Clin Neurosci* 1,12–17.

Hauber W, Schmidt WJ (1990). The NMDA antagonist dizocilpine (MK-801) reverses haloperidol-induced movement initiation deficits. *BehavBrain Res* 41,161–166.

Jackson A, Koek W, Colpaert FC (1992). NMDA antagonists make learning and recall state-dependent. *BehavPharmacol* 3,415–421.

Kalivas PW, Cornish JL (1999). Glutamate transmission in an animal model of cocaine relapse. *Behav Pharmacol* 10(suppl 1),S51.

Knowlton BJ, Mangels JA, Squire LR (1996). A neostriatal habit learning system in humans. *Science* 273,1399–1402.

Kornhuber HH (1974). Cerebral cortex, cerebellum, and basal ganglia: an introduction to their motor functions. In: *Neurosciences III*, Schmitt FO, Worden FG, eds. Cambridge MA: MIT Press, pp. 267–280.

Kornhuber J, Weller M (1997). Psychotogenicity and N-methyl-D-aspartate receptor antagonism: implications for neuroprotective pharmacotherapy. *Biol Psychiatry* 41,135–144.

Kratzer U, Schmidt WJ (1998). The anti-craving drug acamprosate inhibits the conditioned place aversion induced by naloxone-precipitated morphine withdrawal in rats. *Neurosci Lett* 252,53–56.

Kronthaler UO, Schmidt WJ (1998). The mGluRs group II agonist (2S,3S,4S)-alpha-carboxycyclopropyl-glycine induces catalepsy in the rat, which is pronouncedly antagonised by dizocilpine and D,L-amphetamine. *Neurosci Lett* 253,25–28.

Pedersen V, Double K, Schmidt WJ, et al. (1998). Effects of cabergoline and lisuride on motor behavior and dopamine receptor binding in 6-OHDA-lesioned rats. *J Neural Transm* 106,XXV1.

Pedersen V, Schmidt WJ (2000). Expression of c-Fos and c-Jun in the rat basal ganglia mesostriatal and mesolimbic circuits following lesions of nigrostriatal dopaminergic system. *Neurotoxicity Res* 1,1–6.

Robinson TE, Berridge KC (1993). The neural basis of drug craving: an incentive-sensitization theory of addiction. *Brain Res Rev* 18,247–291.

Rodriguez MC, Obeso J, Olanow CW (1998). Subthalamic nucleus-mediated excitotoxicity in Parkinson's disease: a target for neuroprotection. *Ann Neurol* (suppl.) 44,S175–S188.

Sams-Dodd F (1995). Distinct effects of d-amphetamine and phencyclidine on the social behavior of rats. *Behav Pharmacol* 6,55–65.

Schmidt WJ (1984). L-dopa and apomorphine disrupt long- but not short-behavioural chains. *Physiol Behav* 33,671–680.

Schmidt WJ (1986). Intrastriatal injection of DL-2-amino-5-phosphonovaleric acid (AP-5) induces sniffing stereotypy that is antagonized by haloperidol and clozapine. *Psychopharmacology* 90,123–130.

Schmidt WJ (1994). Behavioural effects of NMDA-receptor antagonists. *J Neural Transm* 43,63–69.

Schmidt WJ, Bubser M (1989). Anticataleptic effects of the N-methyl-D-aspartate antagonist MK-801 in rats. *Pharmacol Biochem Behav* 32,621–623.

Schmidt WJ, Kretschmer BD (1997). Behavioural pharmacology of glutamate receptors in the basal ganglia. *Neurosci Biobehav Rev* 21,381–392.

Schmidt WJ, Tzschentke TM, Kretschmer BD (1999). State-dependent blockade of haloperidol-induced sensitization of catalepsy by MK-801. *Eur J Neurosci* 11,3365–3368.

Schultz W, Dayan P, Read Montague P (1997). A neural substrate of prediction and reward. *Science* 275,1593–1599.

Steinpreis RE (1996). The behavioral and neurochemical effects of phencyclidine in humans and animals: some implications for modeling psychosis. *Behav Brain Res* 74,45–55.

Tamminga CA, Holcomb HH, Gao XM, et al. (1995). Glutamate pharmacology and the treatment of schizophrenia: current status and future directions. *Intern Clin Psychopharmacol* 10,29–37.

Tzschentke TM, Schmidt WJ (1998). Does the noncompetitive NMDA receptor antagonist dizocilpine (MK801) really block behavioral sensitization associated with repeated drug administration? *Trends Pharmacol Sci*

19,447–451.

Tzschentke TM, Schmidt WJ (1999). Functional heterogeneity of the rat medial prefrontal cortex: effects of discrete subarea-specific lesions on drug-induced conditioned place preference and behavioral sensitization. *Eur J Neurosci* 11,4099–4109.

Verhagen-Metman L, Del Dotto P, Blanchet PJ, et al. (1998). Blockade of glutamatergic transmission as treatment for dyskinesias and motor fluctuations in Parkinson´s disease. *Amino Acids* 14,75–82.

Wolf ME (1998). The role of excitatory amino acids in behavioral sensitization to psychomotor stimulants. *Progr Neurobiol* 54,679–720.

Zadow B, Schmidt WJ (1994). The AMPA antagonists NBQX and GYKI 52466 do not counteract neuroleptic-induced catalepsy. *Naunyn-Schmiedeberg's Arch Pharmacol* 349,61–65.

5.

Behavioral Models of Tardive Dyskinesia in Rodents

A Chronological Overview

J. Palermo-Neto and R. Frussa-Filho

The term tardive dyskinesia (TD) encompasses a broad spectrum of potentially irreversible involuntary hyperkinetic dyskinesias associated with exposure to long-term neuroleptic treatment. These late-onset involuntary movements, most commonly affecting the orofacial region (i.e., buccolingual-masticatory dyskinesia) but sometimes involving the limbs and trunk, are encountered in a variable proportion of patients receiving such treatment (Jancovic, 1995; Saltz et al., 1997). Because this syndrome represents a major limitation of chronic antipsychotic drug therapy, substantial research has been devoted to identification of the underlying pathophysiological mechanisms of TD for the indication of treatment modalities that might be less likely to induce this movement disorder. Nevertheless, despite data from preclinical and clinical domains, these mechanisms still remain a challenge to research.

A wide range of models has been used to marshal data relevant to each hypothesis for the pathophysiology of TD. These hypotheses span concepts including neurochemical and/or structural abnormalities related to the underlying psychosis or to the drug therapies used to treat them; other models have been used to first try to reproduce the phenomenology of TD and then to search for pathophysiological correlates of such behavior. In this context, data provided by behavioral models using rodents as experimental subjects assumed a distinctive place. This chapter will present and discuss results that support or conflict with the major models of TD. Data centered on behavioral observations of rodents will be specifically reviewed. Results for nonhuman primates have been discussed elsewhere (Crossman, 1987; Kovasic and Domino, 1984; Peacock and Gerlach, 1997).

DOPAMINE RECEPTOR SUPERSENSITIVITY

The dopamine receptor blocking action of the offending agents as well as the transient improvement of TD with the use of higher doses of neuroleptic medications support the notion of up-regulation of dopamine receptors in the basal ganglia. This pathophysiological hypothesis, which has dominated the conceptual approaches to the study of TD, is centered on the notion that the CNS is not static and immutable but rather plastic and adaptable. Indeed there is a close relationship between the supersensitive phenomena and the "withdrawal syndrome" observed after interruption of long-term administration of CNS-depressant drugs (Collier, 1968; Sharpless, 1975). This observation was derived from the classic studies of denervation-induced supersensitivity seen in peripheral muscles. We refer to postsynaptic supersensitivity, also named "denervation" or "disuse" supersensitivity, where the major synaptic change involved is at the level of postsynaptic receptors. Specifically we refer to the hypothesis formulated by Fleming (1976); i.e., the long-term interruption of contact between a neurotransmitter and its related target cells resulted in supersensitive receptors to the endogenously released neurotransmitter or to its related agonists.

Accordingly the supersensitive hypothesis of TD proposes that the nigrostriatal dopaminergic system would develop increased sensitivity to dopamine as a consequence of chronic receptor blockade induced by neuroleptic drugs (Klawans and Rubovits, 1972; Tarsy and Baldessarini, 1974). The reported increment in apomorphine-induced motor activity and rearing behavior in mice and stereotyped behavior in rats after cessation of chronic haloperidol treatment supports this notion (Bernardi et al., 1981; Bernardi and Palermo-Neto, 1983; 1984; Tarsy and Baldessarini, 1974; Thornburg and Moore, 1974). Indeed, the leftward displacement of the dose-response curve constructed for apomorphine-induced stereotyped behavior in rats withdrawn from long-term haloperidol (Bernardi et al, 1981) strengthened the view that the major synaptic change involved is at the receptor level.

Nevertheless in patients the symptoms of TD are present without the requirement of dopamine agonist provocation. Thus we analyzed the effects of neuroleptic withdrawal using an animal model of dopaminergic supersensitivity that would be simple, nondrastic, and reliable in the absence of dopamine receptor agonists. For motor activity in an open field, rats were considered the best candidate (Palermo-Neto, 1982). The simplicity of the apparatus, the easy and rapid measurement of clearly defined behaviors, the generally accepted interpretation of these behaviors (Walsh and Cummins, 1976), and the possibility to analyze the animals for several days after neuroleptic withdrawal in the complete absence of further treatments contributed to our choice. Furthermore, experimental evidence had accumulated relating motor activity and striatal dopaminergic systems and receptors (Buus Lassen, 1976; Schoenfeld and Uretsky, 1972).

In the first experiment (Bernardi and Palermo-Neto, 1979) we examined the effects of abrupt withdrawal from long-term (30 days) haloperidol at increasing doses (up to 10 mg/kg/d, twice daily) on open-field behavior of rats. We observed that abrupt withdrawal from the neuroleptic induced a significant increase in locomotion, rearing, and grooming frequencies of rats observed in the apparatus. This increment was higher 72 hr after the last haloperidol injection. These results were interpreted to be a consequence of striatal dopamine receptor supersensitivity to the endogenously released dopamine. If the decreased motor activity observed 30 min after haloperidol (first open-field session) resulted from dopaminergic receptor blockade (Buus Lassen, 1976), the observed progressive increment in activity in the remaining sessions might be due to supersensitivity of central dopaminergic pathways. This supersensitivity phenomenon was probably induced to counteract the long-term depressant effect of the drug.

To test this possibility, we used the same methodology to compare the effects of single and long-term (30 days) administration of two different doses of haloperidol in rats (Bernardi et al., 1981). A positive correlation was observed between the impairment of motor function induced by the different doses of haloperidol administered as a single dose (2.5 and 10.0 mg/kg) and the increment of motor activity (locomotion and rearing frequencies) registered after abrupt withdrawal from the same neuroleptic doses administered on a long-term basis. Furthermore, no changes were observed in the first open-field session for animals repeatedly treated with 2.5 mg/kg haloperidol, whereas a single 2.5-mg/kg haloperidol injection significantly decreased both locomotion and rearing frequencies. This finding suggests the development of tolerance to haloperidol. Because major tranquilizers cannot induce liver microsomal enzymes (Fandrich and Hadass, 1969) the observed tolerance could only be a consequence of CNS adaptation to the depressant effects of the drug.

The subsequent report that repeated neuroleptic treatment increased the number of dopamine D2 receptors (Burt et al., 1977) strengthened the supersensitive hypothesis of TD. According to these authors, the molecular basis for supersensitivity, and thus for TD, is an increased number of D2 receptor sites in the striatum with no change in their affinity as measured by ^{3}H-neuroleptic binding to striatal membrane homogenates. Nevertheless, this was not the case in all studies. Thus using the stereotyped behavior induced by apomorphine administration as the response, we could analyze in vivo the relative affinity of metoclopramide as reflected by pA_2 values in normal rats and in rats rendered supersensitive to haloperidol (Palermo-Neto et al., 1984).

Specifically pA_2 indicates the dissociation constant of an antagonist and is used not only to classify drugs and receptors but also to study the receptor affinity (Ott et al., 1981). We showed a decrease in dopamine receptor affinity after long-term haloperidol treatment, a concept that was not demonstrated in binding studies conducted in vitro. The pA_2 results were subsequently supported by K_b determination under identical conditions of haloperidol treatment and also using an in vivo methodology (Palermo-Neto and Bernardi, 1984). The significance of the changes in pA_2 and K_b, as opposed both to the supersensitivity to apomorphine in similar quantitative conditions (Bernardi et al., 1981) and to biochemical data provided by in vitro studies, cannot be defined. Nevertheless, it seems relevant to emphasize that affinity and number of receptors are two independent variables not necessarily related to each other (Roscher et al., 1981; Triggle and Triggle, 1976). In this regard, a decrease in antagonist affinity might also explain the development of tolerance to the behavioral effects of haloperidol (see above). At the same time, the increase in the number of dopamine receptor binding sites (Burt et al., 1977) might be related to the increment in activity verified during drug withdrawal. Thus, it may be that the classical pharmacological methods employed in vivo showed new facts not detected in in vitro binding studies. The postsynaptic alterations induced by disuse could be a consequence of several processes that are not exclusive.

The open-field was subsequently used to analyze the effects of withdrawal from long-term bromopride (Felicio et al., 1987, 1989), metoclopramide (Frussa-Filho and Palermo-Neto, 1988), and sulpiride (Frussa-Filho and Palermo-Neto, 1990). In all cases, the withdrawn rats presented increased locomotion and rearing frequencies and decreased immobility duration in the apparatus compared with controls. In this respect, the demonstration that metoclopramide (an antagonist of dopamine D2 receptors used for gastrointestinal disorders and as an antiemetic during cancer chemotherapy) produced dopaminergic behavioral supersensitivity is clinically relevant; indeed, data suggested that caution should be exercised against the long-term use of this drug in clinical practice, in agreement with Miller and Jankovick (1989).

Altogether, these results suggest that supersensitivity of striatal dopamine receptors is involved in the open-field data observed in rats withdrawn from long-term haloperidol, indicating that the open field might be used as a reliable model of TD.

DOPAMINE RECEPTOR SUPERSENSITIVITY AND ALLEGED INCOMPATIBILITIES AND CONTRAPOSITIONS

Some incompatibilities between features of rodent models of dopaminergic supersensitivity and those of clinical TD have been reported (Casey, 1995; Glentjj, 1995; Waddington, 1990, 1997; Wolfarth and Ossowska, 1989). In this respect, animal studies should be considered for their relationship to clinical TD in accordance with the criteria of isomorphism for putative animal models of this movement disorder, as proposed by Jeste and Wyatt (1982a,b).

In patients, TD symptoms gradually develop over many months or years of treatment. In contrast, all animals rapidly develop behavioral and biochemical symptoms of supersensitivity that quickly resolve after neuroleptic discontinuation or gradual removal (Bernardi and Palermo-Neto, 1979). Only a subgroup of patients develop TD, which persists for long periods (Casey, 1990) .

Furthermore, it was reported that dopamine receptor up-regulation was equivalent in chronically treated patients with or without TD (Andersson et al., 1990; Casey and Gerlach, 1986). From another standpoint, if TD is a consequence of dopaminergic receptor supersensitivity, it could be considered to present features opposite those of neuroleptic-induced parkinsonism; thus these two syndromes should not coexist. However, as reviewed by Miller and Chouinard (1993), these two movement disorders can occur together not only in different parts of the body (Crane 1972; Rondot and Bathien, 1986; Wolf et al., 1983) but in the same part of the body (Bitton and Melamed, 1984; De Fraites et al., 1977). Among the most important flaws of this model is that related to the effects of age on TD/behavioral supersensitivity models. Age is the single most frequently implicated risk factor for TD and was shown to increase risk of developing the condition as well as its severity and persistence (Kane 1995; Kane et al., 1985; Saltz et al., 1997; Wolfarth and Ossowska, 1989). Conversely, old animals have a decreased capacity to develop both behavioral supersensitivity to apomorphine-induced stereotyped behavior and dopamine receptor up-regulation after chronic treatment with neuroleptics (Gamble and Waddington, 1981; Misra et al., 1982; Randall et al., 1981; Waddington and Gamble, 1980).

However, a critical analysis of these alleged flaws of the behavioral supersensitivity models of TD in rodents reveals important contrapositions. For example, concerning the time necessary for TD development, note that whereas diagnostic criteria for TD are based on a history of at least 3 months total cumulative neuroleptic exposure (Kane, 1995), increments in apomorphine-induced behaviors can be seen after one dose or after a few days, several weeks, or 1 year of neuroleptic treatment in rodents (Christennsen et al., 1976; Klawans and Rubovits, 1972; Tarsy and Baldessarini, 1973). However, the threshold for TD expression can be altered by challenge with dopamine agonists or antimuscarinic drugs (Carvey et al., 1990). In this regard, note that the increase in spontaneous open-field behavior of rats withdrawn from neuroleptic treatment was never observed before 20 days of treatment, and, even so, extremely high daily doses of haloperidol were necessary to induce behavioral supersensitivity after withdrawal (Bernardi et al., 1981). Although this time is shorter than the 3 months reported necessary for TD development, if the exposures are converted from proportion of life span for rats (2.5 years) to humans (75 years), interpretation is different (Fowler and Wang, 1998). The percentage of life span necessary to induce the movement disorder in humans would be 0.33% (3 months/75 years), a lower result than the 2.19% life span necessary for behavioral supersensitivity development in rats (20 days/2.5 years).

The same rationale can be used with respect to another diagnostic criterion for TD, i.e., persistence of symptoms for at least 4 months (Kane, 1995). The increase in open-field behavior induced by abrupt long-term neuroleptic withdrawal lasted no longer than 10 days (Bernardi and Palermo-Neto, 1979; Frussa-Filho and Palermo-Neto, 1988). These values (4 months for humans and 10 days for rats), when converted to proportions of life span for humans and rats, will be 0.4 and 1.0%, respectively. Note that increased sensitivity of haloperidol-withdrawn rats to apomorphine persisted for at least 100 days, a time equivalent to 8.2 years in humans (I. M. Conceição and R. Frussa-Filho, unpublished data). Even so, the contradictory effects of age on TD and behavioral/ biochemical dopaminergic supersensitivity continue to be among the most important flaws of the behavioral supersensitivity models. However, note that effects of age on behavioral supersensitivity evaluated by spontaneous open-field behavior or by dopamine receptor affinity measured by classical pharmacological methods have not been studied, an important issue given the differences between the in vivo classical pharmacological methods and in vitro binding studies used to evaluate affinity and number of dopamine receptors.

Behavioral and neurochemical changes induced by aging occur in the dopaminergic systems of male and female rats (Dorce and Palermo-Neto, 1991). Specifically, aging decreases animal activity in the open field and increases apomorphine-induced stereotyped behavior. Furthermore, young and aged female rats had higher striatal dopamine and homovanillic acid levels than males, and aging induces a decrease in both striatal dopamine and homovanillic acid levels in males but not in females. These findings suggest that aging reduces nigrostriatal activity and nigrostriatal dopamine levels, leading to supersensitivity of dopamine receptors. Also they indicate that the events related to aging differ between males and females. These results, which agree in some features with others (Godefroy et al., 1989; Roth and Joseph, 1988), might help explain not only the effects of age but also those of gender differences on the age-related pathophysiology of TD. As with age, gender differences in TD incidence and pathophysiology have been extensively discussed (Owens, 1999; Yassa and Jeste, 1997).

Another relevant flaw is the fact that all animals develop behavioral supersensitivity after long-term neuroleptic treatment, whereas only a subgroup of patients develop TD. In this respect, note that in contrast to patients, rodents used in experiments are genetically similar animals maintained under the same experimental conditions (e.g., including the same pharmacological treatments and environmental conditions). Thus many factors affecting TD may be related to the development (or absence of development) of behavioral supersensitivity in rodents. In this context, dose and duration of neuroleptic treatment (Bernardi et al., 1981; Frussa-Filho and Palermo-Neto, 1988) as well as environmental light conditions (Abilio et al., 1999) may be critical for development and expression of behavioral supersensitivity in rodents.

Concerning the coexistence of TD and neuroleptic-induced parkinsonism, whereas long-term treatment with dopaminergic blockers can increase spontaneous open-field behavior and apomorphine-induced stereotypy, it can increase, not modify or decrease, cataleptic behavior (an animal model of neuroleptic-induced parkinsonism) after a challenge neuroleptic injection (Barnes et al., 1990; Ezrin-Waters et al., 1977; Frussa-Filho et al., 1992). Sensitization to cataleptic behavior induced by neuroleptics seems to be closely related to a conditioning phenomenon (Chinen and Frussa-Filho, in press).

Finally, demonstration that dopamine receptor site up-regulation is equivalent in chronically treated patients with or without TD does not invalidate the use of behavioral supersensitivity as a model (Carvey et al., 1990). The increment induced by scopolamine pretreatment in apomorphine-induced stereotyped behavior is smaller in rats withdrawn from long-term haloperidol than in control animals not treated with this neuroleptic (De Souza and Palermo-Neto, 1981). These results suggest that the dopamine/acetylcholine balance was modified during long-term haloperidol. Carvey et al. (1990) presented other data in the same direction. These authors showed that cotreatment of rats with thioridazine or scopolamine attenuated the magnitude of the behavioral supersensitivity to apomorphine induced in rats withdrawn from chronic haloperidol but failed to attenuate dopamine receptor proliferation. According to these authors, dopamine receptor proliferation may not be necessarily correlated with behavioral supersensitivity. It is therefore hypothesized that dopamine receptor proliferation would permit the development of behavioral supersensitivity and possibly of TD. Thus other factors such as striatal muscarinic tone would be relevant to determine whether dopaminergic supersensitivity induced by chronic neuroleptic treatment would be manifest as a behavioral supersensitivity state. A possible development of supersensitivity at the dopamine autoreceptor level was also reported. These hypotheses will be analyzed.

DOPAMINE, COTRANSMITTERS, OTHER NEUROTRANSMITTERS, AND DOPAMINERGIC SUPERSENSITIVITY

The synaptic availability of striatal dopamine can be modulated by cotransmitters and other neurotransmitter systems whose function, if altered, modifies TD symptoms without necessarily modifying dopamine receptor proliferation. In such cases it would be expected that modifications in behavioral supersensitivity evaluated by spontaneous open-field behavior would not be accompanied by alterations in apomorphine-induced stereotyped behavior. In this regard, whereas Tunicliff et al. (1992) showed that withdrawal from repeated treatment with the 5-HT_{1A} agonist buspirone led to marked reductions in synthesis of dopamine in the rat striatum, Queiroz and Frussa-Filho (1997) showed that cotreatment with this drug attenuated supersensitivity evaluated by spontaneous open-field behavior in rats withdrawn from haloperidol but failed to modify apomorphine-induced stereotypy.

In another recent study, Batista and Palermo-Neto (in press) showed that concomitant treatment of rats with haloperidol plus MK801, an antagonist of the Mg^{2+} channel of the NMDA glutamatergic receptor, could not change open-field parameters or apomorphine-induced stereotyped behavior in haloperidol-withdrawn rats. However, when MK801 was administered during withdrawal from long-term haloperidol, open-field behavior increased, but no change in apomorphine-induced stereotypy was evident. Further analysis of striatal dopaminergic activity in this experiment by biochemical measurements showed that MK801 given during haloperidol withdrawal increased striatal dopamine levels and turnover, a fact not observed when the drug was coadministered with haloperidol. By another way, dopamine cotransmitters might also be involved in behavioral supersensitivity models of TD. Cholecystokinin, one of the most abundant peptides in the brain that coexists with dopamine in some neurons (Schalling et al., 1990), can modulate the dopaminergic activity in dopamine-supersensitive rats (Tieppo et al., 1995). Intracerebroventricular administration of CCK-8, a bioactive sulfated terminal octapeptide, reduced stereotypy in haloperidol-supersensitive rats.

These considerations suggest that, like TD, behavioral supersensitivity (especially when evaluated by spontaneous open-field behavior) may be expressed in subjects with equivalent striatal postsynaptic dopamine proliferation depending on dopamine synaptic availability or dopaminergic striatal tone regulated by cotransmitters and/or other neurotransmitter systems.

DOPAMINE AUTORECEPTOR SUPERSENSITIVITY AND DOPAMINERGIC SUPERSENSITIVITY

Unlike other dopaminergic blocking agents, withdrawal from long-term treatment with the butyrophenone droperidol did not significantly increase open-field parameters in rats (Frussa-Filho and Palermo-Neto, 1991). However, as is the case for other dopamine blockers, droperidol withdrawal produced an augmented responsiveness to apomorphine-induced stereotyped behavior. In this respect, apomorphine, at doses that induce stereotypy, is a direct agonist at the postsynaptic dopamine receptor level (Ernst, 1967). In contrast, the open-field behavior depends on the endogenous dopamine action on these receptors; therefore it also depends on dopamine release and reuptake, among many factors, including dopamine autoreceptors. Despite a postsynaptic dopamine proliferation induced by long-term droperidol (behaviorally suggested by the observed increment in apomorphine-induced stereotypy), rats withdrawn from droperidol did not show behavioral supersensitivity, at least as evaluated by locomotion and rearing frequencies in the open field.

Thus according to the open-field model of TD, it would be feasible to think that patients with the same postsynaptic dopamine proliferation may present this movement disorder depending on neuronal dopamine availability at the synaptic level and/or on the dopamine autoreceptor state of activity. Tamminga (1981) proposed that if both auto- and postsynaptic dopamine receptors became equally supersensitive, the synaptic activity would remain balanced, and extrapyramidal motor symptoms of TD would be potentially reduced or perhaps almost absent. Abrupt withdrawal from repeated treatment with a low dose of haloperidol (0.03 mg/kg) induced a significant decrease in open-field behavior of rats, whereas no change was observed in apomorphine-induced stereotypy (Frussa-Filho et al., 1997). Because this low dose of haloperidol was found to increase locomotor activity of rats after one administration, a selective blocking effect was suggested at the dopamine autoreceptor level. Thus it was concluded that long-term blockade at these receptors produced dopamine autoreceptor supersensitivity that resulted in behavioral subsensitivity.

SPONTANEOUS OROFACIAL MOVEMENTS

According to Waddington (1990), an additional and critical flaw of the behavioral supersensitivity models of TD is the absence, in a situation held to reproduce the putative pathophysiology of TD, of spontaneous orofacial movements that are the fundamental characteristics of this disorder. Carvey et al. (1990) indicated that facial musculature of the rodent is exceedingly less complex than that of humans, so one would therefore expect that the threshold to produce spontaneous movements in humans would be lower than that in rodents. Notwithstanding their contraposition, several investigators recognize the importance of evaluating perioral behaviors in rodents, thereby seeking to reproduce the phenomenology of TD to analyze the pathophysiological correlates of such behaviors later (Ellison and See, 1989; Glassman and Glassman, 1980; Gunne et al., 1982; Iversen et al., 1980; Waddington et al., 1983). These rodent models were analyzed in detail in two excellent reviews by Waddington (1990, 1997) and therefore will be only briefly discussed here.

According to Waddington (1990), the most consistently reported occurrence in the phenomenological models of TD is that of vacuous (or abortive or spontaneous) chewing movements (VCM). Neuroleptic-induced VCMs have been described in some experiments; they were reported to develop after months of neuroleptic treatment, persisting for long periods after neuroleptic withdrawal and occurring more markedly in senescent animals (Waddington, 1990, 1997; Waddington et al., 1983). However, as Glenthöj (1995) indicates, evaluating spontaneous perioral movements in rodents during chronic neuroleptic treatment reveals a marked inconsistency. Several authors have reported the emergence of VCMs early during neuroleptic treatment or even after acute treatment with these drugs (Glenthöj and Hemmingsen, 1989; Levy et al., 1987; Rupniak et al., 1986; Steinpreis et al., 1998; Steinpreis and Salamone 1993). Neuroleptic-induced VCM have also been interpreted to be related to acute dystonia (Rupniak, 1986) or parkinsonism (Steinpreis and Salamone, 1993). In this regard, although late onset neuroleptic-induced VCMs are not potentiated by anticholinergic treatment (Waddington, 1990) the early-onset VCMs are alleviated by anticholinergic agents and exacerbated by physostigmine (Rupniak et al., 1983, 1985). Note that challenging with anticholinergic drugs aggravates and/or uncovers preexisting TD (Yassa and Nair, 1997) as well as apomorphine-induced stereotypy in rats withdrawn from long-term haloperidol treatment (De Souza and Palermo-Neto, 1981). This experimental evidence in favor of the behavioral supersensitivity models of TD has been overlooked.

Another relevant criticism of this model of TD is the absence of a clear-cut inhibitory effect of neuroleptic challenge on VCM (Glenth(j, 1995; Waddington, 1990), because symptoms of TD are known to be alleviated by dopamine receptor antagonists (Baldessarini et al., 1980; Kazamatsuri et al., 1972; Klawans, 1973; Klawans et al., 1977; Jeste and Wyatt, 1981, 1982a,b). Finally, in addition to the lack of confident acceptance of neuroleptic-induced VCM as a model of TD originating from the unresolved criticisms, there is also a methodological question; long periods of neuroleptic treatments are necessary for the late-onset appearance of orofacial movements in rodents.

Waddington et al. (1983a,b) reported that after 6 months of continuous treatment with neuroleptics, orofacial movements were manifested in the presence of sufficient amounts of drug to enduringly block stereotyped behavior induced by a modest dose of apomorphine. Thus these movements were evident in the presence of apparently enduring functional blockade of up-regulated dopamine receptors. In addition, after neuroleptic withdrawal after 6 months of treatment, VCMs persisted at least to a point where increases in either D1 or D2 receptor binding were no longer present (Waddington et al., 1983a). Reviewing these and other experimental data, Waddington (1990) concluded that such movements have not had their pathophysiological basis centered on either dopaminergic hyperfunction in general or dopamine receptor supersensitivity in particular.

Despite the alleged absence of intersection and the several criticisms made both to VCM and behavioral supersensitivity models of TD, these models make relevant contributions to the understanding of this movement disorder and to the development of new models to tentatively explain its pathophysiology. The hypotheses formulated so far include the existence of 1) D1/D2 dopamine receptor imbalance (also called the hypothesis of D1-like receptor involvement), 2) γ-aminobutyric acid

(GABA)-ergic deficiencies, and 3) neurotoxicity and structural abnormalities within the basal ganglia. These new hypotheses have been reviewed and detailed elsewhere (Casey, 1995; Ebadi and Srinivasan, 1995; Glenth(j, 1995; Peacock and Gerlach, 1997; Waddington, 1997). We will briefly discuss them by citing examples of contributions of both behavioral supersensitivity and VCM models.

D1/D2 RECEPTOR IMBALANCE

This hypothesis is supported by much data showing the existence of functional interactions between dopamine D1 and D2 receptors (Palermo-Neto, 1997; Waddington, 1989). As reviewed by Casey (1995) and Waddington (1997), this hypothesis can be considered a modification or a variant of the general dopaminergic hypothesis of hyperfunction/receptor supersensitivity, implying a possibly major role of dopamine D1 receptors (Peacock and Gerlach, 1997). According to Casey (1995), the core of this hypothesis is that clozapine has a unique biochemical profile at the D1 and D2 receptor level that may be associated with atypical behavioral and clinical features. Thus this neuroleptic does not produce biochemical or behavioral indications of dopaminergic supersensitivity (Coward et al., 1989). Similarly, clozapine produces little TD in treated patients (Casey, 1989) and has relatively high and moderate occupancy rates at D1 and D2 receptor sites, respectively, as measured by positron emission tomography (Farde et al., 1992). Behavioral data obtained with sulpiride in rats provide additional information (Frussa-Filho and Palermo-Neto, 1990).

Sulpiride, a substituted benzamide drug that differs from classical neuroleptic agents in behavioral (Costall and Naylor, 1975; Eliott et al., 1977; Jenner et al., 1978, 1884) and biochemical (Creese et al., 1979; Elliot et al., 1977) models of dopaminergic studies, increased locomotion and rearing frequencies of rats observed in an open field after withdrawal from long-term treatment (Frussa-Filho and Palermo-Neto, 1990). According to Rupniak et al. (1984), sulpiride induced no increase in D2 receptors in experimental animals but significantly increased D1 receptor function in contrast to traditional neuroleptics such as haloperidol, which increases the D2 but not D1 receptor. Like clozapine, sulpiride elicits few extrapyramidal side effects (Ljungberg and Ungerstedt, 1977). Thus a D1 receptor involvement in this behavioral model of TD is not impossible. These observations have led to the proposal that TD might develop from an imbalance between D1- and D2-mediated effects in the basal ganglia.

These observations seem to be strongly corroborated by a study using selective D1 and D2 receptor antagonists (Marin et al., 1993). Rats received either the selective D1 receptor antagonist SCH 23390, the selective D2 receptor antagonist raclopride, both, or haloperidol, predominantly a D2 antagonist; equivalent cataleptogenic doses of these drugs and drug combinations were employed. Results showed that apomorphine-induced stereotypy was significantly enhanced in rats treated with SCH 23390, raclopride, and haloperidol. In contrast, concomitant administration of SCH 23390 and raclopride had no effect on apomorphine-induced stereotypy.

Similarly, there have been several studies implicating a D1/D2 imbalance in favor of D1 in the pathophysiology of neuroleptic-induced VCM in rodents (Glenth(j, 1995; Peacock and Gerlach, 1997; Waddington et al., 1997). For example, in rats treated for 1 month with haloperidol, VCM was inhibited by the selective D1 antagonist SCH 23390. It was also suppressed by acute challenge with the dopamine synthesis inhibitor α-methyl-*p*-tyrosine; in the treated animals, VCM was reinstated by administering the selective D1 agonist SKF 38393 (Diana et al., 1992).

GABA DEFICIENCY

One pathophysiological hypothesis proposed for TD involves possible GABA deficiencies in the neuronatomical loops of the corticostriatothalamocortical circuits (Fibiger and Lloyd, 1984; Gale, 1980). Specifically the information is funneled from cortical areas into the striatum (though D1 and D2 receptor activation) to internal and external segments of the globus pallidus or substantia nigra and then to specific thalamic nuclei before returning to the cortex (Palermo-Neto, 1997). Thus neuroleptics, secondarily to the blockade of dopamine receptor, may also be able to influence sensitivity of synaptic responses mediated by GABA (Gale, 1980; Gale et al., 1978). Remember that the striatum gives rise to two major GABAergic and inhibitory pathways: the striatonigral (providing direct input to dopaminergic cells within the substantia nigra) and striatopallidal (providing indirect routes between striatum and substantia nigra as it first sends GABAergic inhibitory input to the globus pallidus, which in turn sends GABAergic inhibitory input to the dopaminergic cells of the substantia nigra). Because of this arrangement and because the nigrothalamic projections are GABAergic in nature, the nigrostriatal pathway tends to accentuate thalamic drive (the excitatory glutamatergic input to the cortical mantle), whereas the striatopallidal pathway tends to inhibit or modulate it.

In the basal ganglia, the neuroleptics interact with dopamine receptors located postsynaptically in striatal intrinsic and projection neurons (Seeman, 1980). Thus in rodent models, GABA function was reported to be related (Gale, 1980) or unrelated (Rupniak et al., 1987) to acute and long-term effects of neuroleptics. Of particular importance is the observation by Pan et al. (1985) that receptor binding after unilateral 6-hydroxydopamine striatal lesions in rats showed that GABA receptors were down-regulated in the globus pallidus but inversely up-regulated in the entopeduncular nucleus. Arnt (1985) reported similar data in a study of the hyperactivity of rats after bilateral 6-hydroxydopamine lesions and injection with specific D1 and D2 dopamine receptors. Thus, it seems not only that different populations of striatal neurons project to either region but also that each population appears to be localized in distinct striatal areas where nigral dopaminergic terminals may be differently sensitive to the neurotoxic effects of 6-hydroxydopamine. Scheel-Kruger (1986) has put forward the hypothesis that blockade of striatal dopamine receptors would result in the lack of GABAergic inhibition of efferent GABAergic cells to the substantia nigra pars reticulata and, as a consequence, to a compensatory functional supersensitivity of dopaminergic receptors in this area.

Studies by Gunne et al. (1984, 1986) demonstrated that depressed GABAergic activity in the substantia nigra pars compacta is correlated with enhanced oral activity in neuroleptic-treated rats. Autoradiographic data have shown an increase in the binding sites for GABA receptor-linked Cl^- channels in the ventrolateral caudate putamen of animals with high VCM when compared with animals with low VCM (Sasaki et al., 1997). With respect to the behavioral supersensitivity model, we have shown that haloperidol-withdrawn rats displayed high degrees of stereotyped behavior not only before but also after the ictus activity induced by the GABA antagonist picrotoxin (Sandoval and Palermo-Neto, 1989).

NEUROTOXICITY AND STRUCTURAL ABNORMALITY

Recently the emphasis on TD studies has shifted from neurotransmitter models to other models proposing that TD is a consequence of the neurotoxic effects of free radical byproducts of catecholamine metabolism (Cadet et al., 1986; Jeste and Wyatt, 1981). However, these hypotheses are not conflicting but rather different attempts to define a final common pathway leading to neuronal abnormalities that might be manifested as TD.

According to Parsons (1985), both L-dopa and dopamine are cytotoxic to neuroblastoma, leukemia, and melanoma cell lines; their toxic effects may be related to the rate of auto-oxidation to quinone byproducts and to enzymatic (via monoamine oxidase) and nonenzymatic formation of oxygen free radicals (i.e., superoxide, hydrogen peroxide, and hydroxyl radicals) during their metabolic breakdown (Cohen, 1984; Graham et al., 1978). Free radicals possess many toxic effects; in general, cells, including those of the CNS, depend on detoxifying systems such as enzymes (superoxide dismutase, catalase, and glutathione peroxidase) and free radical scavengers (antioxidants) to protect themselves against oxidative damage (Halliwell and Gutteridge, 1984). The basal ganglia would be particularly vulnerable to membrane lipid peroxidation as a result of the increased catecholamine turnover induced by neuroleptic drugs (Cadet et al., 1986; Lohr, 1991). TD was associated with higher concentrations of lipid peroxidation products in cerebrospinal fluid (Lohr et al., 1990). Thus, as suggested by Jeste and Wyatt (1981), under certain circumstances disturbance of the protective mechanisms might lead to neuropathological changes in structures that contain high concentrations of catecholamines, such as in dopaminergic systems as well as surrounding GABAergic systems and other adjacent neuronal pathways. According to Fibiger and Lloyd (1984), TD might be related to "neuroleptic-induced degeneration of the striatopallidal and/or striatonigral GABAergic systems."

Abnormal free radical activity occurring during neuroleptic treatment may underlie structural changes in the CNS. Several clinical and rodent studies have reported neuropathological alterations in animals chronically treated with neuroleptics (Benes et al., 1985; Nielson and Lyon, 1978; Pakkenberg et al., 1973). A 20% cell loss in the basal ganglia of rats treated chronically with perphenasine enanthate has been reported (Pakkenberg et al., 1973) as well as a 10% cell loss in the ventrolateral striatum of rats treated with flupentixol (Nielson and Lyon, 1978). Additionally, significant neuronal losses, satellitosis, and some glial reactions have been shown in the caudate nuclei of patients who had received chronic neuroleptic treatment. Jellinger (1977) reported that this phenomenon is more marked in individuals who presented with dyskinesias. Electron microscopy has shown that treatment for [gteq]2 months with traditional neuroleptics such as haloperidol increased perforated postsynaptic densities in the head of the caudate nucleus, but this was not seen with clozapine (Meshul et al., 1992a). The D1 antagonist SCH 23390 also produced this effect, but when combined with haloperidol to make D1 and D2 antagonism similar to clozapine, the combination could not alter the structure (Meshul et al., 1992b).

Cohen and Zubenko (1985) demonstrated that striatal cell membranes of rats chronically treated with neuroleptics showed abnormal physicochemical properties; neuroleptics, because of their lipophilicity, might have become incorporated into the membrane, thus altering its properties. In this respect, free radicals have been reported to react with membrane components, leading to membrane destabilization (Diplock, 1983). Finally, chlorpromazine has been shown to increase the brain levels of manganese (Fann et al., 1980), and this ion was reported to potentiate damage caused by free radicals and to be associated with extrapyramidal disorders (Graham, 1984).

Final evidence in favor of the neurotoxicity hypothesis of TD is related to the beneficial effects of the free radical scavenger α-tocopherol (vitamin E) on the manifestation of this movement disorder (Elkashef et al., 1990; Lohr et al., 1987). However, in clinical trials with vitamin E some patients did not show major improvements (Shriqui et al., 1992). According to Casey (1995), more favorable results were obtained with vitamin E in TD patients who were younger and had shorter duration of this movement disorder. Again, both behavioral supersensitivity and VCM models were involved. Gatass et al. (1993) showed that vitamin E coadministration attenuates behavioral supersensitivity evaluated by increased apomorphine-induced stereotyped behavior in haloperidol-withdrawn rats. Similarly, Takeuchi et al. (1998) demonstrated that concomitant administration of vitamin E and haloperidol suppressed the appearance of VCM.

NEW MODELS

Two new promising behavioral models of TD in rodents have been recently proposed. One is the increase in tongue protrusion frequency induced by repeated administration of reserpine (Bergamo et al., 1997; Neisewander et al., 1991a,b, 1994, 1996; Queiroz et al., 1998; Queiroz and Frussa-Filho, 1999; Sussman et al., 1997; Vital et al., 1997). Although reserpine is not classified as a neuroleptic, it was used as an antipsychotic agent and has been associated with the development of TD (Shonecker, 1957; Uhrbrand and Faurdye, 1960). This reserpine-induced oral dyskinesia in rats has several other features that are consistent with this movement disorder, including persistence after interruption of administration and a reported dose-dependent blockade induced by D2 selective antagonists (Neisewander et al.,

1991a,b). As with TD (Wolfarth and Ossowska, 1989), reserpine-induced oral dyskinesia is exacerbated by dopamine agonists such as amphetamine (Neisewander et al., 1996). Furthermore, although reserpine-induced tongue protrusion dyskinesia in rats is of insidious onset (months) after the use of low doses, the response develops rapidly (few days) after high doses (Neisewander et al., 1994); this fact offers an outstanding methodological advantage over long-term neureoleptic administration. Recently Bergamo et al. (1997) verified that when compared with control adult rats, the significant increase in tongue protrusion frequency induced by reserpine was more persistent in old than in adult rats.

The comparison of the effects of different drugs on reserpine-induced oral dyskinesia or behavioral supersensitivity models reveals interesting information. Like TD (Moss et al., 1993; Neppe, 1989, 1990) and behavioral supersensitivity evaluated by spontaneous open-field behavior in haloperidol-withdrawn rats (Queiroz and Frussa-Filho, 1997), reserpine-induced tongue protrusion was attenuated by the anxiolytic agent buspirone (Queiroz and Frussa-Filho, in press). Conversely, the same dose and treatment schedules of the ganglioside GM_1, which were reported to increase behavioral supersensitivity models in rodents (Schröder et al., 1994; Vital et al., 1995), attenuated reserpine-induced orofacial dyskinesia in rats (Vital et al. 1997).

Although mechanisms related to the potentiating effects of GM_1 on behavioral supersensitivity models remain contradictory (Palermo-Neto et al., 1999; Vital et al., 1998), reserpine-induced oral dyskinesia data were interpreted in terms of the free radical hypothesis of TD. Whereas gangliosides can directly scavenge the oxygen free radicals both in vitro and in vivo (Maulik et al., 1993), reserpine may alter oxidative metabolism even more strongly than neuroleptics. Storage of newly synthesized dopamine is prevented by reserpine treatment; therefore dopamine is continuously available for metabolism. We verified that reserpine-induced oral dyskinesia was attenuated by several antioxidant agents, such as melatonin, vitamin E, and *n*-tert-butyl-α-phenyl-nitrone (R. Frussa-Filho, unpublished data). Reserpine did not increase the tongue protrusion frequency in spontaneous hypertensive rats (Queiroz et al., 1998). From a clinical viewpoint, this finding is relevant and agrees with the exceedingly rare literature on reserpine-induced TD in hypertensive patients. From a mechanistic point of view, these results might be related to the presence of alterations in both striatal dopaminergic function (Watanabe et al., 1997) and organic oxidative stress (Ito et al., 1995), previously described in spontaneously hypertensive rats.

The second promising behavioral model is an alternative, instrument-based method for measuring the effects of neuroleptics on orolingual behavior of rats (Fowler and Wang, 1998). Measurements were made of tongue protrusion for each lick, dominant rhythm of tongue movements, and number of individual licks as the rat licked (lapped) water from a force-sensing disk during short time sessions. The effects of chronic haloperidol on one parameter measured (lick rhythm) exhibited some similarities with the clinical descriptions of TD: expression of abnormalities in tongue or jaw, emergence of lick rhythm slowing after 13 days of treatment, and gradual increase in magnitude of this rhythm slowing through the remaining treatment. However, these effects did not worsen upon termination of neuroleptic treatment and were alleviated by anticholinergic treatment.

FUTURE DIRECTIONS AND CONCLUSIONS

Although we have greatly expanded our knowledge of the pathophysiology of TD, there is no direct evidence of a fundamental unifying explanation for the propensity of neuroleptics to induce TD. The number of studies of humans and animals to explain this pathophysiology supports this assumption. Thus 40 years after the first description of neuroleptic-induced involuntary movements (Schonecker, 1957; Uhrbrand and Faursbye, 1960) a definite understanding of the pathophysiology of TD is lacking.

Why is such difficulty encountered in identifying an isomorphic or homologous rodent model of an adverse clinical reaction that can be so prominent in many patients? Trying to answer this question, Waddington (1990) proposed two hypotheses with which we agree and that we present here. First, neuroleptics might exert different pharmacological effects on humans and on nonhuman primates in comparison with rodents; second, some other factor in addition to long-term neuroleptic treatment might be required for symptoms to emerge.

Given our current state of knowledge, the first hypothesis does not seem feasible, but the results observed fit better in the second hypothesis. TD is not seen in all neuroleptic-treated patients despite a similar history of exposure. It seems extremely relevant to remember that neuroleptic drugs are given to humans that have major neuropsychiatric disorders, i.e., patients with already compromised physiological functioning of the CNS. There is a growing body of evidence suggesting a relationship between diseases for which neuroleptic treatment is prescribed and vulnerability to TD (Kane et al., 1985; Owens, 1985; Waddington, 1989; 1990). We agree with Waddington (1990) when he states that it is probably the absence of such an illness dimension that distinguishes the rodent models from the clinical situation. The observations that aging and senescence as well as cortical damage (Waddington, 1990) might precipitate or hasten VCM in neuroleptic-treated animals strongly support the notion that some endogenous or exogenous process of cerebral dysfunction may emerge when neuroleptics are administered long-term.

Differences in dopaminergic sensitivity to the neurotoxic effects of free radical byproducts from catecholamine metabolism or differences in D1/D2 receptor supersensitivity might be involved in patient predisposition to TD. A possible change produced by free radical byproduct-induced neuronal losses in the balance between neurotransmitters within the CNS also cannot be excluded. Given the complexities of neurotransmitter pharmacology and the chemical jungle that is the striatum, to believe that just one hypothesis of TD will explain its pathophysiology or that one animal model will fulfill the necessary requirements for TD validation is an oversimplification.

REFERENCES

Abilio VC, Freitas FM, Dolnikoff MS, et al. (1999). Effects of continuos exposure to light on behavioral dopaminergic supersensitivity. *Biol Psychiatry* 45,1622–1629.

Andersson U, Eckernas SA, Harivig P, et al. (1990). Striatal binding of ^{11}C-NMSP studied with positron emission tomography in patients with persistent tardive dyskinesia: no evidence for altered dopamine D_2 receptor binding. *J Neural Transm* 79,215–226.

Arnt J (1985). Hyperactivity induced by stimulation of separate dopamine D_1 and D_2 receptors in rats with bilateral 6-OHDA lesions. *Life Sci* 37,717–723.

Baldessarini RJ, Cole JO, Davis JM, et al. (1980). Tardive dyskinesia: summary of a task force report of the American Psychiatry Association. *Am J Psychiatry* 137,1163–1172.

Barnes DE, Robson B, Csernansky JG, et al. (1990). Sensitization versus tolerance to haloperidol induced catalepsy: multiple determinants. *Pharmacol Biochem Behav* 36,883–887.

Batista IR, Palermo-Neto J. Effects of Mk-805 on haloperidol-induced behavioral supersensitivity in rats. *Braz J Med Biol Res*, in press.

Benes FM, Paskevich PA, Davidson J, et al. (1985). The effects of haloperidol on synaptic patterns in the rat striatum. *Brain Res* 329,265–274.

Bergamo M, Abilio VC, Queiroz CMT, et al. (1997). Effects of age on a new animal model of tardive dyskinesia. *Neurobiol Aging* 18,623–629.

Bernardi MM, De Sousa H, Palermo-Neto J (1981). Effects of single and long-term haloperidol administration on open-field behavior of rats. *Psychopharmacology* 73,171–175.

Bernardi MM, Palermo-Neto J (1979). Effects of abrupt and gradual withdrawal from long-term haloperidol treatment on open-field behavior of rats. *Psychopharmacology* 65,247–250.

Bernardi MM, Palermo-Neto J (1983). Effect of apomorphine administration on locomotor activity of control and experimental rats withdrawn from long-term haloperidol treatment. *Gen Pharmacol* 14,545–547.

Bernardi MM, Palermo-Neto J (1984). Effect of apomorphine administration on rearing activity of control and experimental rats withdrawn from long-term haloperidol treatment. *Gen Pharmacol* 15,363–365.

Bitton V, Melamed E (1984). Coexistence of severe parkinsonism and tardive dyskinesia as side effects of neuroleptic therapy. *J Clin Psychiatry* 45,28–30.

Burt DR, Creese I, Snyder SH (1977). Antischizophrenic drugs: chronic treatment elevates dopaminergic receptors binding in brain. *Science* 196,326–327.

Buus Lassen J (1976). Inhibition and potentiation of apomorphine-induced hypermotility in rats by neuroleptics. *Eur J Pharmacol* 36,385–393.

Cadet Jl, Lohr JB, Jeste DV (1986). Free radicals and tardive dyskinesia. *Trends Neurosci* 9,107–108.

Carvey PM, Kao LC, Zhang TJ, et al. (1990). Dopaminergic alterations in cotreatments attenuating haloperidol-induced hypersensitivity. *Pharmacol Biochem Behav* 35,291–300.

Casey DE (1989). Clozapine: neuroleptic-induced EPS and tardive dyskinesia. *Psychopharmacology* 99,S47–S53.

Casey DE (1990). Tardive dyskinesia. *West J Med* 153,535–541.

Casey DE (1995). Tardive dyskinesia: pathophisiology. In: *Psychpharmacology: The Fourth Generation of Progress*, Bloom FE, Kupfer DJ, eds. New York: Raven, pp. 1497–1502.

Casey DE, Gerlach J (1986). Is tardive dyskinesia due to dopaminergic hypersensitivity? *Clin Neuropharmacol* 9,134–136.

Chinen CC, Frussa-Filho R. Conditioning to injection procedures and repeated testing increase SCH 23390-induced catalepsy in mice. *Neuropsychopharmacology*, in press.

Christennsen AV, Fjalland B, Moller Nielsen I (1976). On the supersensitivity of dopamine receptors induced by neuroleptics. *Psychopharmacology* 48,1–6.

Cohen G (1984). Oxy-radical toxicity in catecholamine neurons. *Neurotoxicology* 5,77–82.

Cohen BM, Zubenko GS (1985). In vivo effects of psychotropic agents on the physical properties of cell membranes in the rat brain. *Psychopharmacology* 86,365–368.

Collier HOJ (1968). Supersensitivity and dependence. *Nature* 220,228–231.

Costall B, Naylor RJ (1975). Detection of the neuroleptic properties of clozapine, sulpiride and thioridazine. *Psychopharmacology* 43,69–74.

Coward DM, Imperato A, Urwyler S, et al. (1989). Biochemical and behavioural properties of clozapine. *Psychopharmacology* 99,S6–S12.

Crane GE (1972). Pseudo parkinsonism and tardive dyskinesia. *Arch Neurol* 27,426–430.

Creese I, Stewart K, Snyder SH (1979). Species variations in dopamine receptor binding. *Eur J Pharmacol* 60,55–66.

Crossman AR (1987). Primate models of dyskinesia. *Neuroscience* 21,1–40.

De Fraites EG, Davis KL, Berger PA (1977). Coexisting tardive dyskinesia and parkinsonism: a case report. *Biol Psychiatry* 12,267–272.

De Souza H, Palermo-Neto J (1981). The effects of scopolamine pretreatment on stereotyped behavior induced by apomorphine in rats withdrawn from long-term haloperidol administration. *Braz J Med Biol Res* 14,281–284.

Diana M, Collu M, Mura A, et al. (1992) Haloperidol-induced vacuous chewing movements in rats: suppression by alpha-methyl-tyrosine. *Eur J Pharmacol* 211,415–419.

Diplock AT (1983). Biology of vitamin E. *Ciba Found Symp* 101,45–55.

Dorce VAC, Palermo-Neto J (1991). Behavioral and neurochemical changes induced by aging in dopaminergic systems of male and female rats. *Physiol Behav* 56,1015–1019.

Ebadi M, Srinivasan SK (1995). Pathogenesis, prevention, and treatment of neuroleptic-induced movement disorders. *Pharmacol Rev* 47,575–604.

Elkashef AM, Ruskin PE, Bacher N, et al. (1990). Vitamin E in the treatment of tardive dyskinesia. *Am J Psychiatry* 147,505–509.

Elliot PNC, Jenner P, Huising C, et al. (1977). Substituted benzamides as central dopamine antagonists in rodents. *Neuropharmacology* 16,332–342.

Ellison G, See RE (1989). Rats administered chronic neuroleptics develop oral movements which are similar in form to those in humans with tardive dyskinesia. *Psychopharmacology* 98,564–566.

Ernst A (1967). Mode of action of apomorphine and dexamphetamine on gnawing compulsion in rats. *Psychopharmacology* 10,316–324.

Ezrin-Waters C, Muller P, Seeman P (1977). Tolerance of haloperidol catalepsy. *Eur J Pharmacol* 41,321–327.

Fandrich E, Hadass H (1969). Relationship between the perazine concentration in the liver, brain and blood and the pharmacologic effects under chronic perazine medication in rats of different age. *Pharmacopsychiatr Neuropsychopharmacol* 2,109–111.

Fann W, Smith RC, Davis JM, et al. (1980). *Tardive Dyskinesia: Research and Treatment.* New York: SP Medical and Scientific Books, pp. 159–163.

Farde L, Nordistrom AL, Wiesel FA, et al.(1992). Positron emission tomographic analysis of central D_1 and D_2 dopamine receptor occupancy in patients treated with classical neuroleptics and clozapine—relation to extra-pyramidal side effects. *Arch Gen Psychiatry* 49,538–544.

Felicio LF, Nasello AG, Palermo-Neto J (1987). Dopaminergic supersensitivity after long-term bromopride treatment. *Physiol Behav* 41,433–437.

Felicio LF, Palermo-Neto J, Nasello AG (1989). Perinatal bromopride treatment: effects on motor activity and stereotyped behavior of offspring. *Physiol Behav* 45,1081–1085.

Fibiger HC, Lloyd KG (1984). Neurobiological substrates of tardive dyskinesia: the GABA hypothesis. *Trends Neurosci* 7,462–464.

Fleming WW (1976). Variable sensitivity of excitable cells: possible mechanisms and biological significance. *Rev Neurosci* 2,43–90.

Fowler SC, Wang G (1998). Chronic haloperidol produces a time- and dose-related slowing of lick rhythm in rats: implications for rodent models of tardive dyskinesia and neuroleptic-induced parkinsonism. *Psychopharmacology* 137,50–60.

Frussa-Filho R, Abilio VC, Bergamo M, et al. (1997). Behavioural subsensitivity induced by long-term administration of a low dose of haloperidol to rats. *J Pharm Pharmacol* 49,412–415.

Frussa-Filho R, Otoboni JR, Uema FT, et al. (1992). Effects of age and isolation on the evolution of catalepsy during chronic haloperidol treatment. *Braz J Med Biol Res* 25,925–928.

Frussa-Filho R, Palermo-Neto J (1988). Effect of single and long-term metoclopramide administration on open-field and stereotyped behavior of rats. *Eur J Pharmacol* 149,323–329.

Frussa-Filho R, Palermo-Neto J (1990). Effect of single and long-term sulpiride administration on open-field and stereotyped behavior of rats. *Braz J Med Biol Res* 23,463-472.

Frussa-Filho R, Palermo-Neto J (1991). Effect of single and long-term droperidol administration on open-field and stereotyped behavior of rats. *Physiol Behav* 50,825–830.

Gale K (1980). Chronic blockade of dopamine receptors by antischizophrenic drugs enhances GABA binding in substantia nigra. *Nature* 283,569–570.

Gale K, Costa E, Toffano G, et al. (1978). Evidence for a role of nigral gamma-aminobutyric acid and substance P in the haloperidol-induced activation of striatal tyrosine hydroxylase. *J Pharmacol Exp Ther* 206,29–37.

Gamble SJ, Waddington JL (1981). Multiplicity of dopamine-mediated behaviours during six months phenothiazine neuroleptic treatment in young but not aged rats. *Br J Pharmacol* 74,225.

Gattaz WF, Emrich A, Behrens S (1993). Vitamin E attenuates the development of haloperidol-induced dopaminergic hypersensitivity in rats: possible implications for tardive dyskinesia. *J Neural Transm Gen Sect* 92,197–201.

Glassman RB, Glassman HN (1980). Oral dyskinesia in brain damaged rats withdrawn from a neuroleptic: implications for models of tardive dyskinesia. *Psychopharmacology* 69,19–25.

Glenthöj BY (1995). The brain dopaminergic system. Pharmacological, behavioural and electrophysiological studies. *Dan Med Bull* 42,1–21.

Glenthöj BY, Hemmingsen R (1989). Intermittent neuroleptic treatment induces long-lasting abnormal mouthing in the rat. *Eur J Pharmacol* 164,393–396.

Godefroy F, Bassant MH, Weil-Fugassa JW, et al. (1989). Age-related changes in dopaminergic and serotoninergic indices in the rat brain. *Neurobiol Aging* 10,187–190.

Graham DG (1984). Catecholamine toxicity: a proposal for the molecular pathogenesis of manganese neurotoxicity and Parkinson's disease. *Neurotoxicology* 5,83–95.

Graham DG, Tiffany SM, Bell WR Jr, et al. (1978). Auto-oxidation versus covalent binding of quinones as the mechanism of toxicity of dopamine, 6-hydroxydopamine, and related compounds toward C1300 neuroblastoma cells in vitro. *Mol Pharmacol* 14,644–653.

Gunne LM, Andersson U, Bondesson U, et al. (1986). Spontaneous chewing movements in rats during acute and chronic antipsychotic drug administration. *Pharmacol Biochem Behav* 25,897–901.

Gunne LM, Growdon J, Glaeser B (1982). Oral dyskinesia in rats following brain lesions and neuroleptic drug administration. *Psychopharmacology* 77,134–139.

Gunne LM, Haggstrom JE (1983). Reduction of nigral-glutamic acid descarboxylase in rats with neuroleptic-induced oraldyskinesia. *Psychopharmacology* 81,191–194.

Gunne LM, Haggstrom JE, Sjoquist B (1984). Association with persistent neuroleptic-induced dyskinesia of regional changes in brain GABA synthesis. *Nature* 309,347–349.

Halliwell B, Gutteridge JM (1984). Oxygen toxicity, oxygen radicals, transition metals and disease. *Biochem J* 219,1–14.

Ito H, Torii M, Suzuki T (1995). Decreased superoxide dismutase activity and increased superoxide anion production in cardiac hypertrophy of spontaneously hypertensive rats. *Clin Exp Hypertens* 17,803–816.

Iversen SD, Howells RB, Hughes RP (1980). Behavioral consequences of long-term treatment with neuroleptic drugs. *Adv Biochem Psychopharmacol* 24,305–313.

Jancovic, J (1995). Tardive syndromes and other drug-induced movement disorders. *Clin Neuropharmacol* 18,197–214.

Jellinger K (1977). Pathology of intracerebral hemorrhage. *Zentralbl Neurochir* 38,29–42.

Jenner P, Clow A, Reavil G, et al. (1978). A behavioral and biochemical comparison of dopamine receptor blockade produced by haloperidol with that produced by substituted benzamide drugs. *Life Sci* 23,545–550.

Jenner P, Marsden CD (1984). Multiple dopamine receptors in brain and pharmacological actions of substituted benzamide drugs. *Acta Psychiatr Scand* 69(suppl 311),109–123.

Jeste DV, Wyatt RJ (1981). Dogma disrupted: is tardive dyskinesia due to post-synaptic dopamine receptor supersensitivity? *J Clin Psychiatry* 42,455–457.

Jeste DV, Wyatt RJ (1982a). Therapeutic strategies against tardive dyskinesia. *Arch Gen Psychiatry* 39,803–816.

Jeste DV, Wyatt RJ (1982b). *Understanding and Treating Tardive Dyskinesia*. New York: Guilford Press.

Kane JM (1995). Tardive dyskinesia: epidemiological and clinical presentation. In: *Psychopharmacoogy: The Fourth Generation of Progress*, Bloom FE, Kupfer DJ, eds. New York: Raven, pp. 1485–1495.

Kane JM, Woerner M, Lieberman J (1985). Tardive dyskinesia: prevalence, incidence and risk factors. In: *Dyskinesia: Research and Treatment*, Casey DE, Chase TN, Christensen AV, et al., eds. Berlin: Springer-Verlag, pp. 72–78.

Kaufmann CA, Jeste DV, Shelton RC (1986). Noradrenergic and neuroradiologic abnormalities in tardive dyskinesia. *Biol Psychiatry* 21,799–812.

Kazamatsuri H, Chien CP, Cole JO (1972). Treatment of tardive dyskinesia. II. Short-term efficacy of dopamine-blocking agents haloperidol and thiopropazate. *Arch Gen Psychiatry* 27,100–103.

Klawans HL (1973). The pharmacology of tardive dyskinesia. *Am J Psychiatry* 130,83–86.

Klawans HL, D'Amico DJ, Nausieda PA, et al. (1977). The specificity of neuroleptic and methysergide-induced behavioral hypersensitivity. *Psychopharmacology* 55,49–52.

Klawans HL, Rubovits R (1972). An experimental model of tardive dyskinesia. *J Neural Transm* 33,235–246.

Kovacic B, Domino EF (1984). Fluphenazine-induced acute and tardive dyskinesia in monkeys. *Psychopharmacology* 84,310–314.

Levy AD, See RE, Levin ED, et al. (1987). Neuroleptic-induced oral movements in rats: methodological issues. *Life Sci* 41,1499–1506.

Ljungberg T, Ungerstedt U (1977). Different behavioral patterns induced by apomorphine: evidence that the method of administration determines the behavioral response to the drug. *Eur J Pharmacol* 46,41–50.

Lohr JB (1991). Oxygen radicals and neuropsychiatric illness. Some speculations. *Arch Gen Psychiatry*

48,1097–1106.

Lohr JB, Cadet JL, Lohr MA, et al. (1987). Alpha-tocopherol in tardive dyskinesia. *Lancet* 1,913–914.

Lohr JB, Kuczenski R, Bracha HS, et al. (1990). Increased indices of free radical activity in the cerebrospinal fluid of patients with tardive dyskinesia. *Biol Psychiatry* 28,535–539.

Marin C, Parashos SA, Kapitzoglou-Logothetis V, et al. (1993). D_1 and D_2 dopamine receptor-mediated mechanisms and behavioral supersensitivity. *Pharmacol Biochem Behav* 45,195–200.

Maulik N, Das DK, Gorgineni M, et al. (1993). Reduction of myocardial ischemic reperfusion injury by sialylated glycosphingolipids, gangliosides. *J Cardiovasc Pharmacol* 22,74–81.

Meshul CK, Janowsky A, Casey DE, et al. (1992a). Effect of haloperidol and clozapine on the density of "perforated" synapses in caudate, nucleus accumbens, and medial prefrontal cortex. *Psychopharmacology* 106,45–52.

Meshul CK, Janowsky A, Casey DE, et al. (1992b). Coadministration of haloperidol and CCH-23390 prevents the increase in "perforated" synapses due to either drug alone. *Neuropsychopharmacology* 7,285–293.

Miller LG, Jankovick J (1989). Metoclopramide-induced movements disorders. Clinical findings with a review of the literature. *Arch Intern Med* 149,2486–2492.

Miller R, Chovinard G (1993). Loss of striatal cholinergic neurons as a basis for tardive and L-dopa-induced dyskinesias, neuroleptic-induced supersensitivity psychosis and refractory schizophrenia. *Biol Psychiatry* 34,713–738.

Misra CH, Shelat H, Smith RC (1982). Age affects dopamine receptor changes during chronic administration of fluphenazine. *Eur J Pharmacol* 85,343–346.

Moss LE, Neppe VM, Drevets WC (1993). Buspirone in the treatment of tardive dyskinesia. *J Clin Psychopharmacol* 13,204–209.

Neisewander JL, Castañeda E, Davis DA (1994). Dose-dependent differences in the development of reserpine-induced oral dyskinesia in rats: support for a model of tardive dyskinesia. *Psychopharmacology* 116,79–84.

Neisewander JL, Castañeda E, Davis DA, et al. (1996). Effects of amphetamine and 6-hydroxydopamine lesions on reserpine-induced oral dyskinesia. *Eur J Pharmacol* 305,13–21.

Neisewander JL, Lucki I, McGonigle P (1991a). Behavioral and neurochemical effects of chronic administration of reserpine and SKF-38393 in rats. *J Pharmacol Exp Ther* 257,850–860.

Neisewander JL, Lucki I, McGonigle P (1991b). Neurochemical changes associated with the persistence of spontaneous oral dyskinesia in rats following chronic reserpine treatment. *Brain Res* 558,27–35.

Neppe VM (1989). High-dose buspirone treatment in tardive dyskinesia—one case report. *Lancet* 2,8677.

Neppe VM (1990). High dose buspirone treatment in tardive dyskinesia. *143rd Annual Meeting of the American Psychiatry Association*, New York (abstract NR269).

Nielsen EB, Lyon M (1978). Evidence for cell loss in corpus striatum after long-term treatment with a neuroleptic drug (flupenithixol) in rats. *Psychopharmacology* 59,85–89.

Ott L, Weiner D, Cheng H, et al. (1981). Estimating pA_2 values for different designs. *J Pharmacol Meth* 5,75–92.

Owens DGC (1985). Involuntary disorders of movement in chronic schizophrenia: the role of the illness and its treatment. In: *Dyskinesia, Research and Treatment*, Casey DE, Chase TN, Christensen AV, et al., eds. Berlin: Springer, pp. 79–87.

Owens DGC (1999). Tardive dyskinesia. In: *A Guide to the Extrapyramidal Side-Effects of Antipsychotic Drugs*, Owens DGC, ed. London: Cambridge University Press, pp. 166–224.

Pakkenberg H, Fog R, Nilakantan B (1973). The long-term effect of perphenazine enanthate on the rat brain. Some metabolic and anatomical observations. *Psychopharmacology* 29,329–336.

Palermo-Neto J (1982). Supersensitivity, drug withdrawal and open-field behavior. *Psychopharmacol Bull* 18,11–12.

Palermo-Neto J (1997). Dopaminergic systems: dopamine receptors. *Psychiatr Clin North Am* 20,705–721.

Palermo-Neto J, Bernardi MM (1984). Kinetic analysis of central nervous system supersensitivity induced by long-term haloperidol treatment. Part II: KB determination. *Psychopharmacol Bull* 20,681–682.

Palermo-Neto J, Bernardi MM, Saban R (1984). Kinetic analysis of central nervous system supersensitivity induced by long-term haloperidol treatment. I: pA_2 determination. *Pharmacology* 28,203–210.

Palermo-Neto J, Frussa-Filho R, Vital MABF (1999). Kinetic analysis of GM_1 effects on haloperidol-induced dopaminergic supersensitivity. *Gen Pharmacol* 32,265–270.

Pan HS, Penney JB, Young AB (1985). γ-aminobutyric acid and benzodiazepine receptor changes induced by unilateral 6-hydroxydopamine lesions of the medial forebrain bundle. *J Neurochem* 45,1396–1404.

Parsons PG (1985). Modification of dopa toxicity in human tumour cells. *Biochem Pharmacology* 34,1801–1807.

Peacock L, Gerlach J (1997). A reanalysis of the dopamine theory of tardive dyskinesia: the hypothesis of dopamine D_1/D_2 imbalance. In: *Neuroleptic-induced Movement Disorders*, Yassa R, Nair NPV, Jeste DV, eds. New York: Cambridge University Press, pp. 141–160.

Queiroz CMT, Frussa-Filho R (1997). Effects of buspirone on dopaminergic supersensitivity. *Life Sci* 61,371–382.

Queiroz CMT, Frussa-Filho R (1999). Effects of buspirone on a new animal model of tardive dyskinesia. *Progr Neuro-Psychopharmacol Biol Psychiatry* 23,1405–1418.

Queiroz CMT, Piovezan RD, Frussa-Filho R (1998). Reserpine does not induce orofacial dyskinesia in spontaneously hypertensive rats. *Eur J Pharmacol* 336,105–108.

Randall PK, Severson JA, Finch CE (1981). Aging and the regulation of striatal dopaminergic mechanisms in mice. *J Pharmacol Exp Ther* 219,695–700.

Rondot P, Bathien N (1986). Movement disorders in patients with coexistent neuroleptic-induced tremor and tardive dyskinesia: EMG and pharmacological study. *Adv Neurol* 45,361–366.

Roscher AA, Wiesmann UN, Honegger EU (1981). Changes in beta-adrenergic receptors in submaxillary glands of chronically reserpine- or isoproterenol-treated rats. *J Pharmacol Exp Ther* 216,419–424.

Roth GS, Joseph JA (1988). Peculiarities of the effect of hormones and transmitters during aging: modulation of changes in dopaminergic action. *Gerontology* 34,22–28.

Rupniak NMJ, Jenner P, Marsden CD (1983). Cholinergic manipulation of perioral behaviour induced by chronic neuroleptic administration to rats. *Psychopharmacology* 79,226–230.

Rupniak NMJ, Jenner P, Marsden CD (1985). Pharmacological characterization of spontaneous or drug-associated purposeless chewing movements in rats. *Psychopharmacology* 85,71–79.

Rupniak NMJ, Jenner P, Marsden CD (1986). Acute dystonia induced by neuroleptic drugs. *Psychopharmacology* 88,403–419.

Rupniak NMJ, Mann S, Hall MD, et al. (1984). Differential effects of continuos administration for 1 year of haloperidol or sulpiride on striatal dopamine function in the rat. *Psychoparmacology* 84,503–511.

Rupniak NMJ, Prestwick AS, Horton RW, et al. (1987). Alterations in cerebral glutamic acid decarboxylase and (^{3}H(-flunitrazepan binding during continuous treatment of rats for one year with haloperidol, sulpiride, or clozapine. *J Neural Transm* 68,113–125.

Saltz BL, Kane JM, Woerner MG, et al. (1997). Aging and tardive dyskinesia. In: *Neuroleptic-induced Movement Disorders*, Yassa R, Nair NPV, Jeste DV, eds. New York: Cambridge University Press, pp. 13–25.

Sandoval MR, Palermo-Neto J (1989). Behavioral aspects of GABAergic-dopaminergic interactions in the central nervous system. *Eur J Pharmacol* 167,117–125.

Sasaki T, Kennedy JL, Nobrega JN (1997). Localized changes in GABA receptor-gated chloride channel in rat brain after long-term haloperidol: relation to vacuous chewing movements. *Synapse* 25,73–79.

Schalling M, Friberg K, Seroogy K, et al. (1990). Analysis of expression of cholecystokinin in dopamine cells in the ventral mesencephalon of several species and in humans with schizophrenia. *Proc Natl Acad Sci USA* 87,8427–8431.

Scheel-Kruger J (1986). Dopamine-GABA interactions: evidence that GABA transmits, modulates and mediates dopaminergic functions in the basal ganglia and the limbic system. *Acta Neurol Scand* 73(suppl 107).

Schoenfeld R, Uretsky N (1972). Altered response to apomorphine in 6-hydroxydopamine-treated rats. *Eur J Pharmacol* 19,115–118.

Schröder U, Shröder H, Augustin W, et al. (1994). Haloperidol-induced behavioral supersensitivity is increased by monosialoganglioside treatment in rats without affecting spiroperidol binding. *J Pharmacol Exp Ther* 271,1193–1196.

Seeman P (1980). Brain dopamine receptors. *Pharmacol Rev* 32,229–313.

Sharpless SK (1975). Supersensitivity-like phenomena in the central nervous system. *Fed Proc* 34,1990–1997.

Shonecker M (1957). Ein eigentumliches Syndrom im oralen Bereich bei Megaphenapplikation. *Nervenartz* 28,34–35.

Shriqui CL, Bradejn J, Annable L, et al. (1992). Vitamin E in the treatment of tardive dyskinesia: a double blind placebo-controlled study. *Am J Psychiatry* 149,391–393.

Steinpreis RE, Moser L, Parret F, et al. (1998). The effects of the atypical antipsychotic amperozide on vacuous jaw movements in rats: a novel dose-response profile. *Psychopharmacology* 138,107–113.

Steinpreis RE, Salamone JD (1993). Effects of acute haloperidol and reserpine administration on vacuous-jaw movements in three different age groups of rats. *Pharmacol Biochem Behav* 45,323–327.

Sussman AN, Tran-Nguyen TL, Neisewander JL (1997). Acute reserpine administration elicits long-term spontaneous oral dyskinesia. *Eur J Pharmacol* 337,157–160.

Takeuchi H, Ishigooka J, Kobayashi K, et al. (1998). Study on the suitability of a rat model for tardive dyskinesia and the preventive effects of various drugs. *Progr Neuro-Psychopharmacol Biol Psychiatry* 22,679–691.

Taminga CA (1981). Tardive dyskinesia and dopamine receptors. In: *Neuroreceptors: Basic and Clinical Aspects*, Usdin E, Bunney WE, Davis JM, eds. Chichester: John Wiley & Sons, pp. 231–241.

Tarsy D, Baldessarini RJ (1973). Pharmacologically induced behavioral supersensitivity to apomorphine. *Nature* 245,262–263.

Tarsy D, Baldessarini RJ (1974). Behavioral supersensitivity to apomorphine following chronic treatment with drugs which interfere with synaptic function of catecholamines. *Neuropharmacology* 13,927–940.

Thornburg JE, Moore KE (1974). Supersensitivity to dopaminergic agonists following withdrawal of a chronic diet containing haloperidol or pimozide. *Pharmacologist* 16,307–312.

Tieppo CA, Palermo-Neto J, Nasello AG, et al. (1995). Intracerebroventricular administration of cholecystokinin reduces stereotypy in dopamine-supersensitive rats. *Br J Med Biol Res* 28,351–354.

Triggle DJ, Trigle RC (1976). *Chemical Pharmacology of the Synapse: Elementary Considerations of Ligand-Receptor Interactions*. New York: Academic.

Tunnicliff G, Brokaw JJ, Hausz JA, et al. (1992). Influence of repeated treatment with buspirone on central 5-hydroxytryptamine and dopamine synthesis. *Neuropharmacology* 31,991–995.

Uhrbrand L, Faurbye A (1960). Reversible and irreversible dyskinesia after treatment with perphenazine, chlorpromazine, reserpine and ECT. *Psychopharmacology* 1,408–418.

Vital MABF, Florio JC, Frussa-Filho R, et al. (1998). Effects of haloperidol and GM_1 ganglioside treatment on striatal D_2 receptor binding and dopamine turnover. *Life Sci* 62,1161–1169.

Vital MABF, Frussa-Filho R, Palermo-Neto J (1995). Effects of monosialognaglioside on dopaminergic supersensitivity. *Life Sci* 56,2299–2307.

Vital MABF, Frussa-Filho R, Palermo-Neto, J (1997). Effects of monosialoganglioside on a new model of tardive dyskinesia. *Progr Neuro Psychiatry* 21,1169–1179.

Waddington JL (1989). Schizophrenia, affective psychoses and other disorders treated with neuroleptic drugs: the enigma of tardive dyskinesia, its neurobiological determinants, and the "conflict of paradigms." *Int Ver Neurobiol* 31,297–353.

Waddington JL (1990). Spontaneous orofacial movements induced in rodents by very long-term neuroleptic drug administration: phenomenology, pathophysiology and putative relationship to tardive dyskinesia. *Psychopharmacology* 101,432–447.

Waddington JL (1997). Rodent and other animal models of tardive dyskinesia during long-term neuroleptic-drug administration: controversies and implications for the clinical syndrome. In: *Neuroleptic-induced Movement Disorders*, Yassa R, Nair NPV, Jeste DV, eds. New York: Cambridge University Press, pp. 225–237.

Waddington JL, Cross AJ, Gamble SJ, et al. (1983a). Spontaneous orofacial dyskinesia and dopaminergic function in rats after 6 months of neuroleptic treatment. *Science* 220,530–532.

Waddington JL, Cross AJ, Gamble SJ, et al. (1983b). Dopamine receptor function and spontaneous orofacial dyskinesia in rats during 6-month neuroleptic treatments. *Adv Biochem Psychopharmacol* 37,299–308.

Waddington JL, Gamble SJ (1980). Differential effects of aging on distinct features of apomorphine stereotypy in the adult rat. *Neurosci Let* 20,95–99.

Walsh RN, Cummins RA (1976). The open-field: a critical review. *Psychol Bull* 86,482–504.

Watanabe Y, Fujita M, Ito Y, et al. (1997). Brain dopamine transports in spontaneously hypertensive rats. *J Nucl Med* 38,470–474.

Wolf ME, Chevesick J, Lehrer E, et al. (1983). The clinical association of tardive dyskinesia and drug-induced parkinsonism. *Biol Psychiatry* 18,1181–1188.

Wolfarth S, Ossowska K (1989). Can the supersensitivity of rodents to dopamine be regarded as a model of tardive dyskinesia? *Progr Neuro-Psychopharmacol Biol Psychiatry* 13,799–840.

Yassa R, Jeste DV (1997). Gender as a factor in the development of tardive dyskinesia. In: *Neuroleptic-induced Movement Disorders*, Yassa R, Nair, NPV, Jeste DV, eds. London: Cambridge University Press, pp. 26–40.

Yassa R, Nair NPV (1997). Anticholinergic drugs as factors in the development of tardive dyskinesia. In: *Neuroleptic-induced Movement Disorders*, Yassa R, Nair NPV, Jeste DV, eds. New York: Cambridge University Press, pp. 117–125.

6.

Stress and Dopaminergic Function

Jonas Hannestad and Julio Licinio

ABSTRACT

It is well-known that stress influences the activity of dopaminergic neurons in various brain regions, but the neurochemical details of these interactions are not yet fully elucidated. However, some points seem to be relatively certain and are described in this chapter. Stress causes important changes in dopaminergic activity and the resulting behavior and cognitive processes. Stress during intrauterine or early postnatal life can influence the development of an animal's dopaminergic systems. There are important genetic differences in the makeup of the dopaminergic system, and these, together with the changes induced in early life, determine how susceptible adults are to stress and how likely they are to develop stress-related disorders. Antidepressant and anxiolytic drugs reduce the impact of stress on motivation, cognition, and behavior, possibly through modifications of dopaminergic activity. This chapter reviews the available evidence for relationships among the systems activated by stress, including the noradrenergic system, hypothalamus-pituitary-adrenal axis, and dopaminergic system.

INTRODUCTION

In the mammalian brain, phenomena such as motivation, drive, goal-directed behavior and reward, and the underlying cognitive processing and associative learning and translation of these processes into behavioral responses are thought to depend to a large extent on dopaminergic systems (Everitt et al., 1999). The dopaminergic systems involved in these behaviors are easily influenced by external conditions that can be characterized as stressful, and such stressors thus modify the behaviors controlled by dopaminergic activity. This is a necessary evolutionary adaptation, because the continuous changing of external conditions must be considered when an organism is planning and executing motivated behaviors. Thus, an otherwise rewarding object or activity, such as food or sexual activity, cannot be consumed if there is an important stressor occurring at the same time, such as the presence of a predator. The stressor must be dealt with before directing attention to the reward. Therefore, external cues characterized as stressors influence these dopaminergic systems that govern motivated behavior and reward so that their functioning can be adjusted accordingly, allowing the organism to react optimally to the environment, direct attention, and prioritize actions. To date, the neurochemical basis of these interactions is unknown, and the mechanisms by which stress affects dopaminergic systems is not yet fully understood.

Dopamine is a monoamine neurotransmitter synthesized from the amino acid phenylalanine in a two-step biosynthetic pathway in which tyrosine hydroxylase is the rate-limiting enzyme (Deutch and Roth, 1999). Dopamine released into the synaptic cleft can bind to and act through five different signal-transducing receptors, which can be divided into two groups: D1 and D5 dopamine receptors activate adenylate cyclase, whereas D2, D3, and D4 dopamine receptors inhibit this enzyme (Waxham, 1999). The main dopaminergic projections of the mammalian brain arise in the midbrain and project to the basal ganglia and forebrain. Thus the nigrostriatal/mesostriatal pathway originates in the substantia nigra and projects to the striatum, whereas the mesolimbic and mesocortical/mesoprefrontal pathways both originate in the ventral tegmental area and project to the limbic system (specifically the shell of the nucleus accumbens and the amygdala) and frontal cortex, respectively. The nigrostriatal pathway is involved in motor control, and the mesolimbic and mesocortical pathways are involved in reward, motivated behavior, cognition, and selection of significant environmental stimuli to which attention should be directed (Deutch and Roth, 1999).

STRESS AND DOPAMINERGIC PATHWAYS

Stress can be defined as an environmental challenge that must be dealt with because it can interfere with the well-being of the organism and therefore needs directed attention. When an organism is exposed to stress, the activity of noradrenergic, serotonergic, and dopaminergic neuronal systems increases and so does activity of neurons of the hypothalamus that produce corticotropin-releasing hormone (CRH) and cause a subsequent activation of the hypothalamus-pituitary-adrenal (HPA) axis (Dunn, 2000). Many low intensity stressors that do not activate other noradrenergic, indoleaminergic systems, or the HPA axis activate dopaminergic pathways, especially the mesoprefrontal pathway (Horger and Roth, 1996).

All dopaminergic pathways are activated by stress, although the mesocortical pathway is particularly sensitive, and more dopaminergic activity is induced in the prefrontal cortex than in subcortical sites with any given stressor (Finlay and Zigmond, 1997). Some controversy exists regarding which parts of the dopaminergic system are most sensitive to stress. For instance, handling stress increases dopamine turnover in the amygdala more than in the nucleus accumbens or prefrontal cortex, and after cessation of the handling, the levels of dopamine are normalized in the other dopaminergic innervated regions but peak in the nucleus accumbens (Inglis and Moghaddam, 1999). Chronic stress increases motor response to cocaine, which is associated with increased dopamine in accumbens and decreased dopamine in prefrontal cortex (Prasad et al., 1995).

The reaction to stress of the nucleus accumbens is reduced by concurrent activation of the prefrontal cortex (Doherty and Gratton, 1997), and depletion of dopamine in the prefrontal cortex increases stress-induced dopaminergic activity in the nucleus accumbens (King et al., 2000). This means that disruption of prefrontal dopamine innervation enhances stress responsiveness in the mesolimbic system. Psychological stress increases dopamine in the shell of the accumbens but not in the core (Wu et al., 1999). This is consistent with the neuroanatomical data that the shell is part of the limbic system, whereas the core is part of the basal ganglia (Heimer et al., 1991; Zahm and Brog, 1992).

The fine-tuning of dopaminergic activity in the prefrontal cortex is important for decision-making, and a critical range of dopaminergic activity is needed for optimal cognitive functioning (Pani et al., 2000). For example, when an animal is trained to obtain a reward, and at the same time is exposed to stress, the learning process is inefficient (Ghiglieri et al., 1997). Furthermore, spatial working memory is impaired when an animal is exposed to stress and the dopamine turnover in the prefrontal cortex increases (Mizoguchi et al., 2000; Murphy et al., 1996).

An interesting observation is that nonfunctional masticatory activity, such as chewing or gnawing, attenuates the physiological indices of stress. Thus, stress-induced striatal increase in dopaminergic activity is less pronounced if rats display this behavior (Gomez et al., 1999). When rats are exposed to a novel environment the release of dopamine in the prefrontal cortex, nucleus accumbens, and striatum increases. But if they have access to an inedible object to chew, the increase in the prefrontal cortex is reduced, whereas the increase in the other sites is not modified (Berridge et al., 1999). However, it is unknown how this stereotyped motor behavior, which is probably mediated by the nigrostriatal pathway, influences the response to stress in other dopaminergic pathways.

HABITUATION AND RECEPTOR EXPRESSION

The enhancement of dopamine release induced by stress causes habituation and modifications in dopamine receptor expression. These phenomena of habituation and changes in receptor expression depend on the region considered. Thus, repeated restraint stress leads to habituation in the nucleus accumbens; i.e., after several days the dopamine levels no longer increase even though the restraint is applied, whereas the prefrontal cortex reacts with increased dopamine release even after several days of repeated restraint (Cabib and Puglisi-Allegra, 1996).

Tail-pinch causes an increase in dopamine turnover in the medial prefrontal cortex and a decrease in dopamine activity in the nucleus accumbens. Chronic exposure to this stressor causes habituation in the nucleus accumbens with extinction of the increase in dopamine activity. When tail-pinch is combined with chronic mild stress the response shifts to an increase in dopaminergic activity in the nucleus accumbens as opposed to a decrease and a larger increase in the prefrontal cortex than tail-pinch alone (Di Chiara et al., 1999). Feeding increases the dopaminergic activity both in the nucleus accumbens and in the prefrontal cortex, although the increase in the latter is more pronounced. When feeding is combined with mild chronic stress instead of an increase of dopamine in the nucleus accumbens there is a decrease (Di Chiara et al., 1999).

This habituation to stress in the nucleus accumbens could reflect the behavioral change that has been observed in animals from an initial arousal and willingness to cope with the challenge to a state of despair owing to the failure to cope. The habituation that takes place in the nucleus accumbens could in part be explained by the fact that the expression of D1 receptors, but not D2 receptors, decreases after chronic restraint stress (Giardino et al., 1998). However, prior exposure to stress enhances the dopaminergic response in the mesocortical pathway (Finlay and Zigmond, 1997). Thus it seems that in the nucleus accumbens there is a habituation to chronic stress, whereas the prefrontal cortex responds with a sensitization.

As for receptor expression, the observations are not consistent. Other studies find a change in the expression of only D2 receptors and not D1. Thus, stress decreases the mRNA for D2 in the substantia nigra, lateral ventral tegmental area, nucleus accumbens core and shell, and lateral caudate, whereas there are no changes in D1 receptor mRNA expression in these sites (Dziedzicka-Wasylewska et al., 1997).

Lesions to the medial prefrontal cortex cause fear-extinction to take longer, a process mediated by the nucleus accumbens and the mesoprefrontal dopamine neurons that are involved in maintaining response adaptability to stress changes in the environment (Morrow et al., 1999).

IMPACT OF STRESS DURING GESTATION AND EARLY POSTNATAL LIFE

When an animal is stressed during intrauterine or early postnatal life, the makeup of the dopaminergic system is affected for the remainder of its life; thus, the organism is sensitized to stress and possibly predisposed to stress-related disorders (Table 6-1). The effects of prenatal stress in dopaminergic system reactivity may not be apparent at baseline and appear only when an organism is exposed to a stressor (Pani et al., 2000).

When immobilization of the mother is applied during gestation, the gender-dependent differences in the mediobasal hypothalamus dopamine activity disappear, resulting in males with a hypothalamic dopamine makeup that is similar to that of females (Reznikov et al., 1999). The offspring of stressed mothers also show an increase in dopamine turnover in the nucleus accumbens, a modification that is more pronounced on the right side than the left (Alonso et al., 1997). Another study, however, states that most stressors cause more dopamine alterations in left amygdala than in the right (McIntyre et al., 1999).

Perinatal stress, for which cesarean birth is a useful paradigm, sensitizes animals to tail-pinch stress. The response to the first tail-pinch is the same in both groups, but with every exposure there is a higher and longer lasting dopamine response in the nucleus accumbens of the cesarean-born animals compared with those delivered vaginally (Brake et al., 1997).

TABLE 6-1. Effects of maternal stress on offspring

- Offspring of immobilized mothers have changes in the hypothalamic dopamine activity (Reznikov et al., 1999)
- Offspring of stressed mothers show increased dopamine activity in nucleus accumbens (Alonso et al., 1997)
- Cesarean birth sensitizes animals to stress, with higher and longer lasting dopamine response with each exposure (Brake et al., 1997)
- Isolation of rat pup from nest increases mesolimbic dopamine activity and decreases mesostriatal dopamine activity (Kehoe et al., 1998)
- Isolation of rat pup from nest sensitizes it to stressors during adulthood and reduces prefrontal dopamine activity (Zimmerberg and Brown, 1998)
- Lesions to prefrontal cortex in neonates sensitize animal to stress in adulthood (Brake et al., 2000)

Postnatal stress paradigms, such as isolation of the rat pup from the nest for 1 hour daily, produce an increase in the mesolimbic dopaminergic activity and a decrease in the mesostriatal activity. This isolation also enhances the amphetamine-induced dopamine release in the nucleus accumbens (Kehoe et al., 1998). Moreover, separation from the mother causes increased sensitivity to stressors during adulthood and a reduction of dopamine activity in the prefrontal cortex (Zimmerberg and Brown, 1998).

As mentioned above, the medial prefrontal cortex modulates the dopamine response to stress in the nucleus accumbens. Lesions to the medial prefrontal cortex in neonates cause stress to elicit larger and longer lasting dopamine increases in the nucleus accumbens, as well as more corticosterone secretion (Brake et al., 2000).

In summary, subtle differences in exposure to stress during pre-, peri- and early postnatal life can influence the capability of coping with stress for the rest of the organism's life and increase the susceptibility to various stress-related disorders that could have important implications in human clinical psychiatry.

EFFECT OF ANTIDEPRESSANTS AND ANXIOLYTICS

Treatment with antidepressants can often nullify the behavioral changes induced by stress, and chronically stressed animals are often used as a model for human depression and for evaluation of the efficacy of new antidepressant drugs (Pani et al., 2000). Furthermore, behavioral depression is related to decreased dopamine transmission in the nucleus accumbens (Alonso et al., 1994).

When animals are trained to obtain an appetitive stimulus, the acquisition of this knowledge is impaired if stress is applied during the learning process, but if the antidepressants imipramine or fluoxetine are given at the same time, the stress does not impede the learning process (Ghiglieri et al., 1997). In animals that do not receive any particular form of stress, the antidepressant imipramine causes an increase of dopamine D2 receptors in the ventral tegmental area that is not seen with fluoxetine. However, both imipramine and fluoxetine increase dopamine D2 receptor expression in the lateral caudate and shell but not core of the nucleus accumbens (Dziedzicka-Wasylewska et al., 1997).

The application of mild chronic stress to animals causes a reduction of exploratory behavior when they are confronted with spatial novelty. This reduction is not reversed by antidepressant administration. Restraint stress, however, does not cause a reduction of exploratory behavior, and administration of antidepressants reduces this behavior in restrained animals (D'Aquila et al., 2000). Additionally, restraint stress increases grooming behavior, and this increase was abolished by imipramine administration, whereas the same antidepressant increases grooming behavior after chronic mild stress (D'Aquila et al., 2000).

Anxiolytics such as benzodiazepines are another class of psychoactive drugs that influence the dopaminergic response to stress. These drugs do not affect dopaminergic transmission in basal conditions, but they do ameliorate stress-induced alterations in dopamine transmission in a way similar to that of antidepressants (Pani et al., 2000). For example, the decrease in D1 receptors in the nucleus accumbens produced by chronic restraint stress is blocked by concurrent treatment with the benzodiazepine alprazolam (Giardino et al., 1998). New generation anxiolytics, such as ipsapirone and buspirone, also reduce stress-induced dopamine release in the prefrontal cortex (Wedzony et al., 1996).

The effect of antidepressants and anxiolytics on dopaminergic responsiveness to stress can be explained in part by the fact that both serotonergic and γ-aminobutyric acid (GABA)-ergic neurotransmission modulate dopaminergic activity (Mendlin et al., 1999). Chronic social stress reduces serotonin levels in the prefrontal cortex and thus dopaminergic activity (Pani et al., 2000). Both antidepressants and newer anxiolytics, such as buspirone and ipsapirone, modify serotonergic transmission, and this can explain how these drugs can influence dopaminergic reactivity without directly acting on dopamine receptors. Benzodiazepines modify GABA neurotransmission, and because the stress-induced increase of dopamine turnover is activated primarily by GABA (Hawkins et al., 2000), this could explain how benzodiazepines influence dopaminergic responses to stress.

These data have evident and important parallels in clinical medicine and can explain why antidepressants do not exert an effect in a patient who is not suffering depression, whereas the effect in a depressed patient is clinically evident (Table 6-2).

SPECIES AND STRAIN DIFFERENCES

When studies of laboratory animals are interpreted, care must be taken in transferring that knowledge to human clinical medicine. Even between species as similar as mice and rats there are important differences in the influence of stress on the activity of dopaminergic systems. In both species, restraint stress induces an increase of dopamine activity in the hypothalamus. In the amygdala, however, restraint causes a decrease in dopaminergic activity in rats and an increase in mice. There is also an increase in dopamine release in rat striatum and murine locus coeruleus (Konstandi et al., 2000). Therefore, when these two closely related

TABLE 6-2. Antidepressants modulate stress responses and dopaminergic function

- Imipramine and fluoxetine prevent stress-induced inhibition of learning (Ghiglieri et al., 1997)
- Dopamine D2 receptors increase in ventral tegmental area with imipramine and in caudate and accumbens with both imipramine and fluoxetine (Dziedzicka Wasylewska et al., 1997)
- Antidepressants prevent reduction in exploratory behavior produced by mild chronic stress (D'Aquila et al., 2000)
- Antidepressants reduce exploratory behavior in restrained animals (D'Aquila et al., 2000)
- Benzodiazepines ameliorate stress-induced alterations of dopamine activity (Pani et al., 2000)
- Alprazolam prevents increase in D1 receptors in accumbens produced by restraint stress (Giardino et al., 1998)
- Ipsapirone and buspirone reduce stress-induced dopamine release in prefrontal cortex (Wedzony et al., 1996)
- Serotonin modulates dopamine activity in frontal cortex (Mendlin et al., 1999)
- Stress-induced modifications of dopamine are mediated by GABA (Hawkins et al., 2000)

species display important differences in their reaction to stress as assessed by dopamine turnover, it is difficult to apply knowledge obtained from mouse and rat experiments to human beings.

There are also important dopaminergic idiosyncrasies when comparing inbred strains of rats and mice. For instance, the well-studied Fischer and Lewis rats, the former being more reactive and more "anxious" and the latter less reactive and more "laid back," display important differences in their dopaminergic response to restraint stress. Basically, restraint stress causes an increase in dopaminergic activity in the prefrontal cortex, nucleus accumbens, and dorsal striatum of the Fischer rats but not of the Lewis strain, although there are no differences in the basal activity (Lindley et al., 1999). Two other rat strains, which show differences in amygdala excitability, the so-called slow and fast rats, react differently to both psychogenic and neurogenic stressors. Restraint causes the slow rats to not move, whereas the fast rats choose to struggle. However, when confronted with a predator (a ferret), the fast rats are more immobile than the slow rats. Furthermore, the corticosterone level is the same in both strains during restraint, but it increases more in the slow rats than in the fast rats when confronted with the ferret (McIntyre et al., 1999).

WKHA rats are a strain of hyperactive rats with increased dopamine uptake in the prefrontal cortex but no changes in the striatum (Hendley and Fan, 1992). These rats are hyperactive in a novel environment and also hyperreactive to stress and show changes in HPA axis function (Hendley, 2000). The rat strain Flinder's sensitive line (FSL) is used as a model for human depression owing to its sensitivity to stress. The basal level of tyrosine hydroxylase in striatal neurons was similar to a conspecific control but was elevated by immobilization stress in the FSL rats. In the ventral tegmental area the level of TH was higher in the FSL at baseline, but it was unaffected by immobilization (Serova et al., 1998).

With respect to mouse strains, there are also differences between the C57BL/6 and DBA/2 strains in response to stress and in the makeup of their dopaminergic systems (Puglisi-Allegra and Cabib, 1997). When comparing effects of restraint stress on dopamine receptor expression in these two strains, it has been observed that stress increases the expression of dopamine D1 receptors in the nucleus accumbens of the DBA/2 strain and reduces the expression of the same receptor in the striatum of the C57BL/6 strain. As for the D2 receptor, expression increases in the ventral tegmental area only in the C57BL/6, whereas in the DBA/2 strain stress causes this receptor to increase in the nucleus accumbens and decrease in the substantia nigra and ventral tegmental area (Cabib et al., 1998). Also, between the strains C57BL/6 and BALB/c, there are important differences in corticosterone levels and mesocorticolimbic dopamine activity (Shanks et al., 1994).

These differences should tell us much about how important individual differences and genetic polymorphisms can be in human subjects and how this can affect their reactivity to stress and susceptibility to stress-induced diseases. This should also be considered when developing new drugs that target dopaminergic neurotransmission.

HPA AXIS, GLUCOCORTICOIDS, AND DOPAMINE

Stress induces activity in brain catecholaminergic and indoleaminic systems, as well as activation of the HPA axis. It is also well-known that the CRH system and the noradrenergic systems are intimately linked and influence each other. For instance, stimulation of the central nucleus of the amygdala induces release of CRH from the hypothalamus, which is inhibited by norepinephrine depletion (Feldman and Weidenfeld, 1998), and central CRH mediates sympatoadrenal activity during stress (Jezova et al., 1999). The stress-induced activation of dopaminergic systems is probably induced primarily by GABA neurotransmission (Hawkins et al., 2000); however, whether the effect of stress on the dopaminergic systems is mediated also in part by the HPA axis and the nature of the relation between the two is still unclear.

Dopaminergic neurons of the ventral tegmental area express glucocorticoid receptors (Harfstrand et al., 1986), and corticosterone has been shown to increase the amount of tyrosine hydroxylase, the rate-limiting enzyme of dopamine synthesis, in this nucleus (Ortiz et al., 1995). An increase in corticosterone secretion, or a higher sensitivity to this hormone, enhances the activity of mesencephalic dopamine neurons (Piazza and Le Moal, 1996). Administration of CRH into the lateral ventricles causes an induction of dopamine release in the prefrontal cortex, septum, hypothalamus, and brainstem, whereas subcutaneous administration of CRH only causes increased dopamine activity in the prefrontal cortex (Dunn and Berridge, 1987). Intracranial self-stimulation of the medial forebrain bundle increases the turnover of both dopamine and serotonin in the nucleus accumbens as well as HPA axis activity. The increase in dopaminergic activity, but not serotonergic activity, is attenuated by adrenalectomy, and this attenuation is blunted if the adrenalectomized animals receive substitution corticosterone (Nakahara et al., 2000).

As mentioned, the shell of the nucleus accumbens is a part of the limbic system, whereas the core is part of the basal ganglia. The shell is thus more sensitive to stress than the core, showing a larger increase in dopaminergic transmission than in the core (Wu et al., 1999). This hyperresponsiveness of the shell of the nucleus accumbens depends in part on corticosteroids. Depletion of corticosterone by adrenalectomy reduces the extracellular levels of dopamine in the shell, making them equal to levels of the core. Stress-induced or cocaine-induced increases in shell extracellular dopamine are blunted by adrenalectomy (Barrot et al., 2000). The stress-induced increase of dopamine in the nucleus accumbens is suppressed by blockage of corticosterone secretion in predisposed animals, lowering it to the level of resistant animals (Rouge-Pont et al., 1998).

There is evidence that dopamine causes up-regulation of CRH receptors in the intermediate pituitary (Shiver et al., 1992). This last finding suggests that HPA responses to stress can be potentiated by dopamine acting on cells of the pituitary gland, leading to an increase in CRH receptor expression and increased ACTH responses to hypophyseal-portal CRH.

There are other reports that adrenal steroids do not affect dopamine transmission alone (Lindley et al., 1999). For instance, the use of intracerebroventricular CRH antagonists does not prevent the expected increase in monoamines, including dopamine, induced by footshock (Dunn, 2000). Furthermore, there is apparently no link between the dopamine hyperactivity seen in psychotic disorders and concurrent HPA hyperactivity (Duval et al., 2000).

In conclusion, further research is needed to fully identify the pathways and mechanisms of HPA axis-dopaminergic systems interactions.

SOMATIC STRESSORS, NEUROGENIC STRESSORS, AND PSYCHOGENIC STRESSORS

Stressors can be divided into different categories. Psychogenic stressors are perceived and probably processed cognitively. Examples of psychogenic stressors are experimental paradigms such as restraint stress, exposure to novelty, presence of a predator, or presence of a conspecific that has received an electric shock or tail-pinch. Neurogenic stressors are stressors that stimulate the senses and included are air puffs, handling by a researcher, light flicks, or sounds. Somatic stressors include immune system activation and reductions in brain glucose availability, for example, and those that may not be perceived by the animal. The effects of different types of stressors on dopaminergic neurotransmission vary, and it is therefore important to compare similar types of stressors. Thus psychogenic stressors cause an increase in prefrontal dopamine, whereas some types of somatic stressors do not.

Restraint stress causes an increase of norepinephrine and dopaminergic activity in numerous sites of the brain, whereas administration of lipopolysaccharide or interleukin-1, paradigms of immune system activation, causes a localized noradrenergic response in the hypothalamus and activation of the HPA axis but barely any changes in dopamine activity (Dunn et al., 1999). However, interleukin-1 administration increases dopamine activity in the nucleus accumbens and enhances sensitivity to mild neurogenic stressors such as air puffs (Merali et al., 1997). Lipopolysaccharide and interleukin-1 administration does not, however, increase dopamine in the prefrontal cortex, as opposed to even mild psychogenic or neurogenic stressors (Lacosta et al., 1999). Tumor necrosis factor also does not cause any change in dopamine activity (Ando and Dunn, 1999), whereas interleukin-2 and interleukin-6 cause a decrease of dopamine in the nucleus accumbens, and this decrease is enhanced by air puffs (Song et al., 1999). The immunosuppression induced by stress is decreased if dopamine receptors are stimulated by the agonist apomorphine (Idova et al., 1997).

Other stress paradigms occurring in various contexts have effects on dopaminergic function. For example, the somatic stressor glucose deprivation causes striatal dopamine release in both animal and human subjects (Adler et al., 2000).

CONCLUSIONS

There are large bodies of research on central dopaminergic function and on the neuroendocrinology of the stress response. However, a relatively limited amount of work has focused on the interactions between these systems. A reason for the separation between these areas may be due to the fact that dopaminergic function has traditionally been studied by neurobiologists with an ultimate interest in elucidating the biological basis of systems relevant to neurological diseases (e.g., Parkinson's) or schizophrenia. In contrast, the neuroendocrine basis of the responses to stress has been examined by scientists with more of an endocrine background and by those with an interest in depression. Despite these different approaches, available data indicate that these two key neurobiological systems are highly interrelated. Hopefully, as science advances and the connection between these systems is better understood, cross-disciplinary studies will emerge that further our knowledge of the pathways and mechanisms that integrate dopaminergic and neuroendocrine function. Such research may offer new insights into the biological basis of disorders of CNS function, thus leading to novel therapeutic strategies.

REFERENCES

Alder CM, Elman I, Weisenfeld N, et al. (2000). Effects of acute metabolic stress on striatal dopamine releases in healthy volunteers. *Neuropsychopharmacology* 22,545–550.

Alonso SJ, Navarro E, Rodriguez M (1994). Permanent dopaminergic alterations in the nucleus accumbens after prenatal stress. *Pharmacol Biochem Behav* 49,353–358.

Alonso SJ, Navarro E, Santana C, et al. (1997). Motor lateralization, behavioral despair and dopaminergic brain asymmetry after prenatal stress. *Pharmacol Biochem Behav* 58,443–448.

Ando T, Dunn AJ (1999). Mouse tumor necrosis factor-alpha increases brain tryptophan concentrations and norepinephrine metabolism while activating the HPA axis in mice. *Neuroimmunomodulation* 6,319–329.

Barrot M, Marinelli M, Abrous DN, et al. (2000). The dopaminergic hyper-responsiveness of the shell of the nucleus accumbens is hormone dependent. *Eur J Neurosci* 12,973–979.

Berridge CW, Mitton E, Clark W, et al. (1999). Engagement in a non-escape (displacement) behavior elects a selective and lateralized suppression of frontal cortical dopaminergic utilization in stress. *Synapse* 32,187–197.

Brake WG, Flores G, Francis D, et al. (2000). Enhanced nucleus accumbens dopamine and plasma corticosterone stress responses in adult rats with neonatal excitotoxic lesions to the medial prefrontal cortex. *Neuroscience* 96,687–695.

Brake WG, Noel MB, Boksa P, et al. (1997). Influence of perinatal factors on the nucleus accumbens dopamine response to repeated stress during adulthood: an electrochemical study in the rat. *Neuroscience* 77,1067–1076.

Cabib S, Giardino L, Calza L, et al. (1998). Stress promotes major changes in dopamine receptor densities within the mesoaccumbens and nigrostriatal systems. *Neuroscience* 84,193–200.

Cabib S, Puglisi-Allegra S (1996). Different effects of repeated stressful experiences on mesocortical and mesolimbic dopamine metabolism. *Neuroscience* 73,375–380.

D'Aquila PS, Peana AT, Carboni V, et al. (2000). Exploratory behaviour and grooming after repeated restraint and chronic mild stress: effects of desipramine. *Eur J Pharmacol* 30,43–47.

Deutch AY, Bean AJ, Bissette G, et al.(1987). Stress-induced alterations in neurotensin, somatostatin and corticotropin-releasing factor in mesotelencephalic dopamine system regions. *Brain Res* 417,350–354.

Deutch AY, Roth RH (1999). Neurotransmitters. In: *Fundamental Neuroscience*, Zigmond MJ, ed. San Diego: Academic, pp. 198–208.

Di Chiara G, Loddo P, Tanda, G (1999). Reciprocal changes in prefrontal and limbic dopamine responsiveness to aversive and rewarding stimuli after chronic mild stress: implications for the psychobiology of depression. *Biol Psychiatry* 26,1624–1633.

Doherty MD, Gratton A (1997). NMDA receptors in nucleus accumbens modulate stress-induced dopamine release in nucleus accumbens and ventral tegmental area. *Synapse* 26,225–234.

Dunn AJ (2000). Footshock-induced changes in brain catecholamines and indoleamines are not mediated by CRF or ACTH. *Neurochem Int* 37,61–69.

Dunn AJ, Berridge CW (1987). Corticotropin-releasing factor administration elicits a stresslike activation of cerebral catecholaminergic systems. *Pharmacol Biochem Behav* 27,685–691.

Dunn AJ, Wang J, Ando T (1999). Effects of cytokines on cerebral neuro-transmission. Comparison with the effects of stress. *Adv Exp Med Biol* 461,117–127.

Duval F, Mokrani MC, Crocq MA, et al. (2000). Dopaminergic function and the cortisol response to dexamethasone in psychotic depression. *Progr Neuropsychopharmacol Biol Psychiatry* 24,207–225.

Dziedzicka-Wasylewska M, Willner P, Papp M (1997). Changes in dopamine receptor mRNA expression following chronic mild stress and chronic antidepressant treatment. *Behav Pharmacol* 8,607–618.

Everitt BJ, Parkinson JA, Olmstead MC, et al. (1999). Associative processes in addiction and reward. The role of amygdala-ventral striatal subsystems. *Ann NY Acad Sci* 29,412–438.

Feldman S, Weidenfeld J (1998). The excitatory effects of the amygdala on hypothalamo-pituitary-adrenocortical responses are mediated by hypothalamic norepinephrine, serotonin, and CRF-41. *Brain Res Bull* 45,389–393.

Finlay JM, Zigmond MJ (1997). The effects of stress on central dopaminergic neurons: possible clinical implications. *Neurochem Res* 22,1387–1394.

Ghiglieri O, Gambarana C, Scheggi S, et al. (1997). Palatable food induces an appetitive behaviour in satiated rats which can be inhibited by chronic stress. *Behav Pharmacol* 8,619–628.

Gomez FM, Giralt MT, Sainz B, et al. (1999). A possible attenuation of stress-induced increases in striatal dopamine metabolism by the expression of non-functional masticatory activity in the rat. *Eur J Oral Sci* 107,461–467.

Harfstrand A, Fuxe K, Cintra A, et al. (1986). Glucocorticoid receptor immunoreactivity in monoaminergic neurons in rat brain. *Proc Natl Acad Sci USA* 83,9779–9783.

Hawkins MF, Baumeister AA, Larue RH, et al. (2000). Manipulation of central GABAergic and dopaminergic systems alters stress responding in the rat. *Pharmacol Biochem Behav* 66,667–670.

Heimer L, Zahm DS, Churchill L, et al. (1991). Specificity in the projection patterns of accumbal core and shell in the rat. *Neuroscience* 41,89–125.

Hendley ED (2000). WKHA rats with genetic hyperactivity and hyperreactivity to stress: a review. *Neurosci Biobehav Rev* 24,41–44.

Hendley ED, Fan XM (1992). Regional differences in brain norepinephrine and dopamine uptake kinetics in inbred rat strains with hypertension and/or hyperactivity. *Brain Res* 586,44–52.

Horger BA, Roth RH (1996). The role of mesoprefrontal dopamine neurons in stress. *Crit Rev Neurobiol*

10,395–418.

Idova G, Cheido M, Devoino L (1997). Modulation of the immune response by changing neuromediator systems activity under stress. *Int J Immunopharmacol* 19,535–540.

Inglis FM, Moghaddam B (1999). Dopaminergic innervation of the amygdala is highly responsive to stress. *J Neurochem* 72,1088–1094.

Jezova D, Ochedalski T, Glickman M, et al. (1999). Central corticotropin-releasing hormone receptors modulate hypothalamic-pituitary-adrenocortical and sympathoadrenal activity during stress. *Neuroscience* 94,797–802.

Kehoe P, Shoemaker WJ, Arons C, et al. (1998). Repeated isolation stress in the neonatal rat: relation to brain dopamine systems in the 10-day-old-rat. *Behav Neurosci* 112,166–174.

King D, Zigmond MJ, Finlay JM (1997). Effects of dopamine depletion in the medial prefrontal cortex on the stress-induced increase in extra-cellular dopamine in the nucleus accumbens core and shell. *Neuroscience* 77,141–153.

Konstandi M, Johnson E, Lang MA, et al. (2000). Noradrenaline, dopamine, serotonin: different effects of psychological stress on brain biogenic amines in mice and rats. *Pharmacol Res* 41,341–346.

Lacosta S, Merali Z, Anisman H (1999). Behavioral and neurochemical consequences of lipopolysaccharide in mice: anxiogenic-like effects. *Brain Res* 818,291–303.

Lindley SE, Bengoechea TG, Schatzberg AF, et al. (1999). Glucocorticoid effects on mesotelencephalic dopamine meurotransmission. *Neuropsychopharmacology* 21,399–407.

Lindley SE, Bengoechea TG, Wong DL, et al. (1999). Strain differences in mesotelencephalic dopaminergic neuronal regulation between Fischer 344 and Lewis rats. *Brain Res* 832,152–158.

McIntyre DC, Kent P, Hayley S, et al. (1999). Influence of psychogenic and neurogenic stressors on neuroendocrine and central monoamine activity in fast and slow kindling rats. *Brain Res* 840,65–74.

Mendlin A, Martin FJ, Jacobs BL (1999). Dopaminergic input is required for increases in serotonin output produced by behavioral activation: an in vivo microdialysis study in rat forebrain. *Neuroscience* 93,897–905.

Merali Z, Lacosta S, Anisman H (1997). Effects of interleukin-1β and mild stress on alterations of norepinephrine, dopamine and serotonin neurotransmission: a regional microdialysis study. *Brain Res* 761,225–235.

Mizoguchi K, Yuzurihara M, Ishige A, et al. (2000). Chronic stress induces impairment of spatial working memory because of prefrontal dopaminergic dysfunction. *J Neurosci* 20,1568–1574.

Morrow BA, Elsworth JD, Rasmusson AM, et al. (1999). The role of mesoprefrontal dopamine neurons in the acquisition and expression of conditioned fear in the rat. *Neuroscience* 92,553–564.

Murphy BL, Arnsten AF, Goldman-Rakic PS, et al. (1996). Increased dopamine turnover in the prefrontal cortex impairs spatial working memory performance in rats and monkeys. *Proc Natl Acad Sci USA* 93,1325–1329.

Nakahara D, Nakamura M, Oki Y, et al. (2000). Lack of glucocorticoids attenuates the self-stimulation-induced increase in the in vivo synthesis rate of dopamine but not serotonin in the rat nucleus accumbens. *Eur J Neurosci* 12,1495–1500.

Ortiz J, De Caprio JL, Kosten TA, et al. (1995). Strain-selective effects of corticosterone on locomotor sensitization to cocaine and on levels of tyrosine hydroxylase and glucocorticoid receptor in the ventral tegmental area. *Neuroscience* 67,383–397.

Pani L, Porcella A, Gessa GL (2000). The role of stress in the pathophysiology of the dopaminergic system. *Mol Psychiatry* 5,14–21.

Petty F, Jordan S, Kramer GL, et al. (1997). Benzodiazepine prevention of swim stress-induced sensitization of cortical biogenic amines: an in vivo microdialysis study. *Neurochem Res* 22,1101–1104.

Piazza PV, Le Moal ML (1996). Pathophysiological basis of vulnerability to drug abuse: role of an interaction between stress, glucocorticoids, and dopaminergic neurons. *Annu Rev Pharmacol Toxicol* 36,359–378.

Prasad BM, Sorg BA, Ulibarri C, et al. (1995). Sensitization to stress and psychostimulants. Involvement of dopamine transmission versus the HPA axis. *Ann NY Acad Sci* 771,617–625.

Puglisi-Allegra S, Cabib S (1997). Psychopharmacology of dopamine: the contribution of comparative studies in inbred strains of mice. *Progr Neurobiol* 51,637–661.

Reznikov AG, Nosenko ND, Tarasenko LV (1999). Prenatal stress and glucocorticoid effects in the developing gender-related brain. *J Steroid Biochem Mol Biol* 69,109–115.

Serova L, Sabban EL, Zangen A, et al. (1998). Altered gene expression for catecholamine biosynthetic enzymes and stress response in rat genetic model of depression. *Brain Res Mol Brain Res* 63,133–138.

Shanks N, Griffiths J, Anisman H (1994). Central catecholamine alterations induced by stressor exposure: analyses in recombinant inbred strains of mice. *Behav Brain Res* 63,25–33.

Shiver T, Familari M, Aguilera G (1992). Regulation of intermediate pituitary corticotropin-releasing hormone receptors by dopamine. *Endocrinology* 130,2299–2304.

Song C, Merali Z, Anisman H (1999). Variations of nucleus accumbens dopamine and serotonin following systemic interleukin-1, interleukin-2 or interleukin-6 treatment. *Neuroscience* 88,823–836.

Waxham MN (1999). Neurotransmitter receptors. In: *Fundamental Neuroscience*, Zigmond MJ, ed. San Diego: Academic, pp. 261–262.

Wedzony K, Mackowiak M, Fijal K, et al. (1996). Evidence that conditioned stress enhances outflow of dopamine in rat prefrontal cortex: a search for the influence of diazepam and 5-HT1A agonists. *Synapse* 24,240–247.

Wu YL, Yoshida M, Emoto H, et al. (1999). Psychological stress selectively increases extracellular dopamine in the "shell," but not the "core," of the rat nucleus accumbens: a novel dual-needle probe simultaneous microdialysis study. *Neurosci Lett* 275,69–72.

Zahm DS, Brog JS (1992). On the significance of subterritories in the "accumbens" part of the rat ventral striatum. *Neuroscience* 50,751–767.

Zimmerberg B, Brown RC (1998). Prenatal experience and postnatal stress modulates the adult neurosteroid and catecholaminergic stress responses. *Int J Dev Neurosci* 16,217–228.

7.

Is Dopamine in the Prefrontal Cortex Released from Noradrenergic Neurons?

Gian Luigi Gessa, Luca Pani, and Paola Devoto

ABSTRACT

The aim of this study was to investigate whether extracellular dopamine in the prefrontal cortex (PFC) might originate, other than from dopamine neurons, from norepinephrine neurons and/or if such release might occur after treatment with atypical antipsychotics. Changes in extracellular dopamine and norepinephrine concentrations were monitored by microdialysis after treatments that modify norepinephrine and dopamine neuronal activity differently and after typical and atypical antipsychotics. The α_2-adrenoceptor agonist clonidine not only reduced norepinephrine levels, as expected from its ability to suppress norepinephrine neuronal activity, but also reduced dopamine levels. In contrast, the α_2-adrenoceptor antagonist idazoxan not only increased norepinephrine levels but also increased dopamine. Quinpirole produced only a modest reduction of dopamine levels, whereas γ-butyrolactone increased both dopamine and norepinephrine levels. Conversely, haloperidol modified neither norepinephrine nor dopamine. Locally perfused into the PFC, clonidine reduced norepinephrine and dopamine levels, whereas idazoxan increased both norepinephrine and dopamine levels. Conversely, neither quinpirole nor haloperidol modified norepinephrine or dopamine levels. Results indicate that dopamine levels in the dialysate from the PFC are independent of the activity of dopamine neurons but correlate with those of norepinephrine neurons and that norepinephrine and dopamine concentrations in the PFC are controlled by α_2-adrenoceptors, possibly located on norepinephrine nerve terminals. Consistent with their ability to block α_2-adrenoceptors, the atypical antipsychotics clozapine and risperidone increased norepinephrine and dopamine levels. Locally perfused into the PFC, clozapine increased both dopamine and norepinephrine, whereas clonidine perfusion reverted the dopamine and norepinephrine increase produced by systemic clozapine. Results indicate that atypical antipsychotics corelease norepinephrine and dopamine from nerve terminals by blocking α_2-adrenoceptors. Dopamine in the dialysate from the PFC seems to originate from norepinephrine neurons, where it acts as a norepinephrine precursor and cotransmitter.

INTRODUCTION

Numerous studies provide evidence that dopaminergic and noradrenergic innervation are important in prefrontal cortex (PFC) functions, including control of attention, arousal, response to stress, anxiety, fear, mood, cognitive processes, etc (Aston-Jones et al., 1991, 1996; Berridge et al., 1993; Berridge and Foote, 1991; Kalivas, 1993; Mantz et al., 1988; Thierry et al., 1976). Conversely, impaired dopaminergic (Knable and Weinberger, 1997) and noradrenergic (van Kammen et al., 1990) functioning in the PFC appears to be involved in the pathophysiology of negative symptoms of schizophrenia, such as anhedonia, loss of drive, cognitive deficits, etc.

In agreement with this hypothesis, atypical antipsychotics, such as clozapine and olanzapine, have been shown to increase both dopamine and norepinephrine release in the PFC in rats (Li et al., 1998; Pehek et al., 1994) and monkeys (Youngren et al, 1999) and are claimed to ameliorate negative symptoms and cognitive deficits in schizophrenic patients (King, 1998).

PFC is innervated both by noradrenergic neurons that originate in the locus ceruleus and by dopaminergic neurons that originate in the ventral tegmental area. Whereas dopamine terminals are highly localized within specific areas in rats, such as the medial prefrontal cortex, norepinephrine projections are diffuse throughout the PFC. However, although norepinephrine concentration exceeds that of dopamine in all PFC areas, including the medial PFC (Slopsema et al., 1982; Tassin et al., 1978), the rate of dopamine synthesis is the same in areas where dopamine terminals are confined as in areas that receive norepinephrine input but few or no dopamine terminals (Fadda et al., 1984).

Moreover, dopamine synthesis rate in norepinephrine regions is much faster than that of norepinephrine (Neff et al., 1970), suggesting that only a small fraction of the newly synthesized dopamine is converted into norepinephrine in noradrenergic neurons, the rest possibly being deaminated and/or released from norepinephrine nerve terminals.

The aim of this work was to investigate if extracellular dopamine in the PFC originates, other than from dopamine neurons, from norepinephrine neurons and/or if such release might occur after treatment with atypical antipsychotics.

METHODS

Male Sprague-Dawley albino rats (Harlan, Italy) weighing 200–280 g were used in all experiments. All subjects were kept on a 12 hr/12 hr light/dark cycle with food and water available ad libitum. Experimental protocols were approved by the Ethical Committee at the University of Cagliari and performed in strict accordance with the EC regulations for the care and use of experimental animals (CEE 86/609).

Rats were anesthetized with Equithesin (5 ml/kg ip) and placed in a Kopf stereotaxic frame. The skull was exposed, and a hole was drilled through the two temporal bones for transversal insertion across the medial PFC (AP +3.0, V 2 −.6 from bregma, according to Paxinos and Watson atlas) of the dialysis probe (AN 69-HF, Hospal-Dasco, Bologna, Italy; cut-off 20,000 Da, in vitro recovery about 30%). After 20–24 hr, artificial cerebrospinal fluid (147 mM NaCl, 4 mM KCl, 1.8 mM $CaCl_2$, pH 6–6.5) was pumped through the dialysis tube at a constant rate of 1.2

μl/min. Samples were collected every 20 min and directly analyzed by high-performance liquid chromatography with coulometric detection. After collection of at least three consecutive samples differing by no more than 10%, drugs were administered by intraperitoneal injection or by inverse dialysis.

For microdialysis experiments, the raw basal data (pg) were analyzed by chi-square test and then, because no significant difference was found in each group, were normalized to percent of mean basal level of each rat. Statistical significance was evaluated by ANOVA for repeated measures followed by Newman-Keuls test as post hoc.

RESULTS AND DISCUSSION

Mean basal norepinephrine and dopamine extracellular levels, as recovered by transversal microdialysis probe located in the medial PFC, were 0.38 (0.02 and 0.13 (0.01 pg/μl for norepinephrine and dopamine, respectively. Values are the means (SE for 62 animals.

Intraperitoneal administration of the α_2-adrenoceptor agonist clonidine (0.15 mg/kg) reduced norepinephrine levels, as expected from its ability to suppress electrical activity of norepinephrine neurons; however, it also reduced by 60% extracellular dopamine concentrations in the PFC (Fig. 7-1*A*).

In contrast, the α_2-adrenoceptor antagonist idazoxan (1.5 mg/kg ip) not only increased norepinephrine concentrations (up to 160% of basal values), which is consistent with its ability to activate norepinephrine neurons, but also increased dopamine levels in the PFC to 160% (Fig. 7-1*B*).

However, in contrast to their ability to suppress activity of dopamine neurons, the D2 receptor agonist quinpirole (up to 0.5 mg/kg) produced only a modest reduction of dopamine concentration (Fig. 7-2*A*), whereas GBL (up to 500 mg/kg) actually increased both dopamine and norepinephrine concentrations to about 200% of the basal levels (Fig. 7-2*B*). In contrast to its ability to stimulate dopamine neuronal activity, the D2 receptor antagonist haloperidol (0.2 mg/kg ip) failed to modify both norepinephrine and dopamine levels (Fig. 7-2*C*).

Locally perfused into the PFC, clonidine (10-8–10-6 M) reduced to almost zero not only norepinephrine but also dopamine levels (Fig. 7-3*A*), whereas idazoxan (10-6–10-4 M) increased both norepinephrine and dopamine levels up to 280% of the basal levels (Fig. 7-3*B*). Conversely, locally perfused into the PFC, neither quinpirole, up to 10-4 M (Fig. 7-3*C*), nor haloperidol, up to 10-5 M (Fig. 7-3*D*), modified either norepinephrine or dopamine levels.

Results indicate that dopamine concentrations in the perfusate from the PFC are independent of the activity of dopamine neurons, whereas they correlate with the activity of norepinephrine neurons. Moreover our results indicate that norepinephrine and dopamine concentrations in PFC dialysate are controlled by α_2-adrenoceptors in the PFC possibly located on norepinephrine nerve terminals.

Because different atypical antipsychotics have a high affinity for α_2-adrenoceptors, their ability to modify dopamine and norepinephrine extracellular levels in the PFC was studied. Intraperitoneal clozapine and risperidone (10 and 2 mg/kg,

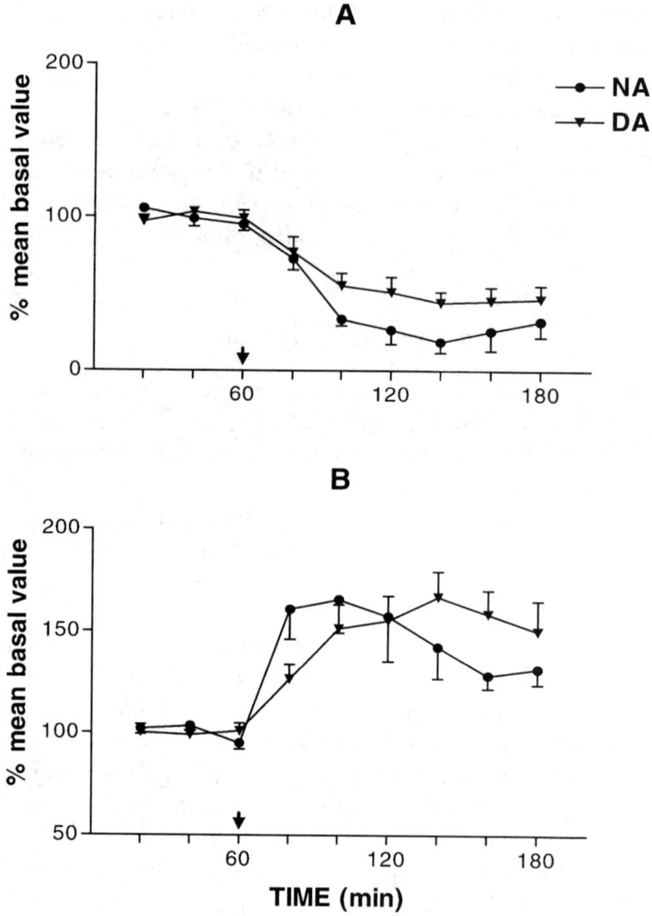

FIG. 7-1. Effect of clonidine (0.15 mg/kg ip) (*A*) and idazoxan (1.5 mg/kg ip) (*B*) on extracellular norepinephrine (*circles*) and dopamine (*triangles*) concentrations in PFC. *Arrow*, time of administration. Data are means (SE for four rats. Norepinephrine and dopamine values were different from baseline by time 100 and 80 min for clonidine and idazoxan, respectively (P <0.01).

respectively) increased both norepinephrine (to 280 and 200%, respectively) and dopamine levels (to 410 and 290%, respectively) (Fig. 7-4A).

Locally perfused into the PFC at 10-6–10-4 M (Fig. 7-4*B*), clozapine increased both norepinephrine and dopamine concentrations to 330% of mean basal values, similarly to idazoxan. Locally perfused into the PFC, clonidine (10^{-6} M) reverted the effect of systemic clozapine and reduced dopamine and norepinephrine concentrations to basal levels (Fig. 7-5). These results suggest that the atypical antipsychotics

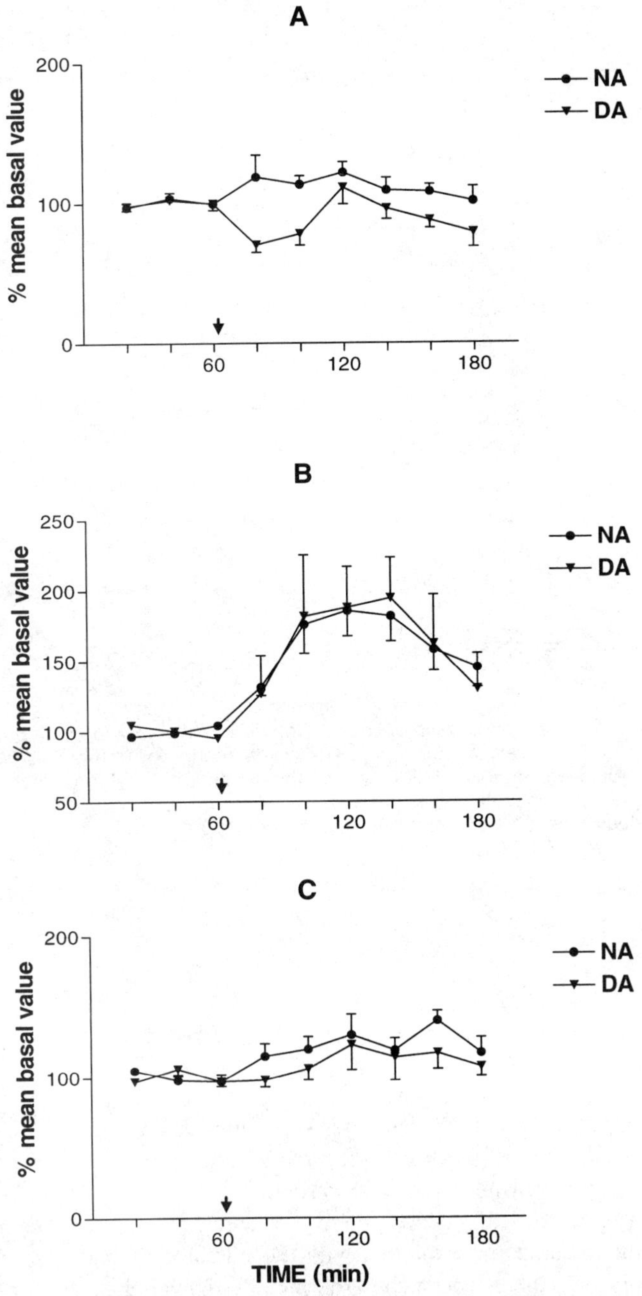

FIG. 7-2. Effect of quinpirole (0.5 mg/kg ip) (*A*), GBL (500 mg/kg ip) (*B*), and haloperidol (0.2 mg/kg ip) (*C*) on extracellular norepinephrine (*circles*) and dopamine (*triangles*) concentrations in PFC. *Arrow*, time of administration. Data are means (SE for at least four rats. Norepinephrine and dopamine values were different from baseline at time 80 min for GBL ($P < 0.01$) and dopamine at times 80 and 100 min for quinpirole ($P < 0.05$).

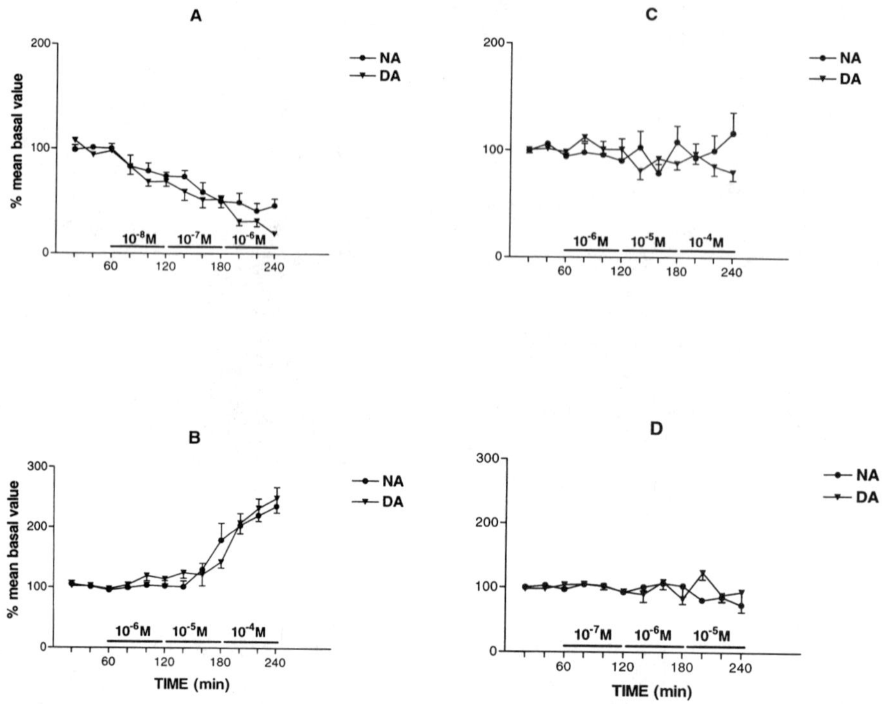

FIG. 7-3. Effect of local perfusion into PFC of clonidine (*A*), idazoxan (*B*), quinpirole (*C*), and haloperidol (*D*) on extracellular norepinephrine (*circles*) and dopamine (*triangles*) concentrations in PFC. Data are means (SE for at least four rats. Each compound was perfused via reverse dialysis at concentrations and times indicated (*black bars*). Norepinephrine and dopamine values were different from baseline by time 100 and 180 min for clonidine and idazoxan, respectively ($P < 0.01$).

clozapine and risperidone induce a corelease of norepinephrine and dopamine from nerve terminals in the PFC by blocking α_2-adrenoceptors, similarly to idazoxan. Because norepinephrine nerve terminals are more densely localized in the superficial cortical layers, where D1 and α_1 receptors are also present, coreleased monoamines may interact with these receptors, and such a mechanism may be involved in the effect of these atypical antipsychotics against the negative symptomatology in schizophrenia and in their antidepressant effect.

In conclusion our results suggest that dialysate dopamine from the PFC may originate, other than from dopamine neurons, from norepinephrine nerve terminals, where it acts as a precursor for norepinephrine and as a cotransmitter.

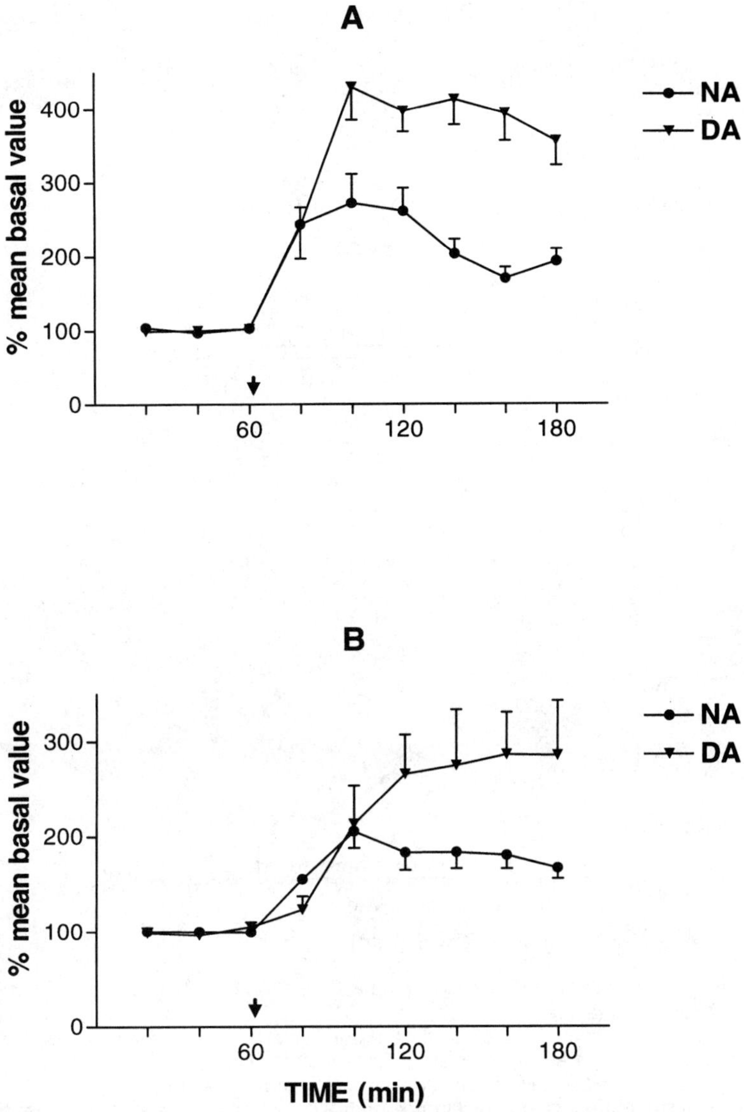

FIG. 7-4. Effect of clozapine (10 mg/kg ip) (*A*) and risperidone (2 mg/kg ip) (*B*) on extracellular norepinephrine (*circles*) and dopamine (*triangles*) concentrations in PFC. *Arrow*, time of administration. Data are means (SE for at least four rats. Norepinephrine and dopamine values were different from baseline by time 80 min ($P < 0.01$).

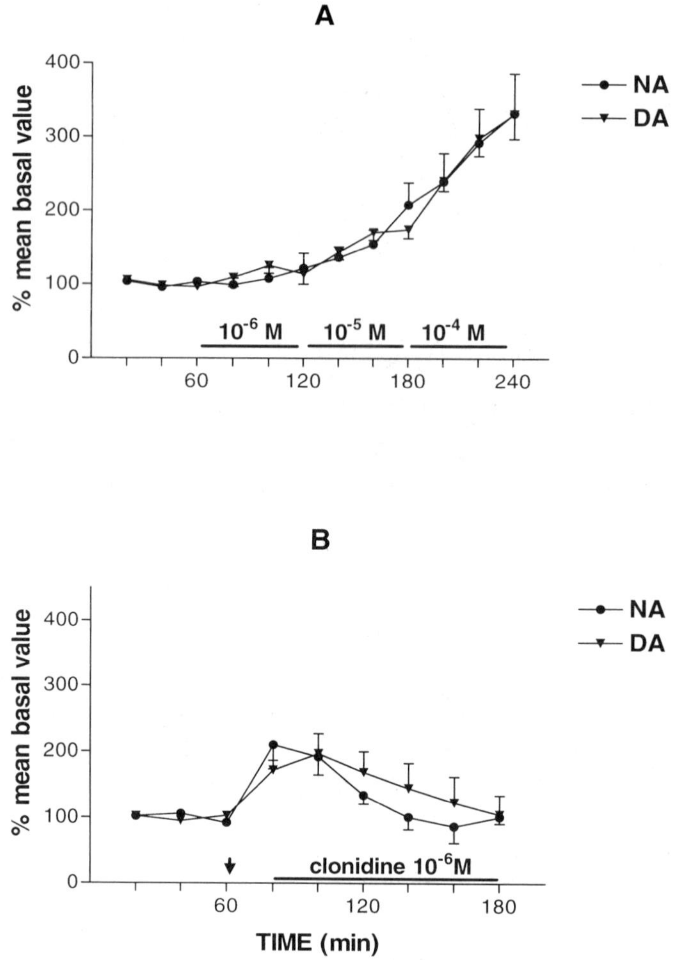

FIG. 7-5. *A*, effect of locally perfused clozapine into PFC on extracellular norepinephrine (*circles*) and dopamine (*triangles*) concentrations in PFC; *B*, reversal of clozapine (10 mg/kg ip) effect by locally infused clonidine. *Arrow*, time of administration. Each compound was perfused via reverse dialysis at concentrations and for times indicated (*black bars*). For clozapine perfusion, norepinephrine and dopamine values were different from baseline by time 140 min ($P < 0.01$). For clonidine perfusion, norepinephrine and dopamine curves were different from clozapine alone (Fig. 7-4*A*) by time 100 min ($P < 0.01$).

REFERENCES

Aston-Jones G, Shipley MT, Chouvet G, et al. (1991). Afferent regulation of locus ceruleus neurons: anatomy, physiology and pharmacology. *Progr Brain Res* 88,47–75.

Berridge CW, Foote SL (1991). Effects of locus ceruleus activation on electroencephalographic activity in neocortex and hippocampus. *J Neurosci* 11,3135–3145.

Fadda F, Gessa GL, Marcou M, et al. (1984). Evidence for dopamine autoreceptors in mesocortical dopamine neurons. *Brain Res* 293,67–72.

Kalivas PW (1993). Neurotransmitter regulation of dopamine neurons in the ventral tegmental area. *Brain Res Rev* 18,75–113.

King DJ (1998). Drug treatment of the negative symptoms of schizophrenia. *Eur J Neuropsychopharmacol* 8,33–42.

Knable MB, Weinberger DR (1997). Dopamine, the prefrontal cortex and schizophrenia. *J Psychopharmacol* 11,123–131.

Li X-M, Perry KW, Wong DT, et al. (1998). Olanzapine increases in vivo dopamine and norepinephrine release in rat prefrontal cortex, nucleus accumbens and striatum. *Psychopharmacology* 136,153–161.

Mantz J, Milla C, Glowinski J, et al. (1988). Differential effects of ascending neurons containing dopamine and noradrenaline in the control of spontaneous activity and of evoked responses in the rat prefrontal cortex. *Neuroscience* 27,517–526.

Neff NH, Spano PF, Groppetti A, et al. (1970). A simple procedure for calculating the synthesis rate of norepinephrine, dopamine and serotonin in rat brain. *J Pharmacol Exp Ther* 176,701–710.

Pehek EA, Yamamoto BY (1994). Differential effects of locally administered clozapine and haloperidol on dopamine efflux in the rat prefrontal cortex and caudate-putamen. *J Neurochem* 63,2118–2124.

Slopsema JS, Van der Gugten J, De Buin JPC (1982). Regional concentrations of noradrenaline and dopamine in the frontal cortex of the rat: dopaminergic innervation of the prefrontal subareas and lateralization of the prefrontal dopamine. *Brain Res* 250,197–200.

Tassin JP, Bockaert J, Blanc G, et al. (1978). Topographical distribution of dopaminergic innervation and dopaminergic receptors of the anterior cerebral cortex of the rat. *Brain Res* 154,241–251.

Thierry AM, Tassin JP, Blanc G, et al. (1976). Selective activation of the mesocortical dopamine system by stress. *Nature* 263,242–244.

van Kammen DP, Peters J, Yao J, et al. (1990). Norepinephrine in acute exacerbations of chronic schizophrenia. *Arch Gen Psychol* 47,161–168.

Youngren KD, Inglis FM, Pivirotto PJ, et al. (1999). Clozapine preferentially increases dopamine release in the rhesus monkey prefrontal cortex compared with the caudate nucleus. *Neuropsychopharmacology* 20,403–412.

8.

Lamina-Specific Alterations in Dopamine Innervation of Prefrontal and Entorhinal Cortices in Schizophrenia

David A. Lewis, Mayada Akil, and Joseph N. Pierri

ABSTRACT

Certain cognitive symptoms of schizophrenia have been proposed to be related to diminished dopamine neurotransmission in the prefrontal cortex. We summarize recent studies demonstrating that the density of axons immunoreactive for the dopamine membrane transporter and tyrosine hydroxylase are significantly decreased in layer 6 of the prefrontal cortex (area 9) of subjects with schizophrenia but that a marker of serotonin axons is unchanged. In the rostral entorhinal cortex, another cortical region implicated in the pathophysiology of schizophrenia, tyrosine hydroxylase-labeled axons are similarly decreased in layer 6 but are also reduced in layer 3. These changes may be specific to the diagnosis of schizophrenia because they were not observed in subjects with other psychiatric disorders. Finally, studies in monkeys chronically treated with haloperidol indicate that the changes in cortical dopamine axons in schizophrenia cannot be attributed to treatment with antipsychotic medications. These findings reveal regional-, laminar-, and neurotransmitter-specific alterations in cortical dopamine axons that appear to be specific to the pathophysiology of schizophrenia.

INTRODUCTION

Abnormalities in dopamine neurotransmission have long been considered to be involved in the pathophysiology of schizophrenia (Carlsson and Lindquist, 1963; Snyder, 1972), although the nature of these abnormalities has been the subject of substantial debate. Recent formulations of the dopamine hypothesis of schizophrenia posit that the psychotic symptoms of this disorder reflect a hyperdopaminergic state in subcortical structures, whereas the cognitive deficits and negative symptoms that are characteristic of schizophrenia have been attributed to a hypodopaminergic state in certain cortical association regions, such as the prefrontal (PFC) and entorhinal cortices (ERC) (Davis et al., 1991; Goldstein and Deutch, 1992; Grace, 1991). Indeed, evidence from model systems suggests that reduced dopamine modulation of neuronal activity in the PFC can contribute to excessive dopamine activity in the striatum (Goldstein and Deutch, 1992; Saunders et al., 1994). However, the integrity of the dopamine innervation of these cortical regions has not been examined in schizophrenia.

The regional and laminar distributions of dopamine axons in the primate PFC and ERC have been characterized using immunocytochemical methods and antibodies directed against dopamine, the dopamine membrane transporter (DAT), or tyrosine hydroxylase (TH), the rate-limiting enzyme in catecholamine biosynthesis (Gaspar et al., 1989; Lewis, 1992; Lewis et al., 1988, 1998; Williams and Goldman-Rakic, 1993). In both monkeys and humans, dopamine afferents innervate all subdivisions of these cortical regions, with labeled axons being particularly dense in the dorsomedial region (area 9) of the PFC and the rostral subdivision (region ER) of the ERC. We have used a similar approach to address the following questions regarding integrity of cortical dopamine systems in schizophrenia: 1) Is the density of axons immunoreactive for TH or DAT altered in the PFC of subjects with schizophrenia? 2) If so, are these alterations specific to dopamine axons, or are markers of other monoaminergic systems also affected? 3) Are changes in dopamine axons also present in other cortical association regions such as subdivision ER of the ERC? 4) Are alterations in cortical dopamine axons specific to the diagnosis of schizophrenia, or are they also observed in subjects with other psychiatric disorders? 5) To what extent can changes in cortical dopamine axons in schizophrenia be attributed to treatment with antipsychotic medications?

METHODS

To address these questions, we examined postmortem tissue specimens from the left hemisphere of 44 human brains (Akil et al., 1999, 2000). Neuropathological examination revealed occasional neuritic plaques in the neocortex of three subjects, but the density of the plaques was insufficient to meet diagnostic criteria for Alzheimer's disease, and none of the subjects had a clinical history of dementia. The cause of death involved brain damage in two subjects, but no neuropathological abnormalities were detected in the regions of interest for this study in either subject.

Sixteen subjects had a diagnosis of schizophrenia or schizoaffective disorder; 22 subjects were considered normal controls (although one had a history of alcohol dependence); and six subjects had a psychiatric illness other than schizophrenia. Consensus DSM-III-R diagnoses were made by an independent panel of experienced clinicians using information obtained from clinical records and structured interviews with one or more surviving relatives of each subject (Glantz and Lewis, 1997). For each study described below (Table 8-1), subjects were studied in pairs matched for gender and race and as closely as possible for age and postmortem interval.

To assess the possible influence of antipsychotic medications on the measures of interest in the human studies, we studied four male cynomolgus (*Macaca fascicularis*) monkeys, each of which was treated for 9–12 months with the typical antipsychotic agent, haloperidol decanoate, and four matched control animals (Akil et al.,

TABLE 8-1. *Characteristics of matched pairs of subjects used in each study*

	PFC—study 1		ERC/PFC—study 2		ERC—study 3	
	Control	Schizophrenic	Control	Schizophrenic	Control	Psychiatric
n	16	16	7	7	6	6
Male : female	10:6	10:6	5:2	5:2	4:2	4:2
Age (yr)	54.6±9.2	53.8±9.4	53.4±12.2	54.7±14.5	44.3±15.6	45.0±14.2
Postmortem interval (hr)	9.2±4.7	9.4±3.9	8.7±2.4	7.5±3.2	8.2±2.6	7.8±3.6

1999). Trough serum levels of haloperidol averaged 4.3 ± 1.1 ng/ml, levels shown to be associated with a therapeutic response in humans (Janicak et al., 1993).

Tissue sections (40 μm) containing PFC area 9 or subdivision ER of the ERC in both human and monkey tissue specimens were processed for immunoreactivity for TH, DAT, or the serotonin transporter (SERT) as previously described (Akil et al., 1999). The relative densities of TH-, DAT-, and SERT-immunoreactive axons were determined by measuring total length of labeled axons per unit area (10,000 μm^2) without knowledge of subject number or diagnostic group. To examine the laminar specificity of any changes in dopamine axons in schizophrenia, we sampled cortical layers 1, deep 3, and 6. These layers were selected for analysis because they contain the highest densities of dopamine axons in monkeys and humans (Gaspar et al., 1989; Lewis, 1992; Lewis et al., 1988; Williams and Goldman-Rakic, 1993) and because the substantial differences in the extrinsic connectivity of these three layers provide a means for interpreting the possible functional significance of any laminar-specific alterations in dopamine innervation. These procedures have been used to characterize differences in TH- and DAT-immunoreactive axons across experimental conditions in animals, and they have been externally validated by comparisons with biochemical measures in both developmental and lesion studies (Erickson et al., 1998; Rosenberg and Lewis, 1995; Venator et al., 1999).

RESULTS

Tyrosine Hydroxylase and DAT Immunoreactive Axons in PFC of Schizophrenic and Matched Control Subjects

Although the intensity of axon labeling was usually less robust with the DAT antibody than with the TH antibody in the same subject, the overall patterns of regional and laminar distribution of labeled axons were the same with both antibodies. Qualitative analyses conducted blind to diagnosis for each of the 16 pairs of schizophrenic and control subjects (Table 8-1, study 1) revealed that the density of DAT-immunoreactive axons was decreased in ten schizophrenic subjects, increased in one, and unchanged in five. In some schizophrenic subjects, the decrease in density of TH- and DAT-immunoreactive axons was marked, especially in the deep layers (Fig. 8-1, *A* and *B*). With one exception, the difference in DAT-immunoreactive axon density between a matched pair of subjects paralleled the difference in TH-immunoreactive axon density.

To determine the magnitude of these differences, we measured innervation density of TH-immunoreactive axons. The mean total length of TH-immunoreactive axons in medial area 9 was nonsignificantly decreased by 10.8% and 13.8% in layers 1 and 3, respectively, of the schizophrenic subjects compared with the matched controls. In contrast, mean total axon length (per 10,000 μm^2) in layer 6 of the schizophrenic subjects was significantly ($F_{3,10} = 5.23$, $P = 0.02$) decreased by 33.6% compared with matched controls (Fig. 8-1*C*). Comparison of individual matched pairs of subjects revealed that in 13 of 16 schizophrenic subjects the mean total axon length in layer 6 was less than in the matched control subject (Fig. 8-2). These differences were not attributable to the effects of gender, race, age, postmortem interval, or tissue storage time (Akil et al., 1999). Correlational analyses also failed to detect any association between magnitude of the decrease in TH-immunoreactive axons in layer 6 of the schizophrenic subjects and age of onset or duration of illness ($r < 0.056$, $P > 0.84$).

To determine whether this reduction in the relative density of labeled axons in layer 6 of schizophrenic subjects was specific to dopamine axons or representative of a more generalized alteration in monoamine-containing afferents to the PFC, we examined SERT-immunoreactive axons in the same 16 pairs of subjects. In contrast to the observations with markers of dopamine axons, the total length of SERT-immunoreactive axons did not differ ($F_{3,10} = 0.56$, $P > 0.40$) between schizo-

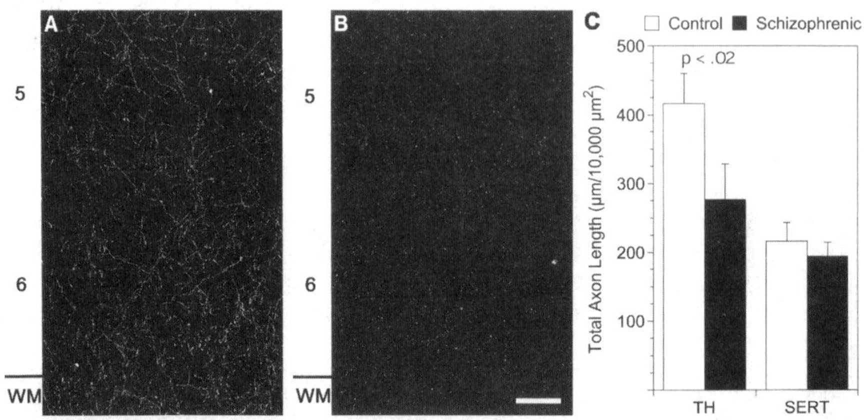

FIG. 8-1. Darkfield photomicrographs of dopamine transporter-labeled axons in PFC area 9 from control subject (A) matched to schizophrenic subject (B). Numbers, cortical layers; WM, white matter. Calibration bar 200 mm. C, bar graph of mean (±SE) total length of TH-immunoreactive and SERT-immunoreactive axons in layer 6 of PFC area 9 in 16 matched pairs of schizophrenic and control subjects. Note that total length of TH-labeled axons is decreased in schizophrenic subjects compared with controls, whereas total length of SERT-labeled axons does not differ across groups. Adapted from Akil et al. (1999).

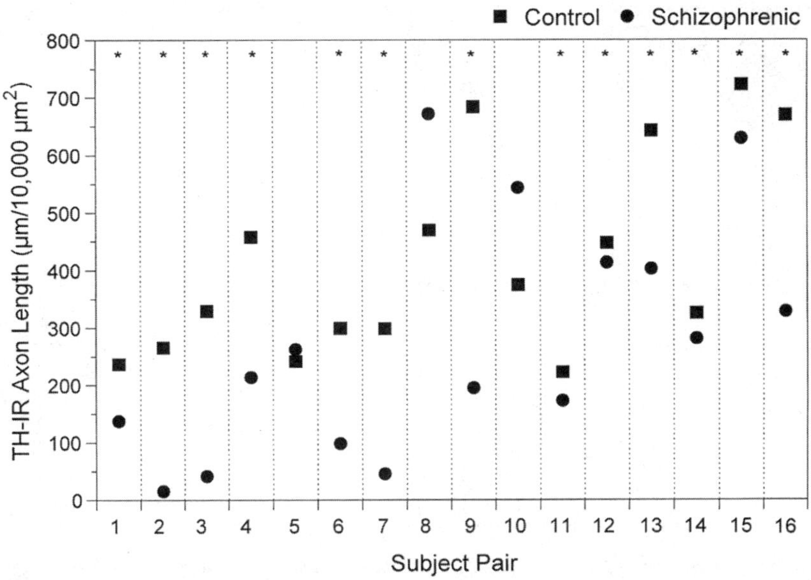

FIG. 8-2. Difference in total length of TH-immunoreactive axons in layer 6 of PFC area 9 for each of 16 matched pairs of schizophrenic and control subjects. Note total length of TH-immunoreactive axons is reduced in 13 schizophrenic subjects (asterisks).

phrenic and control subjects in any layer. In layer 6, mean total length of SERT-immunoreactive axons for each schizophrenic subject was within the range of all control subjects (Fig. 8-1*C*).

Tyrosine Hydroxylase Immunoreactive Axons in ERC of Schizophrenic and Matched Control Subjects

For seven of these same pairs of schizophrenic subjects (Table 8-1, study 1), tissue was available from the rostral subdivision ER of the ERC (Akil et al., 2000). Both qualitative (Fig. 8-3) and quantitative studies, conducted blind to subject, pair, and diagnosis, revealed that density of TH-immunoreactive axons was also decreased in ER of the schizophrenic subjects. Although the mean total axon length of TH-immunoreactive axons (per 10,000 μm^2) did not differ in layer 1 of ER of the schizophrenic and control subjects, mean total axon length in layer 3 of the schizophrenic subjects was significantly decreased ($F_{1,8} = 9.46$, $P = 0.02$) by 67% compared with that in the matched controls (Fig. 8-4*A*). Similarly TH-immunoreactive axon length in layer 6 was reduced ($F_{1,8} = 16.25$, $P = 0.004$) by 62% in the schizophrenic subjects compared with controls. Total length of TH-immunoreactive axons was less in the schizophrenic subject than in the matched control for six of the seven subject pairs in layer 3 and for all seven pairs in layer 6.

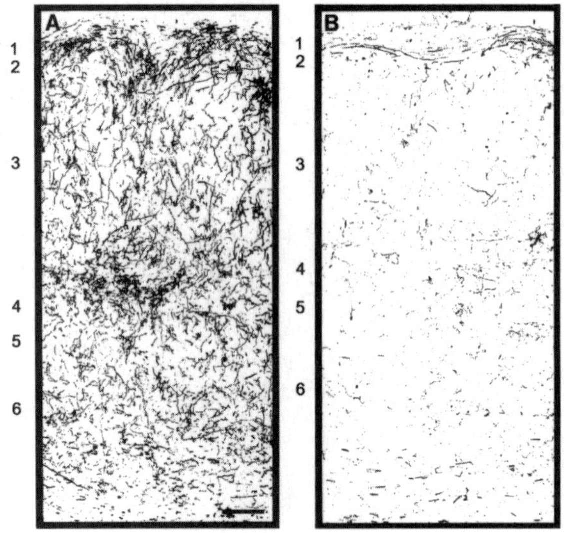

FIG. 8-3. Black-white reversals of darkfield photomicrographs of TH immunoreactivity in subdivision ER of a control subject (A) and schizophrenic subject (B) with the greatest decrease in labeled axons. Calibration bar 300 mm. Adapted from Akil et al. (2000).

To directly compare these observations with those in the PFC, the data for the same seven pairs of subjects from area 9 are shown in Fig. 8-4*B*. TH-immunoreactive axon length showed a different laminar effect in the PFC of the schizophrenic subjects. Although mean total axon length was reduced by 25% and 32% in layers 1 and 3, respectively, of the schizophrenic subjects, neither of these differences was statistically significant ($F_{1,8} < 1.67$, $P > 0.23$). In contrast, mean total axon length in layer 6 of the schizophrenic subjects was significantly ($F_{1,8} = 8.97$, $P = 0.02$) reduced by 62% compared with controls. These regional differences in the cortical layers showing significant decreases in labeled axons in subjects with schizophrenia were supported by correlational analyses. TH-immunoreactive axon length was highly correlated between PFC and ERC in layer 6 ($r = 0.623$, $P = 0.02$) but not in layer 3 ($r = 0.249$, $P = 0.40$).

To evaluate diagnostic specificity of the findings in the ERC, we also conducted a similar analysis in subdivision ER from six matched pairs of nonschizophrenic psychiatric subjects and normal controls (Table 8-1, study 3). Total length of TH-immunoreactive axons did not differ ($F_{1,6} < 0.70$, $P > 0.43$) between subject groups in any of the three layers examined (Fig. 8-5).

Tyrosine Hydroxylase Immunoreactive Axons in PFC and ERC of Haloperidol-Treated Monkeys

To determine the possible influence of antipsychotic agents, we examined TH-immunoreactive axon length in monkeys chronically treated with haloperidol and

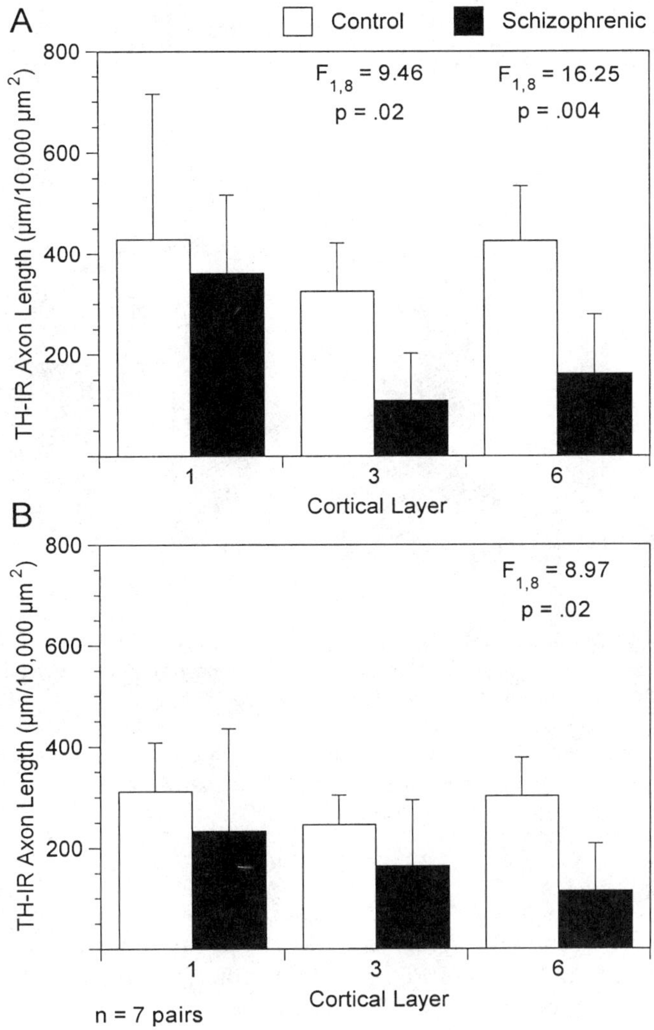

FIG. 8-4. Mean (±SD) total length (in mm) of TH-immunoreactive (TH-IR) axons per 10,000 mm2 in layers 1, 3, and 6 in subdivision ER of ERC (A) and PFC area 9 (B) of same cohort of schizophrenic and matched control subjects. Note that in schizophrenic subjects TH-immunoreactive axon length is significantly decreased in both layers 3 and 6 of ERC but is decreased only in layer 6 in PFC. Adapted from Akil et al. (2000).

matched controls. In the ERC, total TH-immunoreactive axon length in layer 3 did not differ between haloperidol-treated and control animals, whereas a significant ($t = 8.15$, $P = 0.004$) 14% increase in mean total axon length was present in layer 6 of the haloperidol-treated monkeys compared with controls. In the PFC, total length

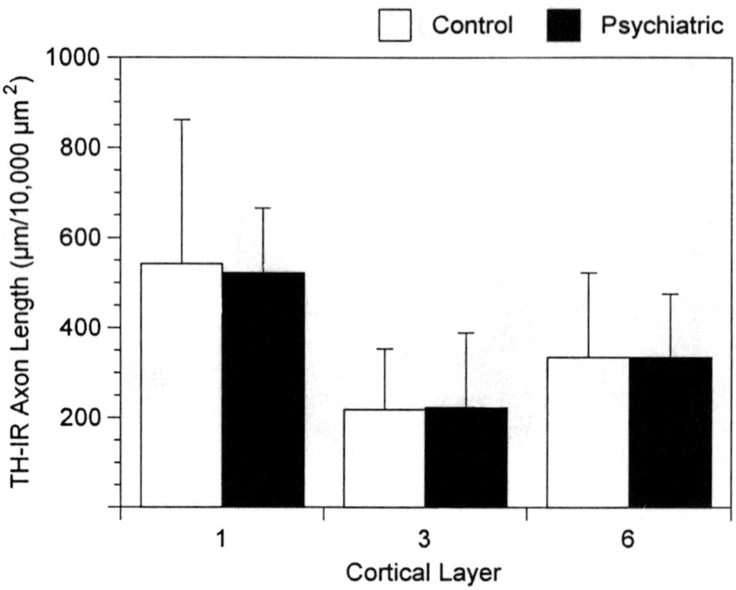

FIG. 8-5. Mean (±SD) total length (in mm) of TH-immunoreactive (TH-IR) axons per 10,000 mm2 in layers 1, 3, and 6 of subdivision ER of ERC in nonschizophrenic psychiatric and matched control subjects. Adapted from Akil et al. (2000).

of TH-immunoreactive axons did not differ between monkeys treated chronically with the antipsychotic agent haloperidol and their matched controls in any layer.

DISCUSSION

The results demonstrate 1) that the relative density of axons immunoreactive for TH or DAT, two critical proteins in dopamine neurotransmission, are significantly decreased in layer 6 of PFC area 9 in subjects with schizophrenia; 2) that PFC axons immunoreactive for SERT, a central protein in serotonin neurotransmission, are not altered in schizophrenia; 3) that density of TH-immunoreactive axons is also decreased in the ERC of schizophrenic subjects, although with a different laminar distribution than in the PFC; 4) that these changes are not a common correlate of psychiatric illness; and 5) that these findings are not likely to be a consequence of the typical treatments used in schizophrenic subjects. Because TH and DAT antibodies have both been shown to specifically label dopamine axons in primate neocortex. (Akil and Lewis, 1993, 1994; Gaspar et al., 1989; Lewis et al., 1987, 1998; Noack and Lewis, 1989), these findings reveal a regional, laminar, and neurotransmitter-specific reduction in the monoaminergic innervation of the cerebral cortex in schizophrenia.

Specificity of Alterations in Markers of Dopamine Axons to Disease Process

The findings of this study appear to directly reflect the pathophysiology of the disease process of schizophrenia and not to represent an epiphenomenon of its treatment or other factors. First, the fact that the density of SERT-immunoreactive axons did not change in concert with the reduction in dopamine axons in the PFC argues against the possibility that the present findings are a consequence of differences in the quality of tissue between the two groups of subjects. Second, failure to detect any differences in the relative density of TH-immunoreactive axons in the ERC of nonschizophrenic psychiatric subjects versus matched controls suggests that the observed decrease in schizophrenic subjects may be specific to the pathophysiology of this disorder. However, note that the psychiatric subjects available for this study were diagnostically heterogeneous. Thus these observations cannot be used to conclude that a decrease in TH-immunoreactive axons is characteristic only of schizophrenia, but they do suggest that this abnormality is not a common feature of all subjects with psychiatric disorders. As described elsewhere (Akil et al., 2000), the presence of a history of alcohol abuse or dependence does not appear to explain our findings.

Although most schizophrenic subjects had been treated at some point with antipsychotic agents, the available evidence suggests that the decreased density of dopamine axons were not the result of that treatment. For example, the PFC study included one schizophrenic who was never medicated, and four subjects who were not receiving medications at the time of death. In each case, density of TH-immunoreactive axons in layer 6 was reduced compared with their matched controls. In addition, we failed to find a difference in TH-immunoreactive axon length in ERC subdivision ER between normal controls and psychiatric subjects, three of whom had been treated with antipsychotic medications at some time (Akil et al., 2000). Chronic treatment of monkeys with haloperidol did not alter relative density of TH-immunoreactive axons in the PFC or ERC.

Pathophysiological Significance

The decreased density of both TH- and DAT-immunoreactive axons in schizophrenic subjects suggests that either 1) the concentrations of both proteins are reduced in a subpopulation of dopamine axons such that these axons are no longer detectable by immunocytochemical techniques or 2) the number of dopamine axons containing these proteins are decreased. Although the first possibility cannot be excluded, the latter might be expected to be associated with alterations in the dopamine neurons of the ventral tegmental area, which furnish many dopamine afferents to the PFC and ERC. The number of neuromelanin-positive (putative dopamine-containing) cells in the medial mesencephalon has been reported to be nonsignificantly decreased by 16% and the somal size of pigmented neurons to be significantly reduced in subjects with schizophrenia (Bogerts et al., 1983). The latter findings could reflect a reduction in the size of the axon arbor of cortically projecting dopamine neurons because somal size and total axon length tend to be positively correlated (Gilbert and Kelly, 1975; Lund et al., 1975).

Either reduced amounts of TH and DAT in dopamine axons or the presence of fewer dopamine axons could be associated with diminished dopamine neurotransmission in the PFC and ERC of schizophrenic subjects. This possibility is consistent with the notion that schizophrenia is associated with a hypodopaminergic state in the cortex (Daniel et al., 1989, 1991; Davis et al., 1991; Goldstein and Deutch, 1992; Weinberger et al., 1988). Cortical dopamine has been shown to be critical in normal cognitive processes (Arnsten et al., 1994; Brozoski et al., 1979; Sawaguchi and Goldman-Rakic, 1991), and subjects with schizophrenia perform poorly on cognitive tasks that appear to be subserved by the PFC and/or ERC (Heckers et al., 1998; Weinberger et al., 1986). Therefore alterations in dopamine neurotransmission in these two cortical regions may contribute to some cognitive deficits exhibited by schizophrenic subjects.

The fact that TH-immunoreactive axons have similar synaptic targets in both ERC (Erickson et al., 2000) and PFC (Sesack et al., 1995) is consistent with a common functional role for dopamine in both cortical regions. In addition, recent animal studies suggest that even relatively modest reductions in density of cortical dopamine axons can be associated with a substantial decrease in indices of dopamine neurotransmission. For example, in contrast to the nigrostriatal dopamine system where residual dopamine terminals can compensate for the loss of most axons in this projection (Snyder et al., 1990), partial lesions of the dopamine mesocortical projection result in significantly decreased extracellular levels of dopamine in the PFC (Venator et al., 1999). We do not know whether the magnitude of the decrease in PFC dopamine axons observed in the present study is sufficient to produce the types of cognitive impairments previously associated with reductions of PFC dopamine in nonhuman primates (Arnsten et al., 1994; Brozoski et al., 1979; Sawaguchi and Goldman-Rakic, 1991). However, the similarities in cognitive deficits observed in these animal studies and in subjects with schizophrenia (Park and Holzman, 1992) suggest that the decrease in markers of PFC dopamine axons observed in the present study could contribute to cortical dysfunction in schizophrenia.

Conversely, our findings of decreased TH- and DAT-immunoreactive axons do not necessarily provide evidence for a hypodopaminergic state in the PFC or ERC of schizophrenic subjects. In fact, the complete absence of DAT and reductions of 90% in TH levels are associated with a markedly hyperdopaminergic state in the DAT knockout mouse (Giros et al., 1996). Recent studies have indicated that PFC function may be impaired by either a deficiency or excess of stimulation at PFC dopamine D1 receptors (Arnsten and Goldman-Rakic, 1998; Murphy et al., 1996; Sawaguchi and Goldman-Rakic, 1991; Williams and Goldman-Rakic, 1995). Layer 6 of the primate PFC contains a high density of dopamine D1-like receptors (Goldman-Rakic et al., 1990), and the density of these receptors has been reported to be decreased in drug-naive schizophrenic subjects (Okubo et al., 1997). Because symptoms of schizophrenia are frequently worsened by stress, which increases PFC dopamine release (Thierry et al., 1976), decreases in pre- and postsynaptic dopamine markers in the PFC may represent a homeostatic response to minimize the impact of excessive levels of PFC dopamine induced by environmental stress.

Multiple studies suggest that schizophrenia may be associated with adverse events occurring during late prenatal or early postnatal life (Pilowsky et al., 1993). Consistent with this view, guinea pigs exposed to placental insufficiency during the second half of gestation have been reported to exhibit neuroanatomical abnormalities reminiscent of those found in the brains of schizophrenic subjects, such as ventriculomegaly and reduced hippocampal volume, as well as a marked reduction in TH-immunoreactive axons in the cerebral cortex (Mallard et al., 1999). Comparisons with developmental studies in nonhuman primates suggest that the regional differences in the cortical layers exhibiting reduced TH-immunoreactive axon length in schizophrenia may reflect an early developmental insult. For example, in macaque monkeys, the density of TH-immunoreactive axons in layer 6 is already at adult levels by the time of birth in both the ERC and PFC (Erickson et al., 1998; Rosenberg and Lewis, 1995). In layer 3, the density of TH-immunoreactive axons peaks by age 6 months in the ERC, but in the PFC, the maximal density of TH-immunoreactive axons in layer 3 is not achieved until after puberty. These regional and laminar differences in developmental time course suggest that cortical dopamine axons may be differentially sensitive to adverse events at different stages of development. Consequently, the abnormalities of the dopamine innervation in ERC layers 3 and 6 and in PFC layer 6 may be consistent with hypotheses positing an early developmental insult in the pathogenesis of schizophrenia.

REFERENCES

Akil M, Edgar CL, Pierri JN, et al. (2000). Decreased density of tyrosine hydroxylase-immunoreactive axons in the entorhinal cortex of schizophrenic patients. *Biol Psychiatry* 47,361–370.

Akil M, Lewis DA (1993). The dopaminergic innervation of monkey entorhinal cortex. *Cereb Cortex* 3,533–550.

Akil M, Lewis DA (1994). The distribution of tyrosine hydroxylase-immunoreactive fibers in the human entorhinal cortex. *Neuroscience* 60,857–874.

Akil M, Pierri JN, Whitehead RE, et al. (1999). Lamina-specific alteration in the dopamine innervation of the prefrontal cortex in schizophrenic subjects. *Am J Psychiatry* 156,1580–1589.

Arnsten AFT, Cai JX, Murphy BL, et al. (1994). Dopamine D1 receptor mechanisms in the cognitive performance of young adult and aged monkeys. *Psychopharmacology* 116,143–151.

Arnsten AFT, Goldman-Rakic PS (1998). Noise stress impairs prefrontal cortical cognitive function in monkeys: evidence for a hyperdopaminergic mechanism. *Arch Gen Psychiatry* 55,362–369.

Bogerts B, Hantsch J, Herzer M (1983). A morphometric study of the dopamine-containing cell groups in the mesencephalon of normals, Parkinson patients, and schizophrenics. *Biol Psychiatry* 18,951–969.

Brozoski TJ, Brown RM, Rosvold HE, et al. (1979). Cognitive deficit caused by regional depletion of dopamine in prefrontal cortex of rhesus monkeys. *Science* 205,929–932.

Carlsson A, Lindquist M (1963). Effect of chlorpromazine and haloperidol on formation of 3-methoxytyramine and normetanephrine in mouse brain. *Acta Pharmacol Toxicol* 20,140–144.

Daniel DG, Berman KF, Weinberger DR (1989). The effect of apomorphine on regional cerebral blood flow in schizophrenia. *J Neuropsychiatry* 1,377–384.

Daniel DG, Weinberger DR, Jones DW, et al. (1991). The effect of amphetamine on regional cerebral blood flow during cognitive activation in schizophrenia. *J Neurosci* 11,1907–1917.

Davis KL, Kahn RS, Ko G, et al. (1991). Dopamine in schizophrenia: a review and reconceptualization.

Am J Psychiatry 148,1474–1486.

Erickson SL, Akil M, Levey AI, et al. (1998). Postnatal development of tyrosine hydroxylase- and dopamine transporter-immunoreactive axons in monkey rostral entorhinal cortex. *Cereb Cortex* 8,415–427.

Erickson SL, Sesack SR, Lewis DA (2000). The dopamine innervation of monkey entorhinal cortex: postsynaptic targets of tyrosine hydroxylase-immunoreactive terminals. *Synapse* 36,47–56.

Gaspar P, Berger B, Fabvret A, et al. (1989). Catecholamine innervation of the human cerebral cortex as revealed by comparative immunohistochemistry of tyrosine hydroxylase and dopamine-beta-hydroxylase. *J Comp Neurol* 279,249–271.

Gilbert CD, Kelly JP (1975). The projections of cells in different layers of the cat's visual cortex. *J Comp Neurol* 63,81–106.

Giros B, Jaber M, Jones SR, et al. (1996). Hyperlocomotion and indifference to cocaine and amphetamine in mice lacking the dopamine transporter. *Nature* 379,606–612.

Glantz LA, Lewis DA (1997). Reduction of synaptophysin immunoreactivity in the prefrontal cortex of subjects with schizophrenia: regional and diagnostic specificity. *Arch Gen Psychiatry* 54,943–952.

Goldman-Rakic PS, Lidow MS, Gallagher DW (1990). Overlap of dopaminergic, adrenergic, and serotoninergic receptors and complementarity of their subtypes in primate prefrontal cortex. *J Neurosci* 10,2125–2138.

Goldstein M, Deutch AY (1992). Dopaminergic mechanisms in the pathogenesis of schizophrenia. *FASEB J* 6,2413–2421.

Grace AA (1991). Phasic versus tonic dopamine release and the modulation of dopamine system responsivity: a hypothesis for the etiology of schizophrenia. *Neuroscience* 41,1–24.

Heckers S, Rauch SL, Goff D, et al. (1998). Impaired recruitment of the hippocampus during conscious recollection in schizophrenia. *Nature Neurosci* 1,318–323.

Janicak PG, Davis JM, Preskorn SH, et al. (1993). *Principles and Practice of Psychopharmacotherapy*. Baltimore: Williams & Wilkins.

Lewis DA (1992). The catecholaminergic innervation of primate prefrontal cortex. *J Neural Transm* 36,179–200.

Lewis DA, Campbell MJ, Foote SL, et al. (1987). The distribution of tyrosine hydroxylase-immunoreactive fibers in primate neocortex is widespread but regionally specific. *J Neurosci* 7,279–290.

Lewis DA, Foote SL, Goldstein M, et al. (1988). The dopaminergic innervation of monkey prefrontal cortex: a tyrosine hydroxylase immunohistochemical study. *Brain Res* 449,225–243.

Lewis DA, Sesack SR, Levey AI, et al. (1998). Dopamine axons in primate prefrontal cortex: specificity of distribution, synaptic targets, and development. In: *Advances in Pharmacology. Catecholamines: Bridging Basic Science with Clinical Medicine*, Goldstein D, Eisenhofer G, McCarty R, eds. San Diego: Academic, pp. 703–706.

Lund JS, Lund RD, Hendrickson AE, et al. (1975). The origin of efferent pathways from the primary visual cortex, area 17, of the macaque monkey as shown by retrograde transport of horseradish peroxidase. *J Comp Neurol* 164,287–304.

Mallard EC, Rehn A, Rees S, et al. (1999). Ventriculomegaly and reduced hippocampal volume following intrauterine growth-restriction: implications for the aetiology of schizophrenia. *Schizophr Res* 40, 11–21.

Murphy BL, Arnsten AFT, Goldman-Rakic PS, et al. (1996). Increased dopamine turnover in the prefrontal cortex impairs spatial working memory performance in rats and monkeys. *Proc Natl Acad Sci USA* 93,1325–1329.

Noack HJ, Lewis DA (1989). Antibodies directed against tyrosine hydroxylase differentially recognize noradrenergic axons in monkey neocortex. *Brain Res* 500,313–324.

Okubo Y, Suhara T, Suzuki K, et al. (1997). Decreased prefrontal dopamine D1 receptors in schizophrenia revealed by PET. *Nature* 385,634–636.

Park S, Holzman PS (1992). Schizophrenics show spatial working memory deficits. *Arch Gen Psychiatry* 49,975–982.

Pilowsky LS, Kerwin RW, Murray RM (1993). Schizophrenia: a neurodevelopmental perspective. *Neuropsychopharmacology* 9,83–91.

Rosenberg DR, Lewis DA (1995). Postnatal maturation of the dopaminergic innervation of monkey prefrontal and motor cortices: a tyrosine hydroxylase immunohistochemical analysis. *J Comp Neurol* 358,383–400.

Saunders RC, Kolachana BS, Weinberger DR (1994). Local pharmacological manipulation of extracellular dopamine levels in the dorsolateral prefrontal cortex and caudate nucleus in the rhesus monkey: an *in vivo* microdialysis study. *Exp Brain Res* 98,44–52.

Sawaguchi T, Goldman-Rakic PS (1991). D1 dopamine receptors in prefrontal cortex: involvement in working memory. *Science* 251,947–950.

Sesack SR, Snyder CL, Lewis DA (1995). Axon terminals immunolabeled for dopamine or tyrosine hydroxylase synapse on GABA-immunoreactive dendrites in rat and monkey cortex. *J Comp Neurol* 363,264–280.

Snyder GL, Keller RW, Zigmond MJ (1990). Dopamine efflux from striatal slices after intracerebral 6-hydroxydopamine: evidence for compensatory hyperactivity of residual terminals. *J Pharmacol Exp Ther* 253,867–876.

Snyder SH (1972). Catecholamines in the brain as mediators of amphetamine psychosis. *Arch Gen Psychiatry* 27,169–179.

Thierry A-M, Tassin JP, Blanc G, et al. (1976). Selective activation of the mesocortical DA system by stress. *Nature* 263,242–244.

Venator DK, Lewis DA, Finlay JM (1999). Effects of partial dopamine loss in the medial prefrontal cortex on local baseline and stress-evoked extracellular dopamine concentrations. *Neuroscience* 93,497–505.

Weinberger DR, Berman KF, Illowsky BP (1988). Physiological dysfunction of dorsolateral prefrontal cortex in schizophrenia. III. A new cohort and evidence for a monoaminergic mechanism. *Arch Gen Psychiatry* 45,609–615.

Weinberger DR, Berman KF, Zec RF (1986). Physiologic dysfunction of dorsolateral prefrontal cortex in schizophrenia. I. Regional cerebral blood flow evidence. *Arch Gen Psychiatry* 43,114–124.

Williams GV, Goldman-Rakic PS (1995). Modulation of memory fields by dopamine D1 receptors in prefrontal cortex. *Nature* 376,572–575.

Williams SM, Goldman-Rakic PS (1993). Characterization of the dopaminergic innervation of the primate frontal cortex using a dopamine-specific antibody. *Cereb Cortex* 3,199–222.

9.

Imaging Dopaminergic Transmission in Schizophrenia

Anissa Abi-Dargham and Marc Laruelle

ABSTRACT

Abnormalities of dopamine function in schizophrenia are suggested by the common antidopaminergic properties of antipsychotic medications. However, direct evidence of a hyperdopaminergic state in schizophrenia had been lacking until recently owing to the difficulty in measuring dopamine transmission in the living human brain. With recent developments, synaptic dopamine in the vicinity of D2 receptors can be measured. Our group and others measured the increase in dopamine transmission after acute amphetamine challenge in untreated patients with schizophrenia and matched healthy subjects. After a brief overview of the techniques, this chapter focuses on the following results: 1) amphetamine-induced dopamine release is elevated in patients with schizophrenia, supporting the idea that schizophrenia is associated with dysregulation of dopamine transmission; 2) after amphetamine, hyperactivity of dopamine transmission is associated with activation of psychotic symptomatology; 3) this dysregulation of dopamine release is not a long-term consequence of previous neuroleptic treatment and is detected in never-medicated patients experiencing a first episode; 4) this exaggerated response to amphetamine exposure is not detected in a patient studied during illness stabilization, suggesting that the hyperdopaminergic state associated with schizophrenia fluctuates over time. In conclusion, a hyperdopaminergic state might be present in schizophrenia during the initial episode and subsequent relapses but not during periods of remission. This finding has important consequences for the development of new treatment strategies for the remission phase.

INTRODUCTION

The "classical" dopamine hypothesis of schizophrenia proposes that hyperactivity of dopamine transmission is responsible for positive symptoms (Carlsson et al., 1963). This hypothesis was supported by the correlation between clinical doses of antipsychotic drugs and their potency to block dopamine D2 receptors (Creese et al., 1976; Seeman and Lee, 1975) and by the psychotogenic effects of dopamine enhancing drugs (Angrist and van Kammen, 1984; Lieberman et al., 1987). Because positive symptoms are more sensitive than negative symptoms to direct manipulation of the dopamine system, hyperactivity of dopamine transmission may be more relevant to positive than negative symptoms (Crow, 1980). These pharmacological effects suggest, but do not establish, a dysregulation of dopamine systems in schizophrenia.

Despite decades of effort to validate this hypothesis, documentation of abnormalities of dopamine function in schizophrenia was lacking. Postmortem studies measuring dopamine and its metabolites in the brain of schizophrenic patients have yielded inconsistent results (Davis et al., 1991). Increased density of striatal D2 and D2-like receptors, reported in most postmortem studies (Lee et al., 1978; Owen et al., 1978; Seeman, 1987), has been difficult to interpret, given that neuroleptic drugs up-regulate these receptors (Burt et al., 1977; Seeman, 1987). Positron emission tomography (PET) and single photon emission computed tomography (SPECT) studies of striatal D2 and D2-like receptor density in neuroleptic-naive patients with schizophrenia have generally been negative (Breier et al., 1997; Farde et al., 1990; Hietala et al, 1994; Laruelle et al., 1996; Pilowsky et al. 1994), but see Wong et al. (1986). A recent meta-analysis of 13 in vivo studies revealed that D2 receptor density might be elevated in schizophrenia, but the effect size was small (0.54) (Laruelle, 1998). The lack of clear evidence for increased dopaminergic indices in schizophrenia might indicate that dopamine transmission is enhanced only relative to other systems, such as the glutamatergic system (Carlsson, 1988). Conversely, the absence of data supporting the dopamine hypothesis of schizophrenia might be due to the difficulty in obtaining a direct measurement of dopamine transmission in the living human brain.

Neuroreceptor imaging with PET and SPECT are classically aimed at measuring neuroreceptor parameters in the living human brain. More recently, several groups have demonstrated that, under specific conditions, in vivo neuroreceptor binding techniques can also be used to measure acute fluctuations in the concentration of transmitters in the vicinity of radiolabeled receptors (Carson et al., 1997; Dewey et al., 1991; Innis et al., 1992; Laruelle et al., 1997). Competition between radiotracers and transmitters for binding to neuroreceptors is the principle underlying this technique. This new application of neuroreceptor imaging allows a direct measurement of synaptic transmission in specific neurotransmitter systems in the brain, a correlation of these measurements with behaviors and symptoms, and an exploration of the role of neurochemical imbalances in the pathogenesis of psychiatric disorders. So far, applications of this new paradigm have been developed to study dopamine transmission at D2 receptors.

Endogenous competition between dopamine and radiolabeled D2 receptor ligands was initially documented in ex vivo studies performed in rodents. Amphetamine, which releases dopamine and thereby increases endogenous dopamine synaptic concentration, reduced in vivo binding of the D2 agonist ^{3}H-*N*-propylnorapomorphine (Köhler et al.. 1981; Ross et al., 1989) and of the D2 antagonist ^{3}H-raclopride (Ross et al., 1989; Young et al. 1991). The opposite effect (i.e., increased tracer accumulation) was induced by drugs that decrease dopamine endogenous concentration such as reserpine and γ-butyrolactone (Ross et al. 1989, 1991; Seeman et al., 1989; Van der Werf et al., 1986; Young et al., 1991).

The development of PET and SPECT neuroreceptor imaging provided a tool for noninvasive measurements of these interactions. In baboons, the binding potential (BP) of various dopamine D2 receptor radiotracers was decreased by drugs that increase dopamine synaptic concentration such as amphetamine (Carson et al., 1997; Ginovart et al., 1999; Innis et al., 1992; Kessler et al., 1993; Laruelle et al., 1997; Logan et al., 1991; Mukherjee et al., 1997), cocaine (Volkow et al., 1999), or GBR-12909 (Dewey et al., 1993). Increased radiotracer uptake was observed after drugs that reduce dopamine availability, such as reserpine (Ginovart et al., 1993) or γ-vinyl-GABA (Dewey et al., 1992).

In humans, decreased specific binding of ^{11}C-raclopride or ^{123}I-iodobenzamide (IBZM) has been reported after acute administration of the dopamine-enhancing drugs methylphenidate (Booij et al., 1997; Volkow et al., 1994), amphetamine (Breier et al., 1997; Laruelle et al., 1995), cocaine (Schlaepfer et al., 1997), and ketamine (Breier et al., 1998; Smith et al., 1998) and even cognitive challenges (Koepp et al., 1998). Increased ^{123}I-IBZM BP has been measured after dopamine depletion with the reversible tyrosine hydroxylase inhibitor α-methyl-para-tyrosine (Laruelle et al., 1997).

We will review the development and validation of a method using SPECT and the specific D2 receptor radiotracer ^{123}I-IBZM to measure amphetamine-induced intrasynaptic dopamine release in humans and its application to schizophrenia.

MEASURING DOPAMINE RELEASE IN LIVING BRAIN: DEVELOPMENT AND VALIDATION

Studies in Baboons

An initial influential observation in this line of research was the observation of increased striatal washout rate of the SPECT D2 receptor radiotracer ^{123}I-IBZM in baboons after amphetamine injection (Innis et al., 1992) (the term "D2 receptors" denotes D2 and D3 but not D4 receptors throughout). Because amphetamine had negligible affinity for ^{123}I-IBZM binding (>10 μM, M. Laruelle, unpublished data), this effect could not be attributed to a direct displacement of ^{123}I-IBZM by amphetamine but rather to a reduction in D2 receptor availability owing to increased dopamine synaptic concentration and increased D2 receptor occupancy by dopamine. To avoid the confounding effects of amphetamine on blood flow, we adopted a tracer constant infusion paradigm (Laruelle et al., 1997). ^{123}I-IBZM was administered as a bolus followed by a constant infusion for the duration of the experiment, which induced a stable baseline to evaluate changes in receptor availability (Fig. 9-1*A*). Under these conditions, amphetamine (0.3–1 mg/kg) decreased the ^{123}I-IBZM striatal specific binding by 10–40% (Fig. 9-1*B*).

BP is the parameter measuring receptor availability (Mintun et al., 1984). BP is equal to the product of receptor density (B_{max}) and affinity ($1/K_D$). Under sustained equilibrium conditions, the decrease in specific-to-nonspecific equilibrium ratio (in this case, the striatal-to-occipital ratio) is equal to the decrease in BP (Kegeles et al., 1999). Because measurements are obtained at equilibrium, these ratios are

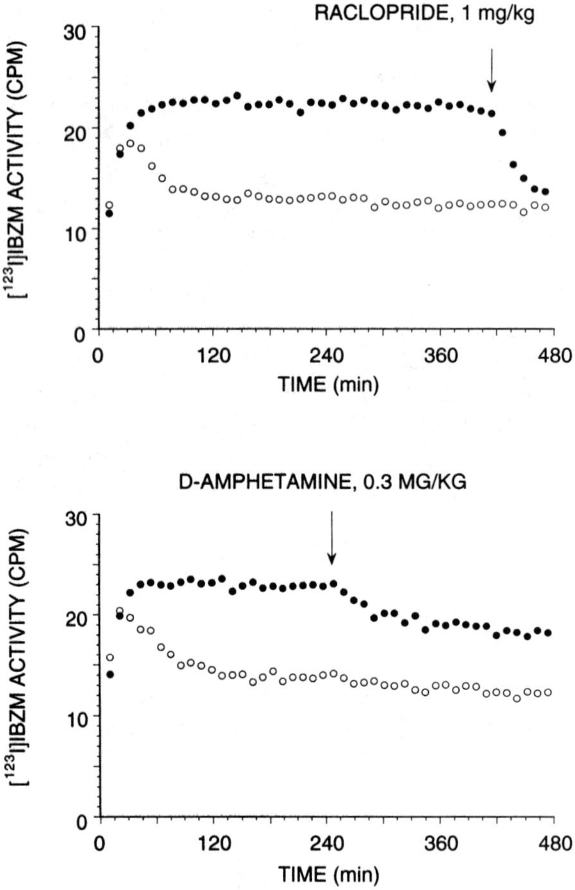

FIG. 9-1. *Top*, striatal (*closed circles*) and occipital (*open circles*) activities during bolus plus constant infusion with ^{123}I-IBZM in a baboon. Constant infusion induced a state of sustained equilibrium (both striatal and occipital activities were stable over time). After the experiment, the D2 receptor antagonist raclopride (1 mg/kg) was injected (*arrow*), which resulted in a decrease of striatal activity (specific binding) to levels observed in occipital region (nonspecific activity). *Bottom*, experiment was repeated in the same baboon, under similar experimental conditions, except for injection of 0.3 mg/kg amphetamine at 240 min (*arrow*), which induced a decrease in striatal activity (specific activity) but did not affect occipital activity (nonspecific activity).

independent of amphetamine effects on cerebral blood flow and peripheral clearance. Thus these experiments established that the reduction in ^{123}I-IBZM-specific binding observed after amphetamine reflects a decrease in D2 receptor BP and not an effect of amphetamine on blood flow and peripheral clearance.

The next step was to establish that the amphetamine-induced reduction in ^{123}I-IBZM BP was mediated by dopamine release. The mediation of the amphetamine effect by dopamine release was demonstrated by establishing that pretreatment with

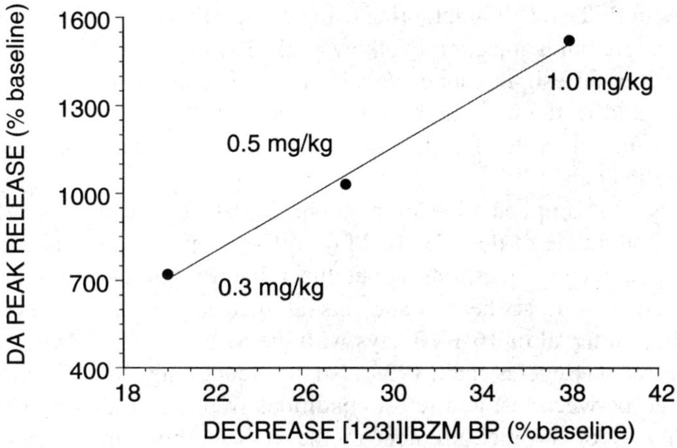

FIG. 9-2. Correlation between amphetamine-induced peak dopamine (DA) release, measured with microdialysis (*y* axis), and decrease in ^{123}I-IBZM D2 BP, measured with SPECT (each point is mean of three experiments). This relationship was linear (y = [minus]190 + 44x, r = 0.99). Constraining the intercept to zero: $y = 39x$. Thus each percent decrement in ^{123}I-IBZM BP corresponded to about a 40% increase over baseline of dopamine concentration.

the dopamine depleter α-methyl-para-tyrosine, a competitive inhibitor of tyrosine hydroxylase, blocked the effect of amphetamine on ^{123}I-IBZM BP (Laruelle et al., 1997). Furthermore, we observed a relationship between dopamine release, measured by microdialysis, and reduction in ^{123}I-IBZM BP, measured by reduction in ^{123}I-IBZM BP with SPECT, after various doses of amphetamine (Fig. 9-2). This observation validated the use of this noninvasive paradigm to measure changes in synaptic dopamine after amphetamine and provided an operational calibration of the SPECT signal. Linear correlation between microdialysis and SPECT measurements revealed that each percent decrement in ^{123}I-IBZM BP corresponded to a 40% increase in peak dopamine concentration. Similar numbers have been published for the effect of amphetamine on ^{11}C-raclopride (Breier et al., 1997). Thus with both radiotracers, the method is relatively insensitive to changes in synaptic dopamine, to the extent that large changes in extracellular dopamine are associated with only small changes in receptor availability.

These experiments in primates established that the reduction in ^{123}I-IBZM BP measured with SPECT after amphetamine challenge provides a noninvasive measurement of the magnitude of the amphetamine-induced increase in synaptic dopamine.

Studies in Healthy Humans

In humans, amphetamine induced a significant decrease in ^{123}I-IBZM BP (range from 5 to 20%) (Laruelle et al., 1995). Similarly, Booij et al. (1997) showed that injection of the dopamine releaser methylphenidate (0.5 mg/kg) resulted in significant decrease in ^{123}I-IBZM BP. Similar studies have been performed in healthy volunteers with PET and ^{11}C-raclopride using constant infusion (Breier et al., 1997) or a double single bolus injection (Volkow et al., 1994).

We also observed a significant correlation between amphetamine-induced euphoria, alertness, and restlessness and the reduction in ^{123}I-IBZM BP ($r^2 = 0.84$, $P = 0.003$), confirming the role of dopamine in mediating these emotions after amphetamine (Laruelle et al., 1995).

After doses of amphetamine or methylphenidate that can be safely used in humans, the magnitude of the ^{123}I-IBZM (or ^{11}C-raclopride) BP reduction is small (5–20% range), raising questions about the reliability of this measurement. To address these questions, six healthy subjects (all male, age 36 ≤ 10 years) were studied twice, at an interval of 16 ± 10 days with the SPECT ^{123}I-IBZM/amphetamine challenge protocol (Kegeles et al., 1999). No differences in ^{123}I-IBZM displacement were observed between test and retest conditions (repeated measure ANOVA, $P = 0.56$). Reliability of the measurement of the amphetamine effect, under the null hypothesis of no difference in the amphetamine effect between test and retest conditions, was excellent, with an intraclass correlation coefficient of 0.89. In other words, the magnitude of the amphetamine effect in a given subject on the test day was a good predictor of the effect on the retest day ($r^2 = 0.76$, $P = 0.023$) (Fig. 9-3). Thus despite the small magnitude of the amphetamine effect, the method is dependable to measure between-subject differences. The data also suggest that, at least in healthy subjects and over 2–3 weeks, this effect is a trait rather than a state factor.

Preliminary studies in healthy controls demonstrated the feasibility and reliability of measuring the reduction in D2 availability after *d*-amphetamine challenge test.

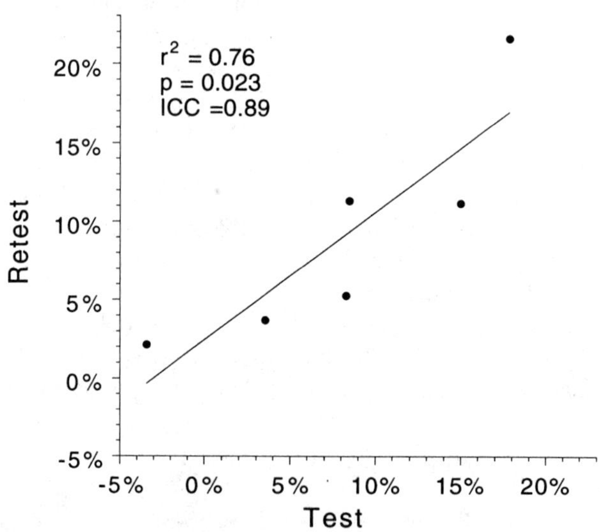

FIG. 9-3. Test/retest reproducibility of amphetamine-induced reduction in ^{123}I-IBZM BP in six healthy subjects (subjects studied twice at 1- to 2-week intervals). ICC, intraclass correlation coefficient.

In addition, these studies demonstrated that the amphetamine effect on ^{123}I-IBZM BP was correlated with behavioral activation experienced by the subjects.

Studies in Patients with Schizophrenia

This imaging technique was used to study amphetamine-induced dopamine release in patients with schizophrenia (n = 34) and matched healthy controls (n = 36) (Table 9-1). The sample includes 15 patients and 15 controls from a first cohort published in 1996 (Laruelle et al., 1996), 15 patients and 15 controls from a second cohort published in 1998 (Abi-Dargham et al., 1998), and a third cohort of six controls and four patients not previously reported. Data were acquired between September 1994 and September 1998.

Methods

Inclusion criteria for patients follow: 1) diagnosis of schizophrenia according to DSM-IV; 2) no other DSM-IV axis I diagnosis; 3) no history of alcohol or substance abuse or dependence; 4) absence of any psychotropic medications for at least 21 days before study (except for lorazepam, which was allowed at a maximal dose of 3 mg/day up to 24 hr before the study); 5) no concomitant or past severe medical conditions; 6) no pregnancy; 7) no current suicidal or homicidal ideation; and 8) ability to provide informed consent. The ability of the patient to provide informed consent was formally evaluated by a psychiatrist not associated with the study. Assent of involved family members was also obtained.

All patients were admitted to an inpatient unit for the duration of the study, including the washout period. Patients were recruited under two modalities: 17 patients were recruited shortly after voluntary admission to the hospital for clinical reasons; another 17 patients were recruited at an outpatient clinic (Veteran's

TABLE 9-1. Demographic composition of groups

	Controls	Patients with schizophrenia	*P*
n	36	34	
Age	40 ± 94	0 ± 9	
Gender (M/F)	32/4	28/6	
Race (C/AA/H)	21/10/3	18/11/5	0.95
Socioeconomic status[a]			
Parental	34.3 ± 9.7	34.4 ± 15.8	0.96
Subject	39.5 ± 12.1	26.0 ± 10.2	< 0.001

C, Caucasian ; AA, African American; H, Hispanic.1
[a]Measured with Hollingshead scale.

Administration Medical Center, West Haven, CT) and admitted to the hospital for the purpose of the study.

Among the patients, seven subjects were neuroleptic naïve and experiencing a first episode of the illness. In previously treated patients, the average neuroleptic-free interval was 104 ± 118 days.

Inclusion criteria for controls follow: 1) absence of past or present neurological, medical, or psychiatric illnesses, including substance or alcohol abuse and dependence; 2) no pregnancy; and 3) informed consent. Groups were matched for age, gender, race, and parental socioeconomic level, assessed by the Hollingshead scale (Hollingshead, 1975). Socioeconomic status of the patients was lower than that of controls (Table 9-1, 9-2).

SPECT experiments were performed as previously described (Laruelle et al., 1995). Briefly, ^{123}I-IBZM with specific activity of >5,000 Ci/mmol and radiochemical purity of >95% was prepared by direct electrophilic radioiodination of the desiodoprecursor BZM. A total ^{123}I-IBZM dose of 10.3 ± 2.5 mCi was given as a bolus followed by a continuous infusion for the duration of the experiment (360 min). The activity given as a bolus was 3.9-fold higher than the activity infused per hour. SPECT data were acquired on the PRISM 3000 (Picker, Cleveland, OH) with high resolution fan beam collimators. Two scanning sessions of 60 min each were obtained for each subject during the ^{123}I-IBZM infusion (before and 1 hr after amphetamine injection).

Group Differences in Amphetamine-induced Dopamine Release

In control subjects, amphetamine-induced reduction in ^{123}I-IBZM BP was 7.5 ± 7.1% (n = 36). Patients with schizophrenia displayed a marked elevation of amphetamine-induced ^{123}I-IBZM displacement (17.1 ± 13.2%, P = 0.0003, Fig. 9-4). The effect size of the difference, calculated as difference of the means divided by the average SD, was 0.95. The variance was larger in the schizophrenic group compared with the controls (variance ratio 3.49, P = 0.004). Because of the difference in variance, we compared the groups with a nonparametric test and obtained the same results (Mann-Whitney, P = 0.0028).

TABLE 9-2. Results: Comparison of controls and patients with schizophrenia

	Controls	Patients with schizophrenia	*P*
n	36	34	
Amphetamine-induced relative decrease in $_{123}$I-IBZM BP (% baseline)	7.5 ± 7.1	17.1 ± 13.2	< 0.001
Amphetamine plasma concentration (ng/ml)	28 ± 11	29 ± 10	0.74

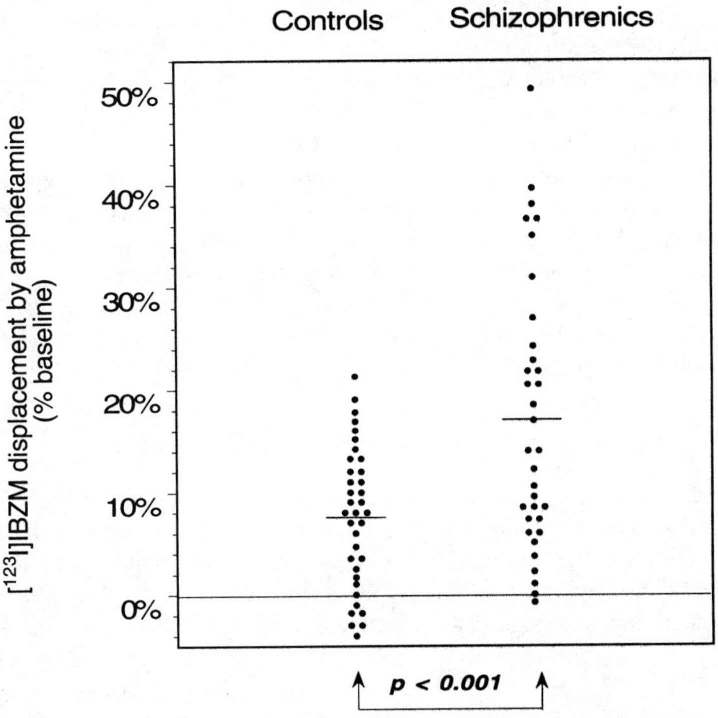

FIG. 9-4. Effect of amphetamine (0.3 mg/kg) on ^{123}I-IBZM binding in healthy controls and untreated patients with schizophrenia. *y* axis, percentage decrease in ^{123}I-IBZM BP induced by amphetamine, which is a measure of increased occupancy of D2 receptors by dopamine after challenge.

This increased effect of amphetamine in patients with schizophrenia was unrelated to differences in amphetamine plasma disposition, because amphetamine plasma levels were similar in both groups (controls 27.7 ± 11.0 ng/ml; patients with schizophrenia 28.7 ± 9.9 ng/ml, $P = 0.73$). Moreover no relationship was found between amphetamine plasma levels and ^{123}I-IBZM displacement, in neither the control ($r = 0.04$, $P = 0.84$) nor patients group ($r = 0.05$, $P = 0.80$).

Relationship between Dopamine Release and Positive Symptoms

The clinical response to the amphetamine challenge was evaluated with the positive and negative symptom scale (PANSS) (Kay et al., 1987). Baseline ratings were obtained 60 min before the first scanning session. Postamphetamine ratings were obtained 30 min after injection of amphetamine. PANSS positive and negative subscales include seven items, each scored from 1 (not present) to 7 (extreme). Thus the total PANSS positive and negative subscales vary from 7 (minimum) to 49 (maximum), i.e., range of 42 points. For each of these subscales, a change of at least four points was considered clinically significant.

In patients with schizophrenia, the amphetamine challenge induced an increase in positive symptoms (positive symptoms subscale of the PANSS increased from 17.5 ± to 20.5 ±7.6, repeated-measure ANOVA, $P = 0.019$). The emergence or worsening of positive symptoms was transient, and patients returned to their baseline symptomatology within a few hours of the challenge. A large between-subject variability was observed in the amphetamine-induced changes in positive symptoms (range from −8 to +13). Sixteen of the 34 patients (47%) were described as "worseners" with positive symptoms; 14 (41%) were described as "no change," and four (12%) were "improvers." We observed a significant correlation between the increase in positive symptoms and the ^{123}I-IBZM displacement ($r = 0.54$, $P = 0.0009$, Fig. 9-5).

Lack of Effect of Previous Neuroleptic Treatment

Twenty-seven patients were previously exposed to antipsychotic drugs, whereas seven patients were antipsychotic-naive. The amphetamine effect on ^{123}I-IBZM BP was similar between the two groups (chronic/previously treated patients 16.2 ±13.5%, n = 27; first episode/neuroleptic-naive patients 20.9 ± 12.2%, n = 7, P = 0.41), and both groups were significantly different from controls (Fig. 9-6, Table 9-3).

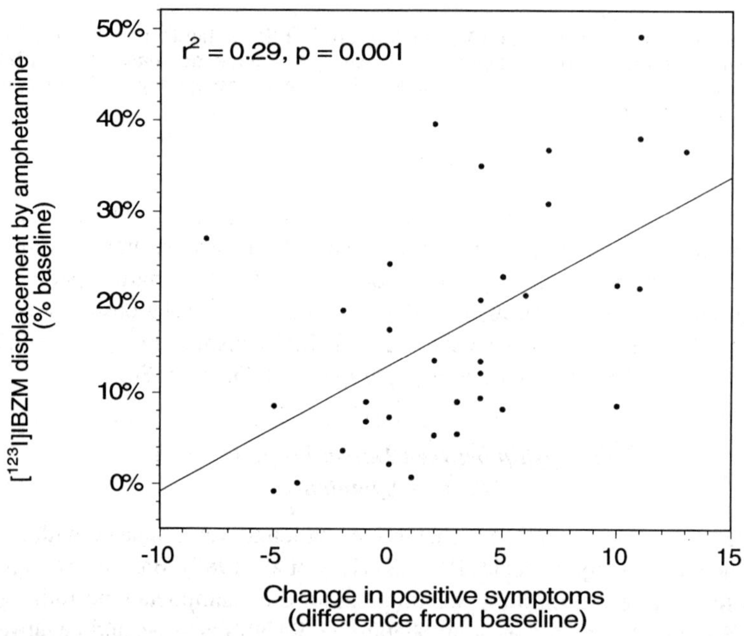

FIG. 9-5. Relationship between striatal amphetamine-induced dopamine release and amphetamine-induced changes in positive symptoms.

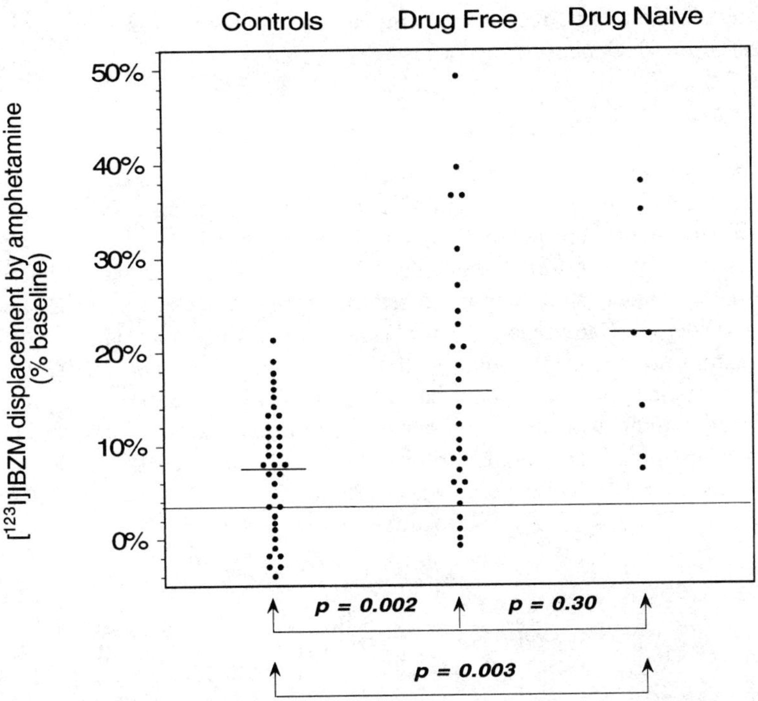

FIG. 9-6. Amphetamine-induced reduction in ^{123}I-IBZM BP in healthy controls, chronic schizophrenic patients previously exposed to antipsychotic drugs, and first episode patients never exposed to antipsychotic drugs.

No association was found between duration of the neuroleptic free period (104 ± 118 days) and amphetamine-induced ^{123}I-IBZM displacement ($r = 0.02$, $P = 0.91$). Furthermore, the number of years of neuroleptic exposure was not associated with the amphetamine effect ($r = 0.14$, $P = 0.48$). Together, these data indicated that the

TABLE 9-3. Results: comparison of controls, chronic/previously treated patients, and first episode/neuroleptic-naive patients

Parameters	Controls	Chronic/previously treated patients	First episode/ neuroleptic-naive patients	*P*
n	36	27	7	
Age	40 ± 9	42 ± 7	29 ± 9	< 0.01
Amphetamine-induced relative decrease in ^{123}I-IBZM BP (% baseline)	7.5 ± 7.1	16.2 ± 13.5	20.9 ± 12.2	< 0.01

exaggerated dopaminergic response to amphetamine exposure was not a prolonged side effect of previous neuroleptic exposure.

Relationship with Clinical Variables

We tested associations between the amphetamine effect on ^{123}I-IBZM BP and several demographic and clinical variables in the patients group to characterize the profile of patients with exaggerated response. Symptom severity at baseline was not predictive of the amphetamine effect (positive symptoms $r < 0.01$, $P = 0.98$; negative symptoms $r = 0.03$, $P = 0.84$). No association was found between amphetamine effect and age ($r = 0.2$, $P = 0.90$), gender ($P = 0.69$), race ($P = 0.15$), subject socioeconomic status ($r = 0.05$, $P = 0.78$), familial socioeconomic status ($= 0.07$, $P = 0.69$), duration of illness ($r < 0.01$, $P = 0.99$), or number of previous hospitalizations ($r = 0.01$, $P = 0.91$).

However, patients who were experiencing an illness exacerbation (admitted for clinical reasons) presented a higher amphetamine-induced ^{123}I-IBZM displacement (23.7 ± 13.2%, $n = 17$) than patients who were in remission and recruited as outpatients (10.5 ± 9.7%, $n = 17$, $P = 0.002$, Table 9-4, Fig. 9-7). Furthermore, ampheta-

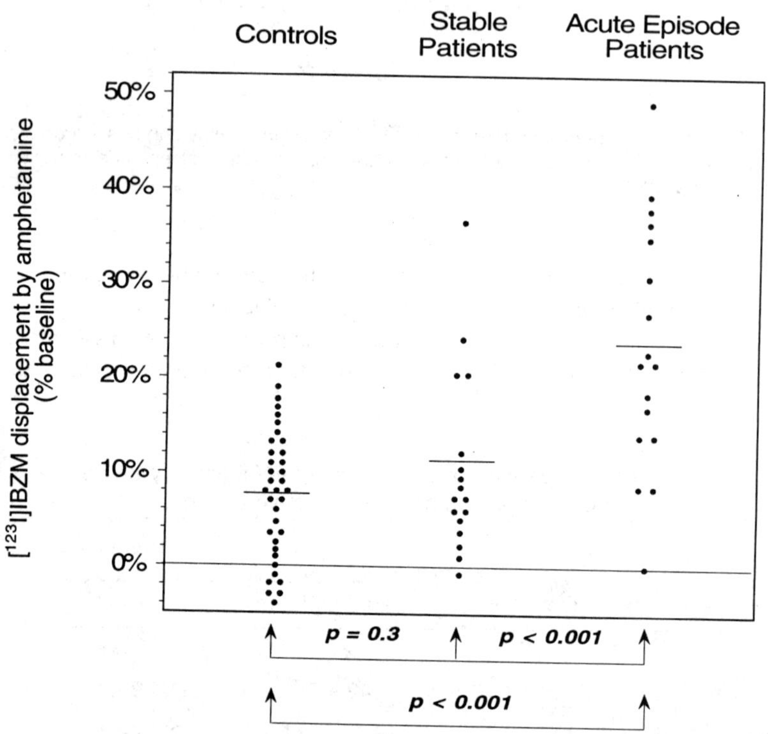

FIG. 9-7. Amphetamine-induced reduction in ^{123}I-IBZM BP in healthy controls, patients with schizophrenia during illness remission, and patients with schizophrenia during acute illness exacerbation.

TABLE 9-4. Results: comparison of controls, patients in remission, and patients in exacerbation

Parameters	Controls	Patients in Remission	Patients in exacerbation	*P*
n	36	17	17	
Age	40 ± 9	42 ± 7	36 ± 10	0.19
Amphetamine-induced relative decrease in ^{123}I-IBZM BP (% baseline)	7.5 ± 7.1	16.2 ± 13.5	23.7 ± 13.2	< 0.001

mine-induced ^{123}I-IBZM displacement in remitted patients (10.5 ± 9.7%, $n = 17$) was not statistically different from controls (7.5 ± 7.1%, $n = 36$, $P = 0.27$). These two groups of patients were not different otherwise in terms of baseline positive symptoms, amphetamine-induced increase in positive symptoms, postamphetamine PANSS positive subscale, and self-reported anxiety levels. Thus the scan data (dopamine release) provided a better discrimination between patients in remission and exacerbation compared with clinical ratings.

DISCUSSION

The main results of this study are that 1) schizophrenia is associated with increased responsiveness of dopamine transmission in the striatum after acute amphetamine exposure; 2) this increased dopamine transmission is associated with transient worsening of positive symptoms; and 3) this exaggerated response is present at onset of illness and during periods of illness exacerbation but is not detected during periods of illness stabilization.

The increased responsiveness of dopamine transmission to amphetamine exposure (0.3 mg/kg) reported in these studies has also been observed with ^{11}C-raclopride after a lower amphetamine dose (0.2 mg/kg) (Breier et al., 1997). Together these findings support the hypothesis that schizophrenia is associated with dysregulation of the dopamine system. The effect size of the difference in the amphetamine-induced displacement between patients and controls (0.95) is considerably larger than the effect size of other alterations described in schizophrenia using brain imaging techniques, such as alterations in ventricular or hippocampal size or alteration of D2 receptor density (Daniel et al., 1991; Laruelle et al., 1998; Lawrie et al., 1998; Nelson et al., 1998). This finding supports the hypothesis that hyperresponsivity of dopaminergic neurons is an important component of the pathophysiology of schizophrenia.

The interpretation of the scan data (increase in ^{123}I-IBZM displacement) in terms of underlying mechanisms (increase in dopamine release) is supported by experimental data acquired in baboons. The hypothesis that the observed increase in ^{123}I-IBZM displacement after amphetamine reflects mostly a dysregulation of dopaminergic neuron reactivity rather than a postsynaptic sensitivity is indirectly supported by several recent investigations demonstrating an increase in ^{18}F-DOPA or ^{11}C-DOPA accumulation in the striatum of patients with schizophrenia (Hietala et al., 1995; Reith et al., 1994), but see Dao-Castellana et al. (1997).

Nevertheless, this interpretation rests on the assumption that the affinity of D2 receptors for dopamine is unchanged in schizophrenia. The sequence of the D2 receptor gene, as well as the D2 receptor affinity for antagonists, is unaltered in schizophrenia (Gejman et al., 1994; Seeman, 1987). Moreover, the binding of dopamine agonists in postmortem striata is not increased in schizophrenia (Cross et al., 1983; Lee et al., 1978). Yet the D2 receptor affinity for agonists is regulated by multiple mechanisms such as coupling to G proteins (Sibley et al., 1982), and we cannot eliminate the possibility of a different in vivo affinity of dopamine for D2 receptors in schizophrenia. The development of radiolabeled D2 receptor agonists as PET radiotracers is needed to address this issue. Until then, interpretation in terms of increased dopamine levels remains tentative. In a strict sense, this study demonstrates that amphetamine leads to a greater stimulation of D2 receptors in schizophrenia compared with controls, and the mechanism underlying this effect (increased dopamine concentration versus increased affinity of D2 receptors for dopamine or some combination of both factors) remains to be established.

The data also indicate that intensity of D2 receptor stimulation by dopamine after amphetamine exposure explains a significant aspect of the variability in psychopathological response to the challenge in schizophrenia. Many studies reviewed by Lieberman et al. (1987) have provided evidence that schizophrenic patients, as a group, display increased sensitivity to the psychotogenic effects of acute psychostimulant administration. In other terms, some, but not all, patients with schizophrenia present emergence or worsening of psychotic symptoms after acute exposure to psychostimulants at doses that do not induce psychosis in healthy subjects. Key features of this response have emerged over the years and were replicated in the present study. The clinical response to acute psychostimulant challenges in schizophrenic patients is highly heterogeneous. About 40% of patients present a worsening of positive psychotic symptoms; 40% show no change; and 20% improve on positive symptoms after acute psychostimulant challenge (Lieberman et al., 1987; van Kammen et al., 1982). This study provides evidence that amphetamine-induced dopamine release is an important determinant of this response.

However, dopamine-mediated stimulation of D2 receptors explained only about 30% of the variance in the positive symptom change, indicating that other factors are involved in the exacerbation of these symptoms after amphetamine. In addition, a psychotic response was never observed in healthy controls, even in the presence of large amphetamine-induced ^{123}I-IBZM displacement, suggesting that dopamine stimulation leads to activation of preexistent and specific dysfunctional neuronal circuits. In other terms, acute dopamine stimulation might activate rather than create the neuronal activity associated with positive symptoms. This view is also consistent with the observation that sustained D2 receptor blockade is necessary to allow the extinction of these putative dysfunctional ensembles.

The data also suggested that this exaggerated dopamine response to amphetamine was mostly observed in the subset of patients who were studied during an episode of illness exacerbation compared with patients in remission. Because no clinical ratings were available for the time before admission, we do not have direct evidence that patients classified as "in exacerbation" experienced a recent increase in symptomatology before admission. However, hospitalization is one of the best indicators of "episode" and "relapse" (Schooler et al., 1997), and it is reasonable to classify these patients as experiencing an active episode of the illness. A prospective study is warranted to further establish the relationship between dopamine dysregulation and illness exacerbation.

This observation is in agreement with previous studies reporting that the psychotic response to psychostimulants is state dependent in patients with schizophrenia (Janowsky et al., 1976; van Kammen et al., 1982), and the vulnerability to psychostimulant-induced psychosis is associated with a higher rate of relapse upon neuroleptic discontinuation (Lieberman et al., 1984, 1987). So the propensity to present a psychotic reaction to a psychostimulant challenge may "reveal" an active phase of the illness not readily identifiable by the clinical symptomatology in the absence of a psychostimulant challenge. The present study shows that the excess dopamine response is state dependent. Studying the same patients during exacerbation and remission is needed to confirm this point.

The mechanism of this increased dopaminergic neuronal reactivity remains unclear. The activity of dopaminergic cells in the ventral tegmental area and substantia nigra is regulated, among others, by glutamatergic projections from the prefrontal cortex primarily through projections to the dopamine cell body area rather than the terminal region (Karreman et al., 1996). Given the evidence for dysfunction of the prefrontal cortex in schizophrenia, it is tempting to speculate that the dysregulation of subcortical dopamine may be secondary to a failure of the prefrontal-ventral tegmental area/substantia nigra projections to properly regulate dopamine release after amphetamine challenge. Preclinical models have been proposed for such a dysregulation. In adult rats, a selective destruction of prefrontal dopamine terminals (Pycock et al., 1980; Roberts et al. 1994), an impairment of cortical GABAergic transmission (Karreman et al., 1996), or an impairment of NMDA transmission (Miller et al., 1996) can lead to a disinhibition of dopamine release. Sensitization to psychostimulants is another well-described phenomenon in rodents that might be relevant to the disorders of dopamine function observed in this study (Lieberman et al., 1997). However, our data suggest that the sensitization model may apply to the mechanism of illness exacerbation as we observe an extinction of this sensitized state during illness remission. This model supports the need for new relapse prevention strategies.

In conclusion, the work summarized here, as well as the work of Breier et al. (1997), support the idea that schizophrenia is associated with episodes of dysregulation of dopamine release that are revealed by the amphetamine challenge imaging technique. Under these conditions, hyperactivity of dopamine transmission is associated with activation of psychotic symptomatology. This dysregulation of dopamine release is not a long-term consequence of previous neuroleptic treatment and is present in never-medicated patients experiencing a first episode of the illness. During periods of illness stabilization, the response of the dopamine system to amphetamine exposure is not different than in control subjects, suggesting that the hyperdopaminergic state associated with schizophrenia fluctuates over time. The mechanism underlying this abnormal response to amphetamine is unclear. A better understanding of this phenomenon might contribute to the development of new treatment strategies.

REFERENCES

Abi-Dargham A, Gil R, Krystal J, et al. (1998). Increased striatal dopamine transmission in schizophrenia: confirmation in a second cohort. *Am J Psychiatry* 155,761–767.

Angrist B, van Kammen DP. (1984). CNS stimulants as a tool in the study of schizophrenia. *Trends Neurosci* 7,388–390.

Booij J, Korn P, Linszen DH, et al. (1997). Assessment of endogenous dopamine release by methylphenidate challenge using iodine-123 iodobenzamide single-photon emission tomography. *Eur J Nucl Med* 24,674–677.

Breier A, Adler CM, Weisenfeld N, et al. (1998). Effects of NMDA antagonism on striatal dopamine release in healthy subjects: application of a novel PET approach. *Synapse* 29,142–147.

Breier A, Su TP, Saunders R, et al. (1997). Schizophrenia is associated with elevated amphetamine-induced synaptic dopamine concentrations: evidence from a novel positron emission tomography method. *Proc Natl Acad Sci USA* 94,2569–2574.

Burt DR, Creese I, Snyder SS (1977). Antischizophrenic drugs: chronic treatment elevates dopamine receptor binding in brain. *Science* 196,326–328.

Carlsson A (1988). The current status of the dopamine hypothesis of schizophrenia. *Neuropsychopharmacology* 1,179–186.

Carlsson A, Lindqvist M (1963). Effect of chlorpromazine or haloperidol on formation of 3-methoxytyramine and normetanephrine in mouse brain. *Acta Pharmacol Toxicol* 20,140–144.

Carson RE, Breier A, deBartolomeis A, et al. (1997). Quantification of amphetamine-induced changes in [C-11]raclopride binding with continuous infusion. *J Cereb Blood Flow Metab* 17,437–447.

Creese I, Burt DR, Snyder SH (1976). Dopamine receptor binding predicts clinical and pharmacological potencies of antischizophrenic drugs. *Science* 19,481–483.

Cross AJ, Crow TJ, Ferrier IN, et al. (1983). Dopamine receptor changes in schizophrenia in relation to the disease process and movement disorder. *J Neural Transm* suppl 18,265–272.

Crow TJ (1980). Molecular pathology of schizophrenia: more than one disease process? *Br Med J* 280,66–68.

Daniel DG, Goldberg TE, Gibbons RD, et al. (1991). Lack of a bimodal distribution of ventricular size in schizophrenia: a Gaussian mixture analysis of 1056 cases and controls. *Biol Psychiatry* 30,887–903.

Dao-Castellana MH, Paillere-Martinot ML, Hantraye P, et al. (1997). Presynaptic dopaminergic function in the striatum of schizophrenic patients. *Schizophr Res* 23,167–174.

Davis KL, Kahn RS, Ko G, et al. (1991). Dopamine in schizophrenia: a review and reconceptualization. *Am J Psychiatry* 148,1474–1486.

Dewey SL, Logan J, Wolf AP, et al. (1991). Amphetamine induced decrease in [^{18}F]-N-methylspiperidol binding in the baboon brain using positron emission tomography (PET). *Synapse* 7,324–327.

Dewey SL, Smith GS, Logan J, et al. (1992). GABAergic inhibition of endogenous dopamine release measured in vivo with ^{11}C-raclopride and positron emission tomography. *J Neurosci* 12,3773–3780.

Dewey SL, Smith GS, Logan J, et al. (1993). Striatal binding of the PET ligand ^{11}C-raclopride is altered by drugs that modify synaptic dopamine levels. *Synapse* 13,350–356.

Farde L, Wiesel F, Stone-Elander S, et al. (1990). D2 dopamine receptors in neuroleptic-naive schizophrenic patients. A positron emission tomography study with [^{11}C]raclopride. *Arch Gen Psychiatry* 47,213–219.

Gejman PV, Ram A, Gelernter J, et al. (1994). No structural mutation in the dopamine D2 receptor gene in alcoholism or schizophrenia. Analysis using denaturing gradient gel electrophoresis. *JAMA* 271,204–208.

Ginovart N, Farde L, Halldin C, et al. (1997). Effect of reserpine-induced depletion of synaptic dopamine on [C-11]raclopride binding to D-2-dopamine receptors in the monkey brain. *Synapse* 25,321–325.

Ginovart N, Farde L, Halldin C, et al. (1999). Changes in striatal D2-receptor density following chronic treatment with amphetamine as assessed with PET in nonhuman primates. *Synapse* 31,154–162.

Hietala J, Syvälahti E, Vuorio K, et al. (1994). Striatal D2 receptor characteristics in neuroleptic-naive schizophrenic patients studied with positron emission tomography. *Arch Gen Psychiatry* 51,116–123.

Hietala J, Syvälahti E, Vuorio K, et al. (1995). Presynaptic dopamine function in striatum of neuroleptic-naive schizophrenic patients. *Lancet* 346,1130–1131.

Hollingshead AB (1975). Four-factor index of social status, New Haven, CT (working paper published by author).

Innis RB, Malison RT, Al-Tikriti M, et al. (1992). Amphetamine-stimulated dopamine release competes in vivo for ^{123}I-IBZM binding to the D2 receptor in non-human primates. *Synapse* 10,177–184.

Janowsky DS, Davis JM (1976). Methylphenidate, dextroamphetamine and levamphetamine. Effects on schizophrenic symptoms. *Arch Gen Psychiatry* 33,304–308.

Karreman M, Moghaddam B (1996). The prefrontal cortex regulates the basal release of dopamine in the limbic striatum: an effect mediated by ventral tegmental area. *J Neurochem* 66,589–598.

Kay SR, Fiszbein A, Opler LA (1987). The positive and negative syndrome scale (PANSS) for schizophrenia. *Schizophr Bull* 13,261–276.

Kegeles LS, Zea-Ponce Y, Abi-Dargham A, et al. (1999). Stability of ^{123}I-IBZM SPECT measurement of amphetamine-induced striatal dopamine release in humans. *Synapse* 31,302–308.

Kessler RM, Votaw JR, de Paulis T, et al. (1993) Evaluation of 5-[^{18}F]fluoropropylepidepride as a potential PET radioligand for imaging dopamine D2 receptors. *Synapse* 15,169–176.

Koepp MJ, Gunn RN, Lawrence AD, et al. (1998) Evidence for striatal dopamine release during a video game. *Nature* 393,266–288.

Köhler C, Fuxe K, Ross SB (1981). Regional in vivo binding of [^{3}H]N-propylnorapomorphine in the mouse brain. Evidence for labelling of central dopamine receptors. *Eur J Pharmacol* 72,397–402.

Laruelle M (1998). Imaging dopamine transmission in schizophrenia. A review and meta-analysis. *Q J Nucl Med* 42,211–221.

Laruelle M, Abi-Dargham A, van Dyck CH, et al. (1995). SPECT imaging of striatal dopamine release after amphetamine challenge. *J Nucl Med* 36,1182–1190.

Laruelle M, Abi-Dargham A, van Dyck CH, et al. (1996). Single photon emission computerized tomography imaging of amphetamine-induced dopamine release in drug free schizophrenic subjects. *Proc Natl Acad Sci USA* 93,9235–9240.

Laruelle M, D'Souza CD, Baldwin RM, et al. (1997). Imaging D-2 receptor occupancy by endogenous dopamine in humans. *Neuropsychopharmacology* 17,162–174.

Laruelle M, Iyer RN, Al-Tikriti MS, et al. (1997). Microdialysis and SPECT measurements of amphetamine-induced dopamine release in nonhuman primates. *Synapse* 25,1–14.

Lawrie SM, Abukmeil SS (1998). Brain abnormality in schizophrenia. A systematic and quantitative review of volumetric magnetic resonance imaging studies. *Br J Psychiatry* 172,110–120.

Lee T, Seeman P, Tourtelotte WW, et al. (1978). Binding of ^{3}H-neuroleptics and ^{3}H-apomorphine in schizophrenic brains. *Nature* 274,897–900.

Lieberman JA, Kane JM, Alvir J (1987). Provocative tests with psychostimulant drugs in schizophrenia. *Psychopharmacology* 91,415–433.

Lieberman JA, Kane JM, Gadaleta D, et al. (1984). Methylphenidate challenge as a predictor of relapse in schizophrenia. *Am J Psychiatry* 141,633–638.

Lieberman JA, Kane JM, Sarantakos S, et al. (1987). Prediction of relapse in schizophrenia. *Arch Gen Psychiatry* 44,597–603.

Lieberman JA, Sheitman BB, Kinon BJ (1997). Neurochemical sensitization in the pathophysiology of schizophrenia: deficits and dysfunction in neuronal regulation and plasticity. *Neuropsychopharmacology* 17,205–229.

Logan J, Dewey SL, Wolf AP, et al. (1991). Effects of endogenous dopamine on measures of [^{18}F]N-methylspiroperidol binding in the basal ganglia: comparison of simulations and experimental results from PET studies in baboons. *Synapse* 9,195–207.

Miller DW, Abercrombie ED (1996). Effects of MK-801 on spontaneous and amphetamine-stimulated dopamine release in striatum measured with in vivo microdialysis in awake rats. *Brain Res Bull* 40,57–62.

Mintun MA, Raichle ME, Kilbourn MR, et al. (1984). A quantitative model for the in vivo assessment of drug binding sites with positron emission tomography. *Ann Neurol* 15,217–227.

Mukherjee J, Yang ZY, Lew R, et al. (1997). Evaluation of d-amphetamine effects on the binding of dopamine D-2 receptor radioligand, F-18-fallypride, in nonhuman primates using positron emission tomography. *Synapse* 27,1–13.

Nelson MD, Saykin AJ, Flashman LA, et al. (1998). Hippocampal volume reduction in schizophrenia as assessed by magnetic resonance imaging: a meta-analytic study. *Arch Gen Psychiatry* 55,433–440.

Owen F, Cross AJ, Crow TJ, et al. (1978). Increased dopamine-receptor sensitivity in schizophrenia. *Lancet* ii,223–226.

Pilowsky LS, Costa DC, Ell PJ, et al. (1994). D2 dopamine receptor binding in the basal ganglia of antipsychotic-free schizophrenic patients. An I-123-IBZM single photon emission computerized tomography study. *Br J Psychiatry* 164,16–26.

Pycock CJ, Kerwin RW, Carter CJ (1980). Effect of lesion of cortical dopamine terminals on subcortical dopamine receptors in rats. *Nature* 286,74–77.

Reith J, Benkelfat C, Sherwin A, et al. (1994). Elevated dopa decarboxylase activity in living brain of patients with psychosis. *Proc Natl Acad Sci USA* 91,11651–11654.

Roberts AC, Desalvia MA, Wilkinson LS, et al. (1994). 6-Hydroxydopamine lesions of the prefrontal cortex in monkeys enhance performance on an analog of the Wisconsin card sort test: possible interactions with subcortical dopamine. *J Neurosci* 14,2531–2544.

Ross SB (1991). Synaptic concentration of dopamine in the mouse striatum in relationship to the kinetic properties of the dopamine receptors and uptake mechanism. *J Neurochem* 56,22–29.

Ross SB, Jackson DM (1989). Kinetic properties of the in vivo accumulation of the dopamine D-2 receptor antagonist raclopride in the mouse brain in vivo. *Naunyn Schmiedeberg Arch Pharmacol* 340,6–12.

Ross SB, Jackson DM (1989). Kinetic properties of the in vivo accumulation of [^{3}H]([minus])-N-n-propylnorapomorphine in the mouse brain. *Naunyn Schmiedeberg Arch Pharmacol* 340,13–20.

Schlaepfer TE, Pearlson GD, Wong DF, et al. (1997). PET study of competition between intravenous cocaine and [C-11]raclopride at dopamine receptors in human subjects. *Am J Psychiatry* 154,1209–1213.

Schooler NR, Keith SJ, Severe JB, et al. (1997). Relapse and rehospitalization during maintenance treatment of schizophrenia. The effects of dose reduction and family treatment. *Arch Gen Psychiatry* 54,453–463.

Seeman P (1987). Dopamine receptors and the dopamine hypothesis of schizophrenia. *Synapse* 1,133–152.

Seeman P, Bzowej NH, Guan HC, et al. (1987). Human brain D1 and D2 dopamine receptors in schizophrenia, Alzheimer's, Parkinson's, and Huntington's diseases. *Neuropsychopharmacology* 1,5–15.

Seeman P, Guan H-C, Niznik HB (1989). Endogenous dopamine lowers the dopamine D2 receptor density as measured by [^{3}H]raclopride: implications for positron emission tomography of the human brain. *Synapse* 3,96–97.

Seeman P, Lee T (1975). Antipsychotic drugs: direct correlation between clinical potency and presynaptic action on dopamine neurons. *Science* 188,1217–1219.

Sibley DR, De Lean A, Creese I (1982). Anterior pituitary receptors: demonstration of interconvertible high and low affinity states of the D2 dopamine receptor. *J Biol Chem* 257,6351–6361.

Smith GS, Schloesser R, Brodie JD, et al. (1998). Glutamate modulation of dopamine measured in vivo with positron emission tomography (PET) and ^{11}C-raclopride in normal human subjects. *Neuropsychopharmacology* 18,18–25.

Van der Werf JF, Sebens JB, Vaalburg W, et al. (1986). In vivo binding of N-n-propylnorapomorphine in the rat brain: regional localization, quantification in striatum and lack of correlation with dopamine metabolism. *Eur J Pharmacol* 87,259–270.

van Kammen DP, Bunney WE, Jr., Docherty JP, et al. (1982). d-Amphetamine-induced heterogeneous changes in psychotic behavior in schizophrenia. *Am J Psychiatry* 139,991–997.

Volkow ND, Fowler JS, Gatley SJ, et al. (1999). Comparable changes in synaptic dopamine induced by methylphenidate and by cocaine in the baboon brain. *Synapse* 31,59–66.

Volkow ND, Wang G-J, Fowler JS, et al. (1994). Imaging endogenous dopamine competition with [^{11}C]raclopride in the human brain. *Synapse* 16,255–262.

Wong DF, Wagner HN, Tune LE, et al. (1986). Positron emission tomography reveals elevated D_2 dopamine receptors in drug-naive schizophrenics. *Science* 234,1558–1563.

Young LT, Wong DF, Goldman S, et al. (1991). Effects of endogenous dopamine on kinetics of [^{3}H]methylspiperone and [^{3}H]raclopride binding in the rat brain. *Synapse* 9,188–194.

10.

Dopamine Function in Neuroleptic-Naive Schizophrenia

Erkka Syvälahti and Jarmo Hietala

ABSTRACT

Postmortem studies have indicated an increase in dopamine D2 receptor density in basal ganglia in schizophrenia, although chronicity and long-term neuroleptic treatment are obvious limitations. In the 1980s, new vistas opened to study these problems in vivo, especially positron emission tomography. These studies suggest no generalized increase in striatal D2 receptor density in drug-naive schizophrenia, although elevations of D2 receptor densities have been reported in some patients. Longitudinal studies reveal a rather high variation of D2 receptor densities in the striatum in schizophrenia when compared with healthy controls, suggesting a labile dopamine pool in schizophrenia. However, alterations in D2 receptor densities in schizophrenia seem not to be psychosis-dependent phenomena. Conversely, recent independent studies have revealed an increase in 6-[^{18}F]-fluorodopa (FDOPA) uptake in basal ganglia in first-admission and more chronic neuroleptic-naive schizophrenic patients. In addition, a highly significant correlation of left striatal FDOPA uptake with depressive symptoms in drug-naive schizophrenic patients has been found, a phenomenon that might reflect human brain reactive or compensatory mechanisms for psychosis. Recent studies on dopamine transporter (DAT) indicate that average 18F-CFT binding potentials between controls and neuroleptic-naive schizophrenics are identical. Thus the reported hyperdopaminergic state in schizophrenia is due to increased activity rather than to increased density of dopaminergic projections to the striatum. Several studies indicate asymmetrical D2 receptor binding in vivo in the human striatum. Recent studies on neuroleptic-naive schizophrenic patients indicate that in contrast to healthy controls, schizophrenic patients show a lack of the normal functional asymmetry in nucleus caudatus but not in putamen regarding the presynaptic dopamine activity in vivo. Lack of normal asymmetry or reversed asymmetry is congruent with the neurodevelopmental hypothesis of schizophrenia. However, the total duration of illness (including prodromal symptoms) correlates negatively with 18F-CFT binding potential in the putamen and tends to correlate negatively in the caudate of drug-naive patients—indicating a progressive loss of striatal DAT–and hence dopaminergic nerve terminals in schizophrenia (a neurodegenerative process?). Thus indirect pharmacological data and modern brain imaging indicate the involvement of dopamine in schizophrenia. These changes should be related to various dimensions of psychopathology in schizophrenia as well as to function of the other neurotransmitter systems linked to the disorder.

INTRODUCTION

The dopamine hypothesis of schizophrenia in its original and simplistic form assumes that overactivity of the brain dopaminergic system is crucial. During the past decades the dopamine hypothesis has been variously reformulated. A recent hypothesis suggests that there might not be a general overactivity of dopaminergic pathways but rather an increased activity in subcortical (limbic) dopamine systems accounting for mainly positive symptoms (e.g., hallucinations, disorganized behavior, thought disorder) and a relative hypoactivity in mesocortical dopamine activity accounting mainly for negative symptoms (e.g., affective flattening, alogia, anhedonia) (Davis et al., 1991). This hypothesis would explain the simultaneous existence of positive and negative symptoms. It is considered that the positive symptoms respond better to current antipsychotic drugs (D2 dopamine receptor antagonists, see below) than the negative symptoms. The division of symptoms to positive and negative is an oversimplification, and previous hypotheses based on this dichotomy such as the type I and type II schizophrenia proposed by Crow (1980) have been largely abandoned. At least three dimensions of symptomatology have been recognized in schizophrenia: psychotic, disorganized, and negative (Andreasen, 1995). It remains to be seen if there are correlates of these dimensions in terms of neurobiology.

A link between schizophrenia and deviations in early brain development is supported by a large body of evidence and is known as the neurodevelopmental hypothesis of schizophrenia (Weinberger, 1995). A deviant development and maturation of the brain may cause a vulnerable set of connections in the neurotransmitter pathways, predisposing to schizophrenic psychosis. In addition, acute symptoms (e.g., auditory hallucinations) have their "neurophysiology" in terms of brain nuclei and transmitters involved. Functional organization of the human brain is such that dopamine or any other neurotransmitter hypothesis must be seen in a larger context as one approach to explore specific aberrations in a set of neural circuits associated with the emergence of clinical disease. We review the evidence for dopamine involvement in schizophrenia with special emphasis on the data achieved in neuroleptic-naive patients.

IS DOPAMINE INVOLVED IN SCHIZOPHRENIA?

Dopamine involvement in schizophrenia has relied mostly on indirect pharmacological evidence because the direct evidence has been circumstantial until quite recently. There are two main lines of pharmacological evidence for schizophrenia. 1) Dopamine-releasing drugs, such as amphetamine, can worsen symptoms in schizophrenia, and prolonged use of amphetamine may trigger a state resembling paranoid schizophrenia. In addition, the dopamine agonist medication (L-DOPA, bromocryptine, pergolide) can cause psychotic symptoms (e.g., in Parkinson's disease). 2) All current antipsychotic drugs act, at least partly, via the dopaminergic system. This is also known as the dopamine (or dopamine D2 receptor hypothesis) of neuroleptic drug action.

Many papers originally implicate and further expand the line of evidence of a link between the dopaminergic system and neuroleptic drug action (Syvälahti, 1994). Several studies have shown a convincing correlation between D2 receptor binding affinity and the daily dose of neuroleptic drugs used in schizophrenia. These drugs occupy about 70–90% of striatal D2 receptors in vivo in schizophrenic patients who have responded to neuroleptic drugs (Farde et al., 1988).

Note that the dopamine hypothesis of neuroleptic action can be true regardless of whether the dopamine hypothesis of schizophrenia holds. However, even dopamine involvement in neuroleptic action can be criticized for the following two reasons.

- Blockade of D2 receptors occurs immediately after a single dose of haloperidol, but antipsychotic effects and some motor side effects occur with a delay of days to a few weeks. Despite many attractive mechanisms proposed (e.g., a dopamine neuron depolarization inactivation hypothesis suggesting a gradual decrease in firing activity of dopamine midbrain nuclei), the detailed mechanisms for this time-dependent adaptation process remain largely unknown.

- Not all schizophrenic patients benefit from classic neuroleptic drugs and merely experience side effects. The atypical antipsychotic drug, clozapine, and possibly some novel atypical antipsychotics are effective in treatment resistance, but these compounds have several effects on a wide variety of neurotransmitter systems. Some patients with predominantly "negative" symptoms may even benefit from dopamine agonist drugs suggested by recent open studies (Benkert et al., 1995). This can also reflect to the heterogeneity issues in the biological substrates of schizophrenia.

POSTMORTEM STUDIES FOR DOPAMINE INVOLVEMENT

Schizophrenia is one of the most extensively studied brain disorders in postmortem studies. The detailed molecular knowledge about dopamine receptor subtypes, the dopamine transporter (DAT), and the enzymes involved in dopamine synthesis and metabolism is increasing quickly and provides new probes to explore the dopamine system in a straightforward manner in postmortem brains. Thus more knowledge on these aspects of schizophrenia is bound to appear in the literature. In addition, modern neuroanatomical postmortem studies on neural connections and neuron morphology in the schizophrenic brain may provide useful data for understanding the pathophysiology of this disorder. However, the limitations of postmortem studies must be remembered. In particular postmortem studies concerning the data on dopamine are seriously biased because most patients have been chronic and treated neuroleptically. When the postmortem literature is reviewed, it is difficult to conclude that dopamine or its metabolites would be consistently altered. The increase in the D2 receptor density in basal ganglia of deceased schizophrenic patients is fairly consistent. This finding, also known as the D2 receptor hypothesis of schizophrenia, probably reflects brain adaptation to neuroleptic drugs rather than a specific change related to schizophrenia (Kornhuber et al., 1989).

DOPAMINE D2 RECEPTOR HYPOTHESIS AND IMAGING STUDIES

Special interest has been devoted to the D2 receptor owing to its likely involvement in antipsychotic effect. As mentioned above, postmortem studies have consistently indicated an increase in D2 receptor density but not affinity in basal ganglia of schizophrenic patients (Seeman et al., 1990). However, this increase may be due to previous neuroleptic medication that is known to cause such an adaptive change in experimental studies and that is also supported by the findings of Kornhuber et al. (1989). Avoiding the limitations of postmortem studies became possible in the 1980s with in vivo emission tomography techniques, especially positron emission tomography (PET). Much hope was held for these techniques to aid in reaching a definite conclusion on the D2 receptor hypothesis of schizophrenia. Note, however, that like the postmortem studies the in vivo studies have their own limitations such as selection bias (common exclusion of agitated, aggressive, and other uncooperative patients) and possible carry-over effects of previous drugs.

Despite an original study reporting a 2- to 3-fold increase in brain D2 receptors (Wong et al., 1986), the prevailing view is that a slight increase may exist in a portion of patients, but there is no generalized increase in striatal D2 receptor density in neuroleptic-naive schizophrenia in vivo (Nordsröm et al., 1995; Syvälahti, 1994). Therefore the increase in striatal D2 receptors in postmortem studies may be mainly iatrogenic, and the D2 receptor hypothesis as such appears to be incorrect (Hietala et al., 1996).

We have recently completed a longitudinal study on striatal D2 dopamine receptor density and emergent psychotic symptoms in drug-naive schizophrenics. The intervals between the first and second PET scanning varied from 6 to 24 months in the four patients studied. Dopamine D2 receptor densities had a rather high variation in the two PET sessions when compared with healthy control subjects, suggesting a more labile dopamine pool in the striatum in schizophrenia. There was, however, no obvious relation of D2 receptor densities to the severity of psychotic symptoms at the test-retest PET scans (Syvälahti et al., 2000). Thus alterations in D2 receptor densities seem not to be clear-cut psychosis-dependent phenomena in schizophrenia.

Another dopamine receptor subtype, the D1 dopamine receptor, has been studied with PET and ^{11}C-SCH 23390 in schizophrenic patients and controls (Sedvall et al., 1995). No major changes in receptor density were observed in these patients. However, one PET study with ^{11}C)-SCH 23390 has found decreased density of dopamine D1 receptors in the prefrontal cortex of drug-naive or drug-free schizophrenic patients that was associated with the severity of negative symptoms and poor performance on the Wisconsin Card Sorting Test measuring the frontal lobe cognitive function (Okubo et al., 1997).

As with D2 dopamine receptors, the failure to observe consistent changes at the dopamine receptor level does not necessarily exclude changes in other indices of the dopamine system, and further studies are needed to establish the precise role of D1 receptors in schizophrenia.

BRAIN IMAGING OF PRESYNAPTIC DOPAMINE FUNCTION

FDOPA Uptake in Basal Ganglia

Recently, imaging studies have explored intracellular processes in the dopaminergic neurons that may be more sensitive to subtle and qualitatively small changes in the function of neurons. Before changes in cell surface receptors, many compensatory events inside the cell may have already happened.

Independent studies with 6-[^{18}F]-fluorodopa (FDOPA) have suggested an increase of the FDOPA uptake in basal ganglia in first-admission (Hietala et al., 1995) and more chronic neuroleptic-naive schizophrenic patients (Reith et al., 1994). Consistent with FDOPA findings, three studies have found increased dopamine release after amphetamine administration in drug-free schizophrenic patients (Abi-Dargham et al., 1998; Breier et al., 1997; Laruelle et al., 1996), suggesting that the quantity of a free, releasable pool of intracellular dopamine is elevated. The accumulation of FDOPA in the striatum portrays tracer uptake to the dopaminergic nerve terminal and intracellular decarboxylation of FDOPA to fluorodopamine (one step in dopamine synthesis). Although it is generally thought that the tyrosine hydroxylase step is rate limiting in the synthesis of dopamine, recent evidence indicates that decarboxylation is also regulated.

Note that although the increase in putamen FDOPA uptake is statistically significant compared with controls, not all patients show increases in FDOPA uptake. Thus a schizophrenic patient with catatonic subtype had a low basal ganglia FDOPA uptake (Hietala et al., 1995), and in these particular subjects presynaptic dopamine function may actually be lower than in healthy subjects (Dao-Castellana et al., 1997; Hietala et al., 1995).

It also seems that another set of clinical symptoms is associated with low presynaptic dopamine function. Recently we found a highly significant correlation of left striatal FDOPA uptake values with depressive symptoms in drug-naive schizophrenic patients, a phenomenon that might reflect human brain reactive or compensatory mechanisms for psychosis (Hietala et al., 1999).

Dopamine Transporter

The DAT is a protein on the plasma membrane of dopaminergic neurons, the main function of which is collection of released dopamine from the synaptic cleft and presynaptic areas back to the presynaptic neuron. This reuptake is a primary means to regulate the synaptic concentration of the released dopamine. CFT (also known as WIN 35,428) is a well-characterized dopamine blocker with structural analogy to a cocaine molecule. Pharmacological studies have shown that CFT can be used as valid indicator of dopaminergic innervation density—not only in vitro and postmortem but in vivo, provided kinetic properties make the compound suitable for PET and single-photon emission computed tomogaphy (SPECT). ^{18}F-CFT is a useful PET tracer for DAT in humans (better than ^{11}C-labeled isotope) owing to its high signal-to-noise ratio and suitability for reliable quantification at equilibrium conditions.

Recent studies have shown that average ^{18}F-CFT binding potentials between controls and neuroleptic-naive schizophrenic patients are identical (Laakso et al., 2000). This indicates that the reported hyperdopaminergic state in schizophrenia using fluorodopa measurements and amphetamine challenge studies (Dao-Castellana et al., 1997; Laruelle et al., 1996) is due to increased activity rather than to increased density of dopaminergic projections to the striatum. In harmony with our data, a recent study in drug-free schizophrenic subjects using SPECT and ^{123}I-CIT found no correlation between DAT density and amphetamine-induced dopamine release, either in patients or controls, confirming that schizophrenia is not associated with general alterations of DAT in the striatum (Laruelle et al., in press). In these patients, the severity of negative symptoms was significantly higher than in patients with normal striatal DAT values, suggesting that in some patients a relative deficit in dopamine nerve terminals might be involved in the pathophysiology of negative symptoms.

Brain Asymmetry and Dopamine

It is well-known that the human brain is organized in a highly asymmetrical way in terms of structure and function. Some previous studies, including Hietala et al. (1994), indicate differences in asymmetries in D2 receptor binding in vivo in striatum. Regarding presynaptic dopamine function, Hietala et al. (1995) and subsequent studies in a larger cohort of neuroleptic-naive schizophrenic patients indicate that the patients show a lack of functional asymmetry in nucleus caudatus but not in putamen. These studies implicate that a reversed or a lack of normal asymmetry may be present in at least half (but not all) of patients congruent with the neurodevelopmental hypothesis of schizophrenia (Weinberger, 1995). It will be of interest to explore whether alterations in FDOPA uptake in the caudate of schizophrenic patients have a functional or structural basis or both.

Some crucial questions follow: 1) Are there clinical symptom correlates? 2) Can the asymmetry be restored by neuroleptic drugs or atypical antipsychotic drugs or is it a stabile sign of once disturbed brain development? 3) Could it be observed in high-risk subjects before the psychotic outbreak?

The DAT studies also indicate disturbed lateralization in schizophrenia. Thus healthy controls showed a significantly higher uptake of ^{18}F-CFT in the right caudate compared with the left caudate, whereas no asymmetry was found in about half of the schizophrenic patients (Laakso et al., 2000). This lack of asymmetry in our study may thus reflect an impaired axonal migration from the midbrain dopaminergic nuclei to the caudate, and it is in harmony with the neurodevelopmental hypothesis.

In our study with neuroleptic-naive schizophrenics, the total duration of illness (including prodromal symptoms) correlated negatively with ^{18}F-CFT binding potential in the putamen and tended to do so in the caudate–suggesting a progressive loss of striatal DAT and hence dopaminergic nerve terminals in schizophrenia. Thus there may also be a neurodegenerative component in the schizophrenic process.

CONCLUSION AND FUTURE NEEDS

The dopamine hypothesis of schizophrenia is one of the oldest biological hypotheses of schizophrenia with many revised versions. However, it is unlikely that any single neurotransmitter hypothesis can satisfactorily explain the biological basis of such a highly heterogeneous disorder. Rather it is evident that the biological vulnerability factors as well as the "acute neurophysiology" of symptoms involve a complex set of imbalances or aberrant connections in neuronal circuits. Dopamine may be one key transmitter substance involved, as evidenced by the labile control of D2 receptor densities as well as increased presynaptic activity in vivo in neuroleptic-naive schizophrenia.

The ongoing and future work on the precise role of dopamine in schizophrenia should focus on first episode/admission neuroleptic-naive schizophrenic patients and their follow-up. Such studies stand the best chance for determining specific changes in the dopaminergic pathways and possibly relating them in a meaningful way to various dimensions of psychopathology seen in schizophrenia.

Brain imaging studies in Turku, Finland, have benefited from the long-lasting experience of developing modern psychosocial treatment (Alanen, 1997) as well as "clinical psychosis teams," which treat patients and families closely from the beginning and try to determine optimal treatment modalities. To help assess the clinical situation and to avoid unnecessary neuroleptic treatment, only benzodiazepines are usually given to the patient during the first treatment days until the diagnosis and treatment options are cleared. During this period PET studies can also be performed to suitable drug-free patients.

Modern imaging techniques represent a powerful means to detect specific neurotransmitter changes in vivo. The obvious involvement of dopamine can be put forward in various testable transmitter imbalance hypotheses, e.g., glutamate-dopamine driven hypothesis (Carlson et al., 1990; Reith et al., 1994). Consequently there is an urgent need to develop methodology for exploration of neurotransmitters other than dopamine [e.g., major amino acid transmitters (glutamate, γ-aminobutyric acid, neurokinins etc.)], and some are now actively tested in imaging centers. Conversely, the changes in brain dopamine function documented in PET studies may not be specific for schizophrenia and may be shared by certain other psychiatric disorders (J. Kajander et al., unpublished data; Pearlson et al., 1995).

REFERENCES

Alanen YO (1997). *Schizophrenia: Its Origin and Need-Adapted Treatment.* London: Karnac Books.

Andreasen NC (1995). Symptoms, signs and diagnosis of schizophrenia. *Lancet* 346,477–481.

Benkert O, Muller-Siecheneder F, Wetzel H (1995). Dopamine agonists in schizophrenia—a review. *Eur J Neuropsychopharmacol* (suppl),43–53.

Breier A, Su T-P, Saunders R, et al. (1997). Schizophrenia is associated with elevated amphetamine-induced synaptic dopamine concentrations: evidence from a novel positron emission tomography method. *Proc Natl Acad Sci USA* 94,2569–2574.

Carlsson, M, Carlsson A (1990). Schizophrenia: a subcortical neurotransmitter imbalance syndrome? *Schizophr Bull* 16,425–432.

Crow TJ (1980). Molecular pathology of schizophrenia: more than one disease process? *Br Med J* 280,66–68.

Dao-Castellana MH, Pailere-Martinot ML, Hantraye P, et al. (1997). Presynaptic dopaminergic function in the striatum of schizophrenic patients. *Schizophr Res* 23,167–174.

Davis KL, Kahn RS, Ko G, et al. (1991). Dopamine in schizophrenia: a review and reconceptualization. *Am J Psychiatry* 148,1474–1486.

Farde L, Nordström AL, Karlsson P, et al. (1995). Positron emission tomography studies on dopamine receptors in schizophrenia. *Clin Neuropharmacol* 18(suppl 1),121–129.

Farde L, Wiesel F-A, Halldin C, et al. (1988). Central D_2 dopamine receptor occupancy in schizophrenic patients treated with antipsychotic drugs. *Arch Gen Psychiatry* 45,71–76.

Hietala J, Syvälahti E (1996). Dopamine in schizophrenia. *Ann Med* 28,557–561.

Hietala J, Syvälahti E, Vilkman H, et al. (1999). Depressive symptoms and presynaptic dopamine function in neuroleptic-naive schizophrenia. *Schizophr Res* 35,41–50.

Hietala J, Syvälahti E, Vuorio K, et al. (1994). Striatal dopamine D_2 receptor binding characteristics in neuroleptic-naive schizophrenics studied with positron emission tomography. *Arch Gen Psychiatry* 51,116–123.

Hietala J, Syvälahti E, Vuorio K, et al. (1995). Presynaptic dopamine function in striatum of neuroleptic-naive schizophrenic patients. *Lancet* 346,1130–1131.

Kornhuber J, Riederer P, Reynolds GP, et al. (1989). ^{3}H-spiperone binding in post-mortem brains of schizophrenic patients: relationship to neuroleptic drug treatment, abnormal movements and positive symptoms. *J Neural Transm* 75,1–10.

Laakso A, Vilkman H, Alakare B, et al. (2000). Striatal dopamine transporter in neuroleptic-naïve schizophrenia studied with PET. *Am J Psychiatry* 157,269–271.

Laruelle M, Abi-Dargham A, van Dyck CH, et al. (1996). Single photon emission computerized tomography imaging of amphetamine-induced dopamine release in drug-free schizophrenic subjects. *Proc Natl Acad Sci USA* 93,9235–9240.

Laruelle M, Abi-Dargham A, van Dyck C, et al. Dopamine and serotonin transporters in patients with schizophrenia: an imaging study with [^{123}I][gb]-C *Biol Psychiatry*, in press.

Nordtröm A-L, Farde L, Eriksson L, et al. (1995). No elevated D2 receptors in neuroleptic-naïve schizophrenic patients revealed by PET and [^{11}C]-methylspiperone. *Psychiatry Res* 61,67–83.

Okubo Y, Suhara T, Suzuki K, et al. (1997). Decreased prefrontal dopamine D1 receptors in schizophrenia revealed by PET. *Nature* 385,634–636.

Pearlson GD, Wong DF, Tune LE, et al. (1995). In vivo D2 dopamine receptor density in psychotic and nonpsychotic patients with bipolar disorder. *Arch Gen Psychiatry* 52,471–477.

Reith J, Benkelfat C, Sherwin A, et al. (1994). Elevated dopa decarboxylase activity in living brain of patients with psychosis. *Proc Natl Acad Sci USA* 91,11651–11654.

Sedvall G, Farde L (1995). Chemical brain anatomy in schizophrenia. *Lancet* 346,743–749.

Seeman P, Niznik HB (1990). Dopamine receptors and transporters in Parkinson's disease and schizophrenia. *FASEB J* 4,2737–2744.

Syvälahti E (1994). Biological factors in schizophrenia. Structural and functional aspects. *Br J Psychol* 164(suppl),9–14.

Syvälahti E, Räkköläinen V, Aaltonen J, et al. (2000). Striatal D2 dopamine receptor density and psychotic symptoms in schizophrenia: a longitudinal study. *Schizophr Res* 43,159–166.

Tune L, Wong DF, Pearlson G, et al. (1993). Dopamine D_2 dopamine receptor density estimates in schizophrenia: a positron emission tomography study with [^{11}C]-N-methylspiperone. *Psychiatry Res* 49,219–237.

Weinberger DR (1995). Schizophrenia: from neuropathology to neurodevelopment. *Lancet* 346,552–557.

Wong DF, Wagner HN, Tune LE, et al. (1986). Positron emission tomography reveals elevated D2 dopamine receptors in drug-naive schizophrenics. *Science* 234,1558–1563.

11.

Pre- and Postnatal Stress as Risk Factors for Major Psychopathology

Induction of "Miswired" Circuitry in Susceptible Individuals

Francine M. Benes

INTRODUCTION

As early as 1959, S. Kety postulated that a combination of a susceptibility gene and environmental factor(s) may contribute to major forms of psychopathology such as schizophrenia. With the knowledge that antipsychotic medications specifically block dopamine receptors (Carlsson, 1978), it seemed reasonable to postulate that an anomalous gene in schizophrenia could potentially be related to the regulation of this system (Kety and Matthysse, 1972). The observation that monozygotic twin pairs show only a 40–50% concordance rate (Gottesman and Shields, 1972; Kety, 1983) has made it clear, however, that environmental factors must be important in determining whether individuals are at risk for exhibiting the schizophrenic phenotype. Is there any evidence that environmental factors actually contribute to the occurrence of schizophrenia and other forms of psychopathology that present during childhood and adolescence?

As a group, patients with schizophrenia (Jacobsen and Kinney, 1980; Parnas et al., 1982) and bipolar disorder (Kinney et al., 1993) have an incidence of obstetrical complications in their birthing records that is much higher than expected. The most prevalent form of perinatal complication is prolonged labor (Jacobsen and Kinney, 1980). It was once believed that hypoxemia might be sufficient to cause schizophrenia, but this no longer appears to be the case because individuals exposed to complete anoxia during birthing may develop cerebral palsy but do not show any increased risk for schizophrenia. Accordingly a "two-factor" model of schizophrenia provides a more useful framework to model for the etiology of schizophrenia and other forms of psychopathology (Parnas et al., 1982).

A key goal of a two-factor model for major psychiatric disorders is to identify changes in neural circuitry and distinguish those associated with a genetically transmitted latent trait from those arising from perinatal disturbances (Benes, 1988). Some investigators have attempted to identify clinically relevant phenotypic markers, such as a disturbance of smooth pursuit eye movements (Holzman et al., 1988) and the schizotypal personality profile (Kety, 1985; Parnas et al., 1982), which are more prevalent among the first-degree relatives of schizophrenics. A similar goal must also be set for histopathologic studies. The discussion will consider how developmental neurobiology can provide a framework for investigating how neural circuitry may be altered in schizophrenia using a "two-hit" model to interpret results.

"MISWIRED" CIRCUITRY IN SCHIZOPHRENIA

Such a model presents a challenge as to how perinatal complications could potentially produce alterations in the circuitry of the brain described in recent postmortem studies of schizophrenia and bipolar disorder. One model of schizophrenia postulates that a prenatal disturbance may have caused a disturbance in the migration of neurons from the subventricular zone outward toward the cortical mantle (Akbarian et al., 1993a,b; Akbarian et al., 1996; Anderson et al., 1996; Benes, 1993; Benes et al., 1992b; Kirkpatrick et al., 1999). Such a mechanism could be associated with changes in the composition of cortical laminae, particularly the outer layers. Such alterations have been implicated by microscopic studies of both the γ-aminobutyric acid (GABA) (Benes et al., 1991, 1992b, 1996, 1997a,b) and glutamate systems (Benes et al., 1987, 1992a; Benes and Bird, 1987; Longson et al., 1996) in layers II and III of the prefrontal, anterior cingulate, and entorhinal cortices.

A recent study of a specialized protein called Reelin that is expressed in Cajal Retzius neurons in layer I of the developing cortex has been found to be markedly decreased in layers I and II of the prefrontal cortex of schizophrenics (Impagnatiello et al., 1998). In adult brain, Reelin is localized in horizontal and bitufted GABAergic neurons, and the decrease of cells expressing this protein is compatible with the idea that a disturbance of early development has affected the population of interneurons found in superficial laminae and resulted in a dysfunction of GABAergic interneurons in layers I, II, and III (Benes, 1997).

Although not all studies have provided support for the idea that there is an overt loss of GABA cells in schizophrenia (Arnold et al., 1995; Akbarian et al., 1995; Selemon et al., 1995), this transmitter system is likely subject to some form of dysfunction, particularly because most neurochemical and cytochemical reports have provided further support for this possibility (Akbarian et al., 1995; Beaseley and Reynolds, 1989; Benes et al., 1992b, 1996, 1997a,b; Bird et al., 1979; Hanada et al., 1987; Perry et al., 1979; Reynolds, 1990; Simpson et al., 1989).

Another recent postmortem study has suggested the possibility that GABA cells may receive hyperinnervations by dopaminergic inputs to layer II (Benes et al., 1997). Specifically, the density of tyrosine-hydroxylase-immunoreactive varicosities in contact with interneurons (nonpyramidal cells) was found to be three times higher than that seen on pyramidal neurons in layer II. There was no difference in the schizophrenics regardless of whether they were treated with neuroleptic drugs. A posthoc analysis of these data subsequently revealed that the findings could best be explained by a shift of dopamine fibers from pyramidal cells to nonpyramidal cells (Benes, 1997), and a miswiring has been proposed as a mechanism, although this would not require an overt loss of GABAergic cells per se.

An important question to ask is whether changes in the circuitry of layer II in the anterior cingulate cortex may represent the expression of a susceptibility gene for schizophrenia or whether perhaps they may reflect an environmental risk factor, such as a perinatal insult.

MODELING FOR EFFECT OF PERINATAL STRESS

A key question is whether changes in layer II of the anterior cingulate cortex are present when the illness begins or whether they are present before the prodrome is initiated, perhaps even as early as the pre- or perinatal period (Benes, 1988, 1997). To distinguish between these two possibilities, it is relevant to consider whether a potential relationship exists between the various histopathologic changes reported and exposure to stress experienced during the perinatal period. The strategies required for assessing the role of the environment in the occurrence of schizophrenia and other mental disorders are quite different from those used to identify susceptibility genes. For environmental factors, animal models can be extremely helpful, even though they have notable limitations (Henn and McKinney, 1987). A critical use of such models can potentially provide meaningful insights into the mechanisms through which abnormal wiring may occur in schizophrenia and probably other mental disorders (See figure 11-1).

By using perinatal stress as a paradigm, it seems reasonable to assume that untoward conditions during embryogenesis or during the birthing process could produce a generalized insult to the brain. Because we know that the time for the development of various cortical regions differs considerably among regions (Gilles, 1983), it is conceivable that a perturbation of brain development at a critical stage could theoretically

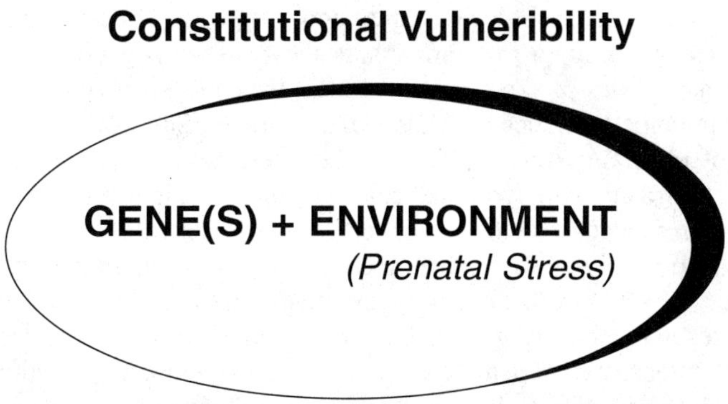

FIG. 11-1. Interaction between genetic and environmental factors as determinants of constitutional vulnerability for psychopathology. Biological constitution is probably a derivative of a genetically defined set of biobehavioral responses that interplay with environmental events. Both elements have analogues at specific corticolimbic circuits. During the life cycle, genetic and environmental factors probably interact in a dynamic fashion to give rise to what we identify phenotypically as the selective "vulnerability" for a particular form of mental illness. A nonspecific factor, such as stress, may influence the extent to which a selective vulnerability is phenotypically expressed. Reproduced with permission from Benes (1997).

result in preferential changes in one region but not another. Although many different obstetrical complications have been described in the birthing records of schizophrenics, stress would be a common denominator of all. In this regard, one potential source of injury to the brain could come from elevated levels of adrenal steroids, hormones that are released as part of the general adaptive response to stress (Sapolsky, 1992).

This possibility is particularly intriguing because these hormones have been found to be toxic to the developing brain. For example, during prenatal development, high circulating levels of glucocorticoid hormone have been associated with a reduced number of neurons (Balazs and Cotterrell, 1972; Cotterrell et al., 1972). Normally the DNA content of the brain continues to increase until the second postnatal week (Ardeleanu and Sterescu. 1978); however, with exposure to high levels of adrenal steroid hormones, decreased nucleic acid content, and presumably the number of surviving neurons, have been reported (Cotterrell et al., 1972). Exposure to stress in utero has been associated with a reduced number of hippocampal pyramidal cells as well as their dendritic processes (Uno et al., 1990). Such a change could potentially contribute to a decrease of avoidance learning that has been observed in animals treated with glucocorticoid hormones (DeKloet et al., 1988) and is thought to bear some relationship to abnormal sprouting in the hippocampus, an effect that seems to worsen with age (DeKosky et al., 1984). Adrenal steroid hormones also influence the normal functioning of nonneuronal cells, such as astroglia (Scheff et al., 1986) and microglia (Vijayan and Cotman, 1987) in injured brain tissue. Note that prenatal exposure to stress is associated with persistently high levels of activity in the hypothalamo-pituitary-adrenal axis (Takahashi and Kalin, 1991) and potentiates the response to stress during the pubertal period and even much later during adulthood (Fride et al., 1986). Overall, prenatal exposure to stress appears to be associated with an interference with the maturation of neurons and with an enhancement of the stress response during adulthood. Do these effects provide a useful model for understanding postmortem changes seen in schizophrenia?

A preliminary series of experiments was conducted to identify whether perinatal stress could potentially induce changes in the neural circuitry of the anterior cingulate cortex of rat brain. Toward this end, the interaction of tyrosine hydroxylase-immunoreactive fibers with pyramidal cells and nonpyramidal neurons was assessed in pregnant dams injected with 10 mg corticosterone or vehicle for 3 days before parturition (Benes, 1997). After birth, the offspring were subsequently exposed to either corticosterone or vehicle during the postweanling and early adult periods. Those rats receiving corticosterone both pre- and postnatally showed a marked increase in the density of dopamine terminals forming appositions with nonpyramidal neurons in the medial prefrontal cortex, a homologue of the anterior cingulate region of human and primate brain. There was no change in the density of fibers in contact with pyramidal cells, nor were there differences observed in rats receiving corticosterone only during the postnatal period.

Taken together, the results have suggested that exposure to nonspecific stress in utero may sensitize animals to subsequent exposure to stress during adulthood. Because exposure to stress is known to be associated with a marked increase in the release of dopamine in rat medial prefrontal cortex (Roth et al., 1988; Thierry et al., 1976), prenatal exposure to stress may be capable of inducing a structural change in cortical dopamine fibers that would tend to enhance further the release of dopamine. Direct effects of steroids on the expression of tyrosine hydroxylase mRNA (Iuvone and Dunn, 1986; Stone et al., 1978; Stone and McCarty, 1983) could also be related to the changes described above and are consistent with the idea that prenatal exposure to stress can potentiate the subsequent response of animals to stress during the adult period. In cortical circuits where there is a preexisting reduction of GABAergic activity, such a change could lead to even further decreases of inhibitory activity and thereby cause a severe decompensation in the activity of this circuitry. Because glucocorticoids can directly increase the activity of the $GABA_A$ receptor (Lambert et al., 1987; Majewska et al., 1985), such an effect could potentially overcome at least some component of a GABAergic defect in schizophrenia. In fact, there is some possibility that the increase of this receptor in schizophrenics (Benes et al., 1992b, 1996a, 1997) could be related in some way to the effect of stress.

It is well-established that stress can induce a pronounced and selective increase in the release of dopamine in the medial prefrontal cortex (Roth et al., 1988; Thierry et al., 1976). Dopamine probably exerts an inhibitory effect on GABA cells (Penit-Soria et al., 1987; Retaux et al., 1991a,b). In schizophrenia, if there is a pre-existing increase of dopaminergic inputs to interneurons (see above), the stressful conditions would tend to result in an exceptionally high increase of dopamine release. Because GABA cells are believed to be dysfunctional in schizophrenia, then an excessive release of dopamine under stressful conditions could be sufficient to cause the intrinsic circuitry within layer II to decompensate. In this context, note that the dopamine innervation of the anterior cingulate cortex continues to increase until the early adult period in rats (Benes et al., 1996; Kalsbeek et al., 1988; Verney et al., 1982). On this basis, it seems likely that under normal conditions, the interaction between dopamine fibers and GABA cells is probably increasing until the start of the adult period (Benes et al., 1996). Given this natural plasticity of the cortical dopamine projections during the postnatal period, it does not seem surprising that the concurrence of stress could be associated with the formation of a miswired circuit.

CONCLUSIONS

In 1949 Hebb was the first to suggest that the influence of environment on the occurrence of mental illness "must be a function of experience and of the constitution that does the experiencing." Based on the above discussion, it can be postulated that constitutional vulnerability involves, in part, the exposure to stress during the pre- and/or postnatal periods and the associated alterations in the circuitry in key locations within the corticolimbic system. Some histopathologic changes that are detected in schizophrenic brain with modern neuroscientific techniques may reflect the presence of an anomolous gene, but others may represent changes that are environmentally induced. Based on rodent experiments, stress early in life may sensitize an individual to the subsequent exposure to stress during adolescence and adulthood.

Through such a combination of effects, a miswiring of dopaminergic inputs to corticolimbic circuitry may be induced during the critical stages of childhood and adolescence when particular forms of psychopathology are apt to present.

REFERENCES

Akbarian S, Bunney WE, Potkin SG, et al. (1993). Altered distribution of nicotinamide-adenine dinucleotide phosphate-diaphorase cells in frontal lobe of schizophrenics implies disturbances of cortical development. *Arch Gen Psychiatry* 50,227–230.

Akbarian S, Huntsman MM, Kim JJ, et al. (1995). $GABA_A$ receptor subunit gene expression in human prefrontal cortex: comparison of schizophrenics and controls. *Cereb Cortex* 5,550–560.

Akbarian S, Kim JJ, Potkin SG, et al. (1995). Gene expression for glutamic acid decarboxylase is reduced without loss of neurons in prefrontal cortex of schizophrenics. *Arch Gen Psychiatry* 52,258–278.

Ardeleanu A, Sterescu N (1978). RNA and DNA synthesis in developing rat brain: hormonal influences. *Psychoneuroendocrinology* 3,93.

Arnold SE, Franz BR, Gur RC, et al. (1995). Smaller neuron size in schizophrenia in hippocampal subfields that mediate cortical-hippocampal interactions. *Am J Psychiatry* 152,738–748.

Balazs R, Cotterrell M (1972). Effect of hormonal state on cell number and functional maturation of the brain. *Nature* 236,348–350.

Beasley CL, Reynolds GP (1996). Parvalbumin-immunoreactive neurons are reduced in the prefrontal cortex of schizophrenics. *Schizophr Res* 24,349–355.

Benes FM (1997). Corticolimbic circuitry and the development of psychopathology during childhood and adolescence. In: *Development of the Prefrontal Cortex: Evolution, Neurobiology, and Behavior*, Krasnegor NA, Lyon GR, Goldman-Rakic PS, eds. Baltimore: Paul H. Brookes, pp. 211–239.

Benes FM (1997). Is there evidence for neuronal loss in schizophrenia? *Int Rev Psychiatry* 9,429–436.

Benes FM (1988). Post-mortem structural analyses of schizophrenic brain. Study designs and the interpretation of data. *Psychiatr Dev* 6,213–226.

Benes FM (1997). The role of stress and dopamine-GABA interactions in the vulnerability for schizophrenia. *J Psychiatr Res* 31,257–275.

Benes FM, Bird ED (1987). An analysis of the arrangement of neurons in the cingulate cortex of schizophrenic patients. *Arch Gen Psychiatry* 44,608–616.

Benes FM, Farol PA, Majocha RE, et al. (1991). Evidence for axonal loss in regions occupied by senile plaques in Alzheimer cortex. *Neuroscience* 42,31–35.

Benes FM, Khan Y, Vincent SL, et al. (1996d). Differences in the subregional and cellular distribution of GABA-A receptor binding in the hippocampal formation of schizophrenic brain. *Synapse* 22,338–349.

Benes FM, Majocha R, Bird ED, et al. (1987a). Increased vertical axon numbers in cingulate cortex of schizophrenics. *Arch Gen Psychiatry* 44,1017–1021.

Benes FM, McSparren J, Bird ED, et al. (1991a). Deficits in small interneurons in prefrontal and anterior cingulate cortex of schizophrenic and schizoaffective patients. *Arch Gen Psychiatry* 48,996–1001.

Benes FM, Sorensen I, Vincent SL, et al. (1992a). Increased density of glutamate-immunoreactive vertical processes in superficial laminae in cingulate cortex of schizophrenic brain. *Cereb Cortex* 2,502–512.

Benes FM, Todtenkopf MS, Taylor JB (1997). Differential distribution of tyrosine hydroxylase fibers on neuronal subtypes in layer II of anterior cingulate cortex of schizophrenic brain. *Synapse* 25,80–92.

Benes FM, Vincent SL, Alsterberg G, et al. (1992b). Increased GABA-A receptor binding in superficial layers of cingulate cortex in schizophrenics. *J Neurosci* 12,924–929.

Benes FM, Vincent S, Marie A, et al. (1996a). Upregulation of GABA-A receptor binding on pyramidal neurons of prefrontal cortex in schizophrenic subjects. *Neuroscience* 75,1021–1031.

Benes FM, Vincent SL, Molloy R, et al. (1996a). Increased interaction of dopamine-immunoreactive varicosities with GABA neurons of rat medial prefrontal cortex occurs during the post-weanling period. *Synapse* 23,237–245.

Benes FM, Wickramasinghe R, Vincent SL, et al. (1997). Uncoupling of $GABA_A$ and benzodiazepine receptor binding activity in the hippocampal formation of schizophrenic brain. *Brain Res* 755,121–129.

Bird ED, Spokes EGS, Iversen LL (1979). Increased dopamine concentration in limbic areas of brain from patients dying with schizophrenia. *Brain* 102,347–360.

Carlsson A (1978a). Does dopamine have a role in schizophrenia? *Biol Psychiatry* 13,3–21.

Carlsson A (1978b). Antipsychotic drugs, neurotransmitters, and schizophrenia. *Am J Psychiatry* 135,164–173.

Carlsson A (1978c). Mechanism of action of neuroleptic drugs. In: *Psychopharmacology: A Generation of Progress*, Lipton M A, DiMascio A, Killam KF, eds. New York: Raven, pp. 1057–1070.

Cotterrell M, Balazs R, Johnson AL. (1972). Effects of corticosteroids on the biochemical maturation of rat brain: postnatal cell formation. *J Neurochem* 19,2151–2167.

deKloet E, Rosenfeld P, van Eekelen J, et al. (1988). Stress, glucocorticoids and development. *Progr Brain Res* 73,101–120.

DeKosky S, Scheff S, Cotman C (1984). Elevated corticosterone levels: a possible cause of reduced axon sprouting in aged animals. *Neuroendocrinology* 38,33–38.

Fride E, Dan Y, Feldon H, et al. (1986). Effects of prenatal stress on vulnerability to stress in prepubertal and adult rats. *Physiol Behav* 37,681–687.

Gilles FH (1983). Telencephalic medium and the olfacto-cerebral outpouching. In: *The Developing Human Brain. Growth and Epidemiologic Neuropathology*, Gilles FH, Leviton A, Dooling EC, eds. Boston: John Wright-PSG, pp. 59–114.

Gottesman II, Shields J (1972). *Schizophrenia and Genetics: A Twin Study Vantage Point*. New York: Academic.

Hanada S, Mita T, Nishinok N, et al. (1987). ^{3}H-muscimol binding sites increased in autopsied brains of chronic schizophrenics. *Life Sci* 40,259–266.

Henn FA, McKinney WT. (1987). Animal models in psychiatry. In: *Psychopharmacology: The Third Generation of Progress*, Meltzer HY, ed. New York: Raven, pp. 687–695.

Holzman PS, Kinglem E, Matthysse S, et al. (1988). A single dominant gene can account for eye tracking dysfunctions and schizophrenia in offspring of discordant twins. *Arch Gen Psychiatry* 45,641–647.

Impagnatiello F, Guidotti AR, Pesold C, et al. (1998). A decrease of reelin expression as a putative vulnerability factor in schizophrenia. *Proc Natl Acad Sci USA* 95,15718–15723.

Iuvone P, Dunn A (1986). Tyrosine hydroxylase activation in mesocortical 3,4-dihydroxyphenylethylamine neurons following footshock. *J Neurochem* 47,837–844.

Jacobsen B, Kinney DK (1980). Perinatal complications in adopted and non-adopted schizophrenics and their controls: preliminary results. *Acta Psychiatr Scand* 238,103–123.

Kalsbeek A, Voorn P, Buijs RM, et al. (1988). Development of the dopaminergic innervation in the prefrontal cortex of rat. *J Comp Neurol* 269,58–72.

Kety S (1983). Mental illness in the biological and adoptive relatives of schizophrenic adoptees: findings relevant to genetic and environmental factors in etiology. *Am J Psychiatry* 140,720–727.

Kety S (1985). Schizotypal personality disorder. An operational definition of Bleuler's latent schizophrenia. *Schizophr Bull* 11,590–594.

Kety S, Matthysse S (1972). Prospects for research on schizophrenia. An overview. *Neurosci Res Bull* 10,456–467.

Kirkpatrick B, Conley RC, Kakoyannis A, et al. (1999). Interstitial cells of the white matter in the inferior parietal cortex in schizophrenia: an unbiased cell-counting study. *Synapse* 34,95–102.

Lambert JJ, Peters JA, Cottrell GA (1987). Actions of synthetic and endogenous steroids on the GABA-A receptor. *Trends Pharmacol Sci* 8,224–227.

Longson D, Deakin JWF, Benes FM (1996). Increased density of entorhinal glutamate-immunoreactive vertical fibers in schizophrenia. *J Neural Transm* 103,503–507.

Majewska MD, Bisserbe J-C, Eskay LR (1985). Glucocorticoids are modulators of GABA-A receptors in brain. *Brain Res* 339,178–182.

Parnas J, Schulsinger F, Teasdale W, et al. (1982). Perinatal complications and clinical outcome. *Br J Psychiatry* 140,416–420.

Penit-Soria J, Audinat E, Crepel F (1987). Excitation of rat prefrontal cortical neurons by dopamine: an in vitro electrophysiological study. *Brain Res* 425,363–374.

Perry TL, Buchanan J, Kish SJ, et al. (1979). Gamma-aminobutyric acid deficiency in brains of schizophrenic patients. *Lancet* 1,237–239.

Retaux S, Besson MJ, Penit-Soria J (1991a). Opposing effects of dopamine D2 receptor stimulation on the spontaneous and the electrically evoked release of [^{3}H]GABA on rat prefrontal cortex slices. *Neuroscience* 42,61–71.

Retaux S, Besson MJ, Penit-Soria J (1991b). Synergism between D1 and D2 dopamine receptors in the inhibition of the evoked release of [^{3}H]GABA in the rat prefrontal cortex. *Neuroscience* 43,323–329.

Reynolds GP, Czudek C, Andrews H (1990). Deficit and hemispheric asymmetry of GABA uptake sites in the hippocampus in schizophrenia. *Biol Psychiatry* 27,1038–1044.

Roth RH, Tam SY, Ida Y, et al. (1988). Stress and the mesocorticolimbic dopamine systems. *Ann NY Acad Sci* 537,138–147.

Sapolsky RM (1992). *Stress, the Aging Brain, and the Mechanisms of Neuron Death.* Cambridge, MA: MIT Press.

Scheff S, Joff S, Anderson K (1986). Altered regulation of lesion-induced synaptogenesis by adrenalectomy and corticosterone in young adult rats. *Exp Neurol* 93,456–470.

Selemon LD, Rajkowska G, Goldman-Rakic PS (1995). Abnormally high neuronal density in the schizophrenic cortex: a morphometric analysis of prefrontal area 9 and occipital area 17. *Arch Gen Psychiatry* 52,805–818.

Simpson MD, Slater P, Deakin JF, et al. (1989). Reduced GABA uptake sites in the temporal lobe in schizophrenia. *Neurosci Lett* 107,211–215.

Stone E, Freedman L, Morgano L (1978). Brain and adrenal tyrosine hydroxylase activity after chronic footshock stress. *Pharmacol Biochem Behav* 9,551–553.

Stone E, McCarty R (1983). Adaptation to stress: tyrosine hydroxylase activity and catecholamine release. *Neurosci Biobehav Rev* 7,29–34.

Takahashi LK, Kalin NH (1991). Early developmental and temporal characteristics of stress-induced secretion of pituitary-adrenal hormones in prenatally stressed rat pups. *Brain Res* 558,75–78.

Thierry AM, Tassin JP, Blanc G, et al. (1976). Selective activation of the mesocortical DA system by stress. *Nature* 263,242–244.

Uno H, Lohmiller L, Thieme C, et al. (1990). Brain damage induced by prenatal exposure to dexamethasone in fetal rhesus macaques. I. Hippocampus. *Dev Brain Res* 53,157–167.

Verney C, Berger B, Adrien J, et al. (1982). Development of the dopaminergic innervation of the rat cerebral cortex. A light microscopic immunocytochemical study using anti-tyrosine hydroxylase antibodies. *Dev Brain Res* 5,41–52.

Vijayan V, Cotman C (1987). Hydrocortisone administration alters glial reaction to entorhinal lesion in the rat dentate gyrus. *Exp Neurol* 96,307.

12.

Dopamine and Related Factors in Schizophrenia and Other Psychoses

Recent Molecular Genetics Studies in China

Dongfeng Zhou, Rulun Zhou, Xianzhang Hu, Xiangyang Zhang, Jianhua Fan, Feng Wei, and Yucun Shen

INTRODUCTION

It has long been suspected that dopamine may be involved in the biology of mental disorders. It is thought that the dopamine system may be up-regulated in schizophrenia. 5-Hydroxytryptamine (5-HT) is an important neurotransmitter in the CNS that is involved in the regulation of sleep and wakefulness. Most antipsychotics such as chlorpromazine act through the dopamine system; some drugs used to treat mental disorders appear to function by means of the 5-HT system, whereas other drugs function by way of both dopamine and 5-HT. Zotepine, resperidone, and olanzapine, the atypical antipsychotics used in schizophrenia, interrupt dopamine receptors but have antiserotonin effects in the CNS.

Dopamine receptors have been divided into five subgroups: D1–D5. Each subgroup has been mapped and cloned (Civelli et al., 1991). Many studies have been published concerning their relationship with the biological background of schizophrenia. In tests that used both familial and sporadic samples and by analyses of both association and linkage methods, most results were negative. There were, however, some positive findings regarding possible contributions of dopamine receptor genes, such as a relationship between dopamine D2 and schizophrenia (Arinami et al., 1996).

We believe there are four reasons for the overwhelming number of negative reports: 1) the heterogeneity of schizophrenia may make the samples diverse in their genetic background; 2) the sample scale may not be large enough to ensure a definite result; 3) different diagnosis criteria were adopted and application of the same standard may not be the same; and 4) the dopamine system itself may be just one of several pathways involved in schizophrenia.

In our studies, we collected familial and sporadic schizophrenic patients and tested both dopamine receptors and some enzymes or neurotransmitters that may serve as cofactors of dopamine receptors at the gene level. Considering the relationship between the dopamine system and CNS inflammatory mediators, we tested some cytokines such as interleukin (IL)-2, -6, and -8 and superoxide dismutase. We also tested those candidate genes in mental disorders such as alcoholism. This chapter summarizes this research.

MATERIALS AND METHODS

Sample Collection

Familial samples for schizophrenia consist mainly of nuclear families that include at least two schizophrenic siblings and their parents. The first stage collection took place in 1991. The present symptoms examination was used in interviews, and diagnosis was made according to ICD-9/10 and the Chinese criteria for mental disorders, second release. The second stage collection took place in 1998. For the second collection the family investigation for genetics of schizophrenia and diagnosis instrument for genetics of schizophrenia were adopted, and the diagnosis was made according to DSM-IV. More than 100 families were collected through coordination of several sites in China. Familial samples for alcoholism were separately collected in the Beijing area; the diagnosis of alcoholism was made according to DSM-IV.

Sporadic samples of schizophrenia were collected since 1994 for genetic studies. Different research programs used samples collected on their own because they use different criteria.

Different controls were correspondingly collected in China. All samples are Chinese Han. The Han are the world's largest ethnic group and comprise about 91% of the entire population of China.

Genotyping

Genome DNA was obtained through standard techniques from 5–10 ml peripheral blood extracted from each subject. Primers for polymerase chain reaction were synthesized according to literature reports [dopamine D2 receptor (DRD2), monoamine oxidase (MAO)-A, catechol-*O*-methyltransferase (COMT), 5-HT, cholecystokinin (CCK)] and were self-designed (DRD2 promoter). Polymerase chain reaction was performed in a total volume of 25 μl containing 10 ng genomic DNA, 2.5 pmol/μl of each primer, 50 mM KCl, 10 mM Tris-HCl (pH 9.0), 1.5 mM MgCl2, 200 μM each of dATP, dCTP, dGTP, and dTTP (for detection of dinucleotide polymorphism: 50 μM each of dATP, dGTP, and dTTP and 10 μCi α-^{32}P-dCTP), and 0.5 units Taq polymerase. Amplification was performed for 30–35 cycles. Polymerase chain reaction products were subjected to enzyme digestion for restriction fragment length polymorphism genotyping (Cfra 13 I for DRD2, EcoR V for MAO-A, Nla III for COMT, Msp I or Hpa II for 5-HT, Pst I for CCK, and Mae III for DRD2 promoter).

Variable numbers of tandem repeats (VNTR) such as the $(CA)_n$ polymorphisms of DRD2 are detected by separating the polymerase chain reaction products through electrophoresis on 12% polyacrylamide gels for VNTR genotyping. DNA ladders and some previously determined standard DNA samples were used in restriction fragment length polymorphism genotyping and microsatellite genotyping, to determine fragment sizes of our subjects. Genes and corresponding polymorphisms are listed in Table 12-1.

TABLE 12-1. Genes and corresponding polymorphisms

Gene	Polymorphism
DRD2	Ser311Cys
DRD2	$(CA)_n$
D2P	A241G
MAO-A	EcoR V
COMT	Val108Met
5-HT_{2a}	T102C
CCK	Pst I

Biochemical Analysis

All biochemical tests were made using the corresponding assay kits. Tests of IL-6 and IL-8 were performed by enzyme-linked immunosorbent assay, and tests of IL-2 and superoxide dismutase were conducted with radioactive labeled bioantibodies.

Statistical Analysis

General information and genotype were used to establish a simple database. We used Epi Info Version 6.04b from the World Health Organization, SPSS release 8, and some small programs established by our colleagues for statistical software. We performed association analysis, linkage analysis, and linkage disequilibrium analysis using our genotyping results.

RESULTS

We have measured the dopamine D2 Ser311Cys polymorphism in 105 schizophrenics and 108 controls. The distribution of Ser311/Cys311 allele had no significant difference between samples and controls, whereas the schizophrenics with Cys311 tended to have a lower age of onset and a positive family history. The Ser311→Cys311 variant may affect the onset of some subtypes of schizophrenia.

The allele frequencies of the VNTR polymorphism of DRD2 gene have been tested in 28 Chinese schizophrenic families and eight control families. The schizophrenic families consisted of 112 individuals, including 63 who were affected; the average age of the 112 individuals was 42.5 ± 14.3 years. The control families consisted of 45 normal individuals with an average age of 40.8 ± 13.6 years. Four fragments that have 13 to 16 times the number of CA repeats [$(CA)_{13}$, $(CA)_{14}$, $(CA)_{15}$, and $(CA)_{16}$] have been detected. Association analyses showed that there were statistical differences in the distribution of the four alleles between the two groups of familial members. The difference was mainly between schizophrenic siblings and normal siblings and in $(CA)_{14}$ and $(CA)_{15}$ alleles.

The Mae III polymorphism of dopamine receptor 2 promoter gene (DRD2P) was tested in 42 Han pedigrees where there were at least two schizophrenic-affected siblings according to ICD-10 criteria and at most only one living parent with a history of schizophrenia. The samples include 85 parents, 94 schizophrenic siblings, and 46 nonaffected siblings. The transmission disequilibrium test showed no transmission disequilibrium among affected siblings. But we found that more "–241A" allele, which could not be cut off by Mae III, was transmitted to nonaffected siblings.

The EcoR V polymorphism of MAO-A, which was suggested to affect activity of CNS dopamine function, was tested in the 42 familial samples. Results show that the T941G polymorphism shows transmission disequilibrium among the schizophrenics. The 941G/941G genotype is significantly positively correlative to symptoms such as delusions, thought disorders, or emotional disorders.

The distribution of alleles or genotypes of the COMT gene is not significantly different among groups of parents, unaffected siblings, and affected siblings, between genders, and among the subtypes of schizophrenia. The transmission disequilibrium test does not show transmission disequilibrium in affected siblings but in unaffected siblings. There are significant relations between COMT genotypes and delusion, affective disorders, depersonalization, disorganized behaviors, thought form disorders, and irritation.

The 5-HT_{2a} receptor T102C polymorphism was tested in 42 nuclear pedigrees with at least two schizophrenic-affected siblings according to ICD-10. The distribution of alleles is not significantly different among the groups of parents, unaffected siblings, and affected siblings, between genders, and among the subgroups of schizophrenia. Transmission disequilibrium test analysis did not show transmission disequilibrium in these families.

To investigate the CCK-A receptor, the function of which is closely related to that of dopamine in CNS, 84 sporadic male schizophrenics and 70 male normal controls were tested with a Pst I polymorphism at the boundary region of intron 1 and exon 2 of CCK-A gene. There is significant difference between patients with hallucination-delusion syndrome and those without ($P = 0.036$). There was also significant difference in genotype frequency between schizophrenic patients with and without the first- and second-level family psychiatric history.

To investigate CNS dopamine function, we measured basal prolactin and its response to paroxetin stimulating test in plasma before and after 12 weeks of typical antipsychotic haloperidol and atypical antipsychotic risperidone in schizophrenics. We found the prolactin level in the patients before treatment was lower than in normal controls, and after treatment with both drugs, the prolactin level and its response to paroxetin were increased significantly from those before and from those in controls. Results suggest that CNS dopamine function is elevated and that after antipsychotics it is suppressed.

We also tested the VNTR polymorphism of DRD2 and EcoR V polymorphism of MAO-A in nine high-risk alcoholic families that possess at least two alcoholics and eight control families paired in age, gender distribution, and living standards. For DRD2, distribution of the alleles, especially the $(CA)_{15}$ allele in the alcoholic families, shows statistical difference contrasted to that of controls. For MAO-A, the allele frequency of MAOA*1 was significantly higher in the alcoholic families than in controls ($P < 0.01$, odds ratio 2.37). The allele frequency of MAOA*1 in males is also significantly higher in alcoholic families than in controls ($P < 0.05$, odds ratio 2.56). The nonalcoholic males in alcoholic families also show higher frequency of MAOA*1 compared with those in control families.

Among 78 sporadic schizophrenics, it was found that IL-2 ($P = 0.0001$) and IL-8 ($P = 0.006$) showed a negative association with schizophrenia, whereas IL-6 ($P = 0.024$) showed a positive association with schizophrenia. In 33 schizophrenic inpatients, superoxide dismutase levels showed positive association with N factor ($P = 0.025$) and G factor ($P = 0.012$) of the positive and negative symptom scale.

DISCUSSION

Schizophrenia has a complex biological background. The relationship between the dopamine system and schizophrenia has been extensively studied, and it is accepted that schizophrenia is associated with some dysfunction of dopaminergic neurotransmission. Nevertheless most tests about the dopamine system at the genetic level yield negative results. We may consider several reasons for this situation: 1) schizophrenia may not be a single disease—it may be a syndrome or a disease complex; 2) the heterogeneity background of schizophrenia results in various subtypes; and 3) the dopamine system is just a small part of the whole pathway in the etiology of schizophrenia. Alternatively, the dopamine system may have a key role in the pathogenesis of schizophrenia, in conjunction with various factors. In our studies we examined cytokines as other factors that may be involved in schizophrenia.

There has been evidence that the DRD2 is involved in human psychoses, especially schizophrenia (Seeman, 1992; Seeman and Lee, 1975). A series of linkage studies, however, has so far provided no support for a major gene that may cosegregate with schizophrenia (Grassi et al., 1996; Kalsi et al., 1995; Moises et al., 1991). Some analysts still thought that a gene of major effect may exist within the dopamine D2 region, although the result was negative (Mulcrone et al., 1995). For the locus D11S35, positive results were derived from an association study (Hattori et al., 1993) as well as from a linkage study (Maziade et al., 1995). However, most previous studies examined Caucasians as research subjects, and accumulated data have shown salient differences among ethnic groups.

In our study, we tested the Ser311Cys polymorphism. This polymorphism lies in the middle of the third intracellular loop of the short form of the DRD2, which can modulate or participate in receptor-G-protein interaction. Replacement of Ser311 with Cys311 can affect regulation of desensitization and internalization of the receptor. It may also produce a conformational change of the receptor protein by forming a new disulfide bond. After considering the pharmacological importance of DRD2, this polymorphism should be highly suspected. Although our test did not get a positive result, we think it may be valuable to expand our sample scale and make a further division. For the VNTR test, the main difference was in schizophrenic siblings and controls for the frequencies of $(CA)_{13}$ and $(CA)_{14}$ alleles of DRD2. In the schizophrenic families, $(CA)_{16}$ allele frequency showed a difference between fathers and mothers. Within these families, we had two affected fathers and five affected mothers; the latter were more than the former, but definitive conclusions cannot be reached because of the limited sample scale.

Polymorphism of the MAO-A gene was investigated in 42 pedigrees with at least two schizophrenic siblings. There was no significant difference of frequencies of alleles or genotype among parents, unaffected siblings, and affected siblings. However, more 941G allele transmission in affected siblings was found through transmission disequilibrium test analysis. This suggested that there is association between schizophrenia and polymorphism of MAO-A gene or between a locus in linkage disequilibrium with it. Hotamisligil and Breakefield (1991) suggested that the EcoR V polymorphism may be involved in regulation of the activity of MAO-A in which the EcoR V positive type showed a higher activity (odds ratio 6.0). Biochemical research (Cesura and Pletscher, 1992) illustrated that the substrates of MAO-A consist mainly of norepinephrine and 5-HT, whereas the clinical pharmacological data showed that the antihypertensive drug reserpine takes effect by exhausting both CA and 5-HT. It is therefore reasonable to regard 5-HT as a candidate gene.

The Mae III polymorphism, which is caused by an A to G mutation in the –241 position, showed a positive association with schizophrenia. This result was reached through a transmission disequilibrium test. DRD2 is the target for a wide range of neuroleptic drugs (Crese et al., 1976). This test shows a different result compared with that from the Ser311Cys analysis. This time, the sample exceeded 100 sib-pair families, but the Ser311Cys test only used about 100 sporadic schizophrenics. Concerning the sample scale, we think the present results are more definitive based on the larger sample size.

The frequent negative findings regarding the relationship between dopamine and schizophrenia have many possible reasons. The enzymes in the metabolism of dopamine are involved in the dopamine pathway. Besides MAO, COMT is another candidate. In our results, the high activity Val158 allele of COMT itself, or its adjacent genes, may be involved in protecting individuals from schizophrenia.

We did not find that the distributions of 5-HT_{2a} receptor alleles are significantly different among the groups of parents, nonaffected siblings, and affected siblings. The same type of finding was observed between different genders and between the subtypes of schizophrenia on the frequency of the 5-HT_{2a} receptor gene. (Table 12-2).

We plan to replicate our findings in a larger sample. In the present study of CCK-A, unlike the previous findings (Grassi et al., 1996), we found no significant association of the CCK-A receptor gene with auditory hallucinations in a Chinese population. This suggests at least two possibilities: 1) the genes for schizophrenia may not specifically determine a single psychotic symptom; 2) ethnic cultures may influence clinical expression of a schizophrenic illness. Because both the hallucination-delusion syndrome and auditory hallucinations are the positive symptoms common in

TABLE 12-2. Summary of studies

Ref.	No. of schizophrenics	No. of controls	Ethnic group	*P*
Williams (1996)	571	639	European	0.008
Tay (1997)	101	103	Chinese	0.015
Chen (19963)	177	98	Chinese	NS
Shinkai (1998)	106	109	Japanese	NS

schizophrenia, it could be hypothesized that the CCK-A receptor gene may be associated with the positive symptoms of schizophrenia. In a recent study conducted with a large sample, we also found that the CCK-A receptor gene was significantly associated with the hallucination-delusion syndrome in a Caucasian population (W. Jun et al., unpublished data). Further investigation will be conducted with a larger sample in both Caucasian and Chinese populations to determine if the CCK-A receptor gene is associated with other psychotic symptoms.

Dopamine interacts with various informational substances in the CNS. The role of cytokines has been examined in schizophrenia. For example, IL-2 can affect dopamine levels in the CNS (Licinio et al., 1993; Petitto et al., 1977). In addition to cytokines, free radicals have also been thought to be involved in schizophrenia (Reddy et al., 1991). Available evidence supports the concept that free radicals may increase dopamine levels (Cadet and Lohr, 1987). Our results on IL-2, -6, and -8 and superoxide dismutase also suggest such a possibility.

REFERENCES

Arinami T, Itokawa M, Aoki J, et al. (1996). Further association study on dopamine D2 receptor variant S311C in schizophrenia and affective disorders. *Am J Med Genet (Neuropsychiatr Genet)* 67,133–138.

Cadet Jl, Lohr JB (1987). Free radicals and the developmental pathobiology of schizophrenic burnout. *Integr Psychiatry* 5,40–48.

Cesura AM, Pletscher A (1992). The new generation of monoamine oxidase inhibitors. *Progr Drug Res* 38,171.

Chen CH, Lee YR, Liu MY, et al. (1996). Identification of a BglI polymorphism of catechol-O-methyltransferase(COMT) gene and association study with schizophrenia. *Am J Med Genet* 67,556–559.

Civelli O, Bunzow JR, Grandy DK, et al. (1991). Molecular biology of dopamine receptors. *Eur J Pharmacol* 207,277–286.

Coon H, Byerley W, Holik J, et al. (1993). Linkage analysis in schizophrenia with five dopamine receptor genes in nine pedigrees. *Am J Hum Genet* 52,327–334.

Crese I, Burt DR, Snyder SH (1976) . Dopamine receptor binding predicts clinical and pharmacological potencies of antischizophrenic drugs. *Science* 192,481–483.

Grassi E, Mortilla M, Amaducci L, et al. (1996). No evidence of linkage between schizophrenia and D2 dopamine receptor gene locus in Italian pedigrees. *Neurosci Lett* 206,196–198.

Hattori M, Kuwata S, Tokunaga K, et al. (1993). Association study of schizophrenia with D11S35 and dopamine D2 receptor gene loci using dinucleotide repeat polymorphisms. *Psychiatry Genet* 3,247–252.

Hotamisligil GS, Breakefield XO (1991). Human monoamine oxidase A gene determines levels of enzyme activity. *Am J Hum Genet* 49,383.

Kalsi G, Mankoo BS, Curtis D, et al. (1995). Exclusion of linkage of schizophrenia to the gene for the dopamine D2 receptor (DRD2) and chromosome 11q translocation sites. *Psychol Med* 25,531–537.

Licinio J, Seibyl JP, Altemus M, et al. (1993). Elevated CSF levels of interleukin-2 in neuroleptic free schizophrenia patients. *Am J Psychiatry* 150,1408–1410.

Maziade M, Raymond V, Cliche D, et al. (1995). Linkage result on 11Q21-22 in Eastern Quebec pedigrees densely affected by schizophrenia. *Am J Med Genet (Neuropsychiatr Genet)* 60,522–528.

Moises HW, Gelernter J, Giuffra LA, et al. (1991). No linkage between D2 dopamine receptor gene region and schizophrenia. *Arch Gen Psychiatry* 48,643–647.

Mulcrone J, Whatley SA, Marchbanks R, et al. (1995). Genetic linkage analysis markers in Israeli pedigrees. *Am J Med Genet* 60,103–108.

Petitto JM, McCarthy DB, Rinker CM, et al. (1977). Modulation of behavioral and neurochemical measures of forebrain dopamine function in mice by species-specific interleukin-2. *J Neuroimmunol* 73,183–190.

Reddy R, Mahadik SP, Mukherjee S, et al. (1991). Enzymes of the antioxidant defense system in chronic schizophrenic patients. *Biol Psychiatry* 30,409–412.

Seeman P (1992). Dopamine receptor sequences. *Neuropsychopharmacology* 7,261–284.

Seeman P, Lee T, (1975). Antipsychotic drugs: direct correlation between clinical potency and presynaptic action on dopamine neurons. *Science* 188,1217–1219.

Shinkai T, Ohmori O, Kojima H, et al. (1998). 5-HT2a receptor gene and schizophrenia. *Hum Hered* 48,212–215.

Tay AHN, Lim LCC, Lee WL, et al. (1997). Association between allele 1 of T102C polymorphism, 5-hydroxytryptamine-2a receptor gene and schizophrenia in Chinese males in Singapore. *Hum Hered* 47,298–300.

Williams J, Spurlockj G, Mcguffin P, et al. (1996). Association between schizophrenia and T102C polymorphism of the 5-hydroxytryptamine type 2a-receptor gene. *Lancet* 347,1294–1296.

13.

Dopamine System

Reward and Behavior

Richard P. Ebstein, Jonathan Benjamin, Inga Gritsenko, and Moshe Kotler

ABSTRACT

We discuss the concept of reward, as understood from animal experiments, and extend this concept to humans. We also examine human genetics studies suggesting that common dopaminergic polymorphisms contribute to individual differences in personality traits and the propensity for substance abuse, kindred phenomena grounded in the mesolimbic motive circuit. The mesolimbic dopamine system constituting the motive circuit is strongly implicated in the habit-forming properties of several abused drugs, suggesting a common ground for addictions. Addictive drugs would then appear to mimic aspects of the natural reinforcers and interact with identical brain reward mechanisms. The motivational and reinforcement value that people attribute to appetitive environmental events clearly differs among individuals. Differences in personality traits (especially novelty seeking and harm avoidance) reflect and partially determine individual motivational states and the value individuals attach to environmental reward cues. Many recent genetics studies suggest that common dopaminergic polymorphisms explain some variance in personality traits. Novelty seeking is a personality trait that seems to govern how much stimulation is needed from environmental events to reach optimal arousal. Thrill seekers need more stimulation than the average; some obtain stimulation by bungee jumping and others in less socially acceptable ways such as substance abuse. Genetics studies illuminate the neural basis of these differences in individual motivational states and suggest that common polymorphisms in the DRD4, dopamine transporter, serotonin transporter promoter region, and catechol-*O*-methyltransferase enzyme influence dopaminergic tone in the brain.

INTRODUCTION

It would seem a daunting task to clarify the physiological, anatomical, and neurochemical bases of the complex phenomenon of reward-directed behavior. Nevertheless marked progress has been made in all three areas in the past decade. Several recent reviews summarize current knowledge regarding the central role played by dopaminergic neurons in this "motive" circuit and the particular importance of these systems in the phenomenon of addiction (Kalivas and Nakamura, 1999; Robbins and Everitt, 1996; Schultz, 1997; Wise, 1996a). We will discuss the concept of reward, as understood from animal experiments, and attempt to extend this concept to humans. We will also discuss recent human genetics studies suggesting that common dopaminergic polymorphisms contribute to individual differences in personality traits and the propensity for substance abuse, kindred phenomena grounded in the mesolimbic motive circuit.

PLEASURE IN PEOPLE VERSUS INCENTIVE-MOTIVATION AND REINFORCEMENT IN RATS

Robbins and Everitt (1996) suggest that one eventual goal of behavioral neuroscience is the elucidation of the neurobiological basis of subjective phenomena, e.g., what constitutes pleasure in humans. Most current ideas of pleasure (a "human" notion) and its correlate concept, reward, are based on animal experiments. There is a gap between the Skinnerian operational definition of a reinforcer (event that increases the probability of an instrumental response) and subjective human states such as pleasure, although these terms likely refer to the same phenomenon. Indeed, Robbins and Everitt prefer to restrict the terminology to more objective concepts such as the neural basis of incentive-motivation and reinforcement because they feel reward has too many subjective connotations.

REWARD—AN ENVIRONMENTAL EVENT WITH MOTIVATIONAL VALUE

Reward (or incentive-motivation and reinforcement, per Robbins and Everitt) can be considered as the motivational value that an organism attaches to an environmental event (e.g., encounters with a member of the opposite sex or with a food supply) that is important to the welfare and survival of the individual or species—see Schultz (1997). Rewards are typically appetitive events (as opposed to aversive events that also have motivational values). Appetitive objects induce two forms of behavioral reactions: an initial preparatory approach behavior, which can be similar for different objects and serves to more closely inspect the appetitive object and prepare for its consumption, and a final consummatory behavior that is more specific (sex versus drinking) for the particular appetitive object encountered. The neurochemical and neuroanatomical bases of approach and consummatory reward-directed behaviors might be distinct.

NUCLEUS ACCUMBENS—THE MOTIVE CIRCUIT'S COMPUTER

Our understanding of the neuroanatomical substrate of brain reward mechanisms has been elucidated by the discovery of intracranial self-stimulation that allowed mapping of positively and negatively reinforcing brain sites in the mesocortical limbic system (amygdala, septum, and prefrontal cortex as well as the catecholaminergic neuronal projections from the brainstem). The nucleus accumbens (now known to be divided into core and shell components) is viewed as a primary anatomical locus for integrating cortical (amygdala and prefrontal cortex) and subcortical (ventral tegmental area-substantia nigra zona compacta) information via γ-aminobutyric acid

(GABA)-ergic, glutamatergic, and particularly dopaminergic input. The ventral pallidum is viewed as the primary output nucleus communicating with classic motor systems. Thus this limbic-ventral-striatopallidal system presumably provides a neural mechanism by which motivation gets translated into action. Reinforcement can be viewed as a form of interaction between the excitatory amino acid (glutamatergic) inputs from these limbic afferents and the ascending dopamine system, which together determine output of the ventral striatal GABAergic medium spiny neurons projecting to the globus pallidus (ventral pallidum).

DOPAMINE NEURONS IN MOTIVE CIRCUIT RESPOND TO NOVELTY AND THE UNPREDICTABLE

Schultz (1997) focuses on the neurophysiological responses of individual dopaminergic neurons to primary rewards and reward-predicting stimuli. Schultz emphasizes that the learning process in appetitive behavior (preparatory-approach) depends on the unpredictability of primary appetitive events. Only unpredicted primary appetitive events are effective for conditioning; no further learning occurs when the reward is entirely predicted. Deviations or errors between the predicted and the actually experienced reward drive learning.

Individual dopamine neurons in the pars compacta of the substantia nigra and ventral tegmental area (neurons that project to nucleus accumbens) do not distinguish between different primary food rewards and reward predicting, appetitive conditioned audio or visual stimuli. Most interesting is that these dopamine neurons are activated by repeated novel stimuli. Responses of the dopamine neurons depend entirely on the unpredictability of stimuli and respond to reward stimuli only when the reward occurs outside of a task or during learning. By contrast, a fully predicted reward does not activate dopamine neurons. In situations requiring repeated learning, dopamine neurons are activated by primary rewards during each learning phase but cease responding to the reward when the learning curve reaches its asymptote and the reward becomes fully predictable. Consequently, dopamine neurons are seen to constitute a scalar, global reinforcement signal that is broadcast simultaneously to most postsynaptic neurons in the striatum and to a large proportion of neurons in the frontal cortex.

The three most important inputs modulating activation and depression of dopamine neurons to appetitive stimuli appear to be 1) excitatory, cholinergic, and glutamergic input from the nucleus pedunculopontius, 2) a monosynaptic GABAergic inhibitory input from the striatum, and 3) a double inhibitory, net activating influence from the striatum, which releases dopamine neurons from tonic inhibition, involving GABAergic inhibitory striatonigral projections to inhibitory pars reticulata output neurons, with local collaterals to dopamine neurons.

NEURAL SUBSTRATE OF REWARD MECHANISMS MEDIATES ADDICTIVE BEHAVIOR

Addiction offers a good model of addictive behavior, and further understanding of the neural substrate of reward mechanisms was due to the discovery that the reinforcing effects of psychomotor stimulant drugs such as amphetamine and cocaine were primarily mediated by dopamine dependent mechanisms of the ventral striatum (Wise, 1996b). In early addiction research the predominant concept of addiction was that compulsive drug self-administration was due to the drug's ability to alleviate aversive withdrawal symptoms (negative reinforcement model). Recent theories underscore the role of drugs in positive reinforcement and euphoria. Studies with self-stimulation demonstrated that drugs such as amphetamine that do not entail physical dependence were addictive owing to their positive reinforcement value that is mediated by dopamine release in the motive and brain reward circuits. The mesolimbic dopamine system is strongly implicated in the habit-forming properties of several classes of abused drugs (alcohol, nicotine, opiates, stimulants, phenylcyclidine, and cannibinoids), suggesting a common ground for addictions. Addictive drugs then appear to mimic aspects of the natural reinforcers and interact with identical brain reward mechanisms.

Withdrawal from the various drugs that activate the mesolimbic dopamine system and potentiate the rewarding effects of lateral hypothalamic electrical stimulation causes rebound depression of the mechanism of positive reinforcement. Such withdrawal symptoms involving depression of the brain motive circuitry are common denominators of addictive drugs and may contribute to drug seeking behavior. Experimental evidence for this concept is based on microdialysis experiments showing that dopamine depletion can accompany withdrawal from chronic intoxication with cocaine, amphetamine, opiates, and ethanol.

REWARD MECHANISMS IN HUMANS: RELATIONSHIP TO PERSONALITY TRAITS AND COGNITION

Rat and mouse studies provide a bland view of behavior in which individual differences between organisms have rarely been examined. Conversely, a critical issue regarding correlated human behaviors is the neural basis for *differences* among people. The motivational and reinforcement values that people attribute to particular environmental events and stimuli clearly differ among individuals. Such personality traits combine with situational manipulations to produce motivational states that in turn affect cognitive performance (Revelle, 1989). To some extent individual differences in learning affectively valenced material are thought to occur at the encoding stage and may be related to differential sensitivities to rewards and punishments. The encoding of environmental demands reflects differences in biological sensitivities to cues for rewards and punishment as suggested by Gray (1981) as well as the prior contents of memory. In the past two decades it has become possible to assess such differences and attribute them to underlying neural mechanisms.

Zuckerman (1994) cogently discusses the notion that sensation seeking [or novelty seeking (NS)] is a primary drive in animals and humans. Sensation seeking has its expression in human personality and furthermore is closely linked to brain reward mechanisms. Arousal theories propose that low intensities of stimulation tend to evoke approach reactions, and high intensities of stimulation evoke withdrawal reactions. Approach-withdrawal has also been identified as a fundamental trait in human neonates and infants and may be the first manifestation of sensation seeking in humans. Any stimuli (not necessarily primary reward objects such as sex or food) possess motivational value, a property not only of stimulus intensity but also of arousal potential. Arousal potential represents the capacity of stimuli to command attention, excite the nervous system, or influence behavior. Arousal potential is particularly dependent on novelty, degree of change from preceding stimulation, suddenness of change, surprise, incongruity, and uncertainty. The motive circuit in the brain provides the neuroanatomical and neurochemical basis for the reward value of arousing stimuli.

It has been suggested that stable, individual differences in optimal levels of stimulus arousal preference serve as the foundation for basic human personality traits. For example, Eysenck (1967) proposed that extroverts require higher levels of stimulation compared with introverts and because such a high level is not provided by routine environments they tend to seek sensation. Introverts reach optimal levels of arousal at lower levels of stimulation than the population average. Differences between extroverts and introverts are presumed to be due to individual variations in background, nonstimulated, or tonic levels of arousal. Such tonic levels of arousal may be determined at least partially by common genetic polymorphisms.

Gray (1981) generalized from a model of rat learning to propose a neuropsychological basis for anxiety and a revision of Eysenck's theory of introversion-extroversion and neuroticism. In brief, Gray proposed that individuals differ in their sensitivities to cues for reward with a behavioral activation system and the sensitivity to cues for punishment with a behavioral inhibition system. He associates impulsivity with the activation system and anxiety with the inhibition system.

SELF-REPORT PERSONALITY QUESTIONNAIRES MEASURE NOVELTY SEEKING

Impulsive, unsocialized sensation seeking is a major factor discovered in factor analyses of scales used in psychobiological research and appears as a higher order factor in most self-report questionnaires (Zuckerman, 1994). Zuckerman's sensation seeking is strongly convergent with Eysenck's P dimension, conscientiousness in the "big five" (impulsiveness in the big five is a subscale of neuroticism), and the trait of NS in the tridimensional personality questionnaire (TPQ) of Cloninger (1987). Factor analyses suggest that sensation seeking together with impulsivity and asocial tendencies constitute the third dimension of personality that Eysenck called "psychoticism." Risk taking for the sake of novel experience is part of the definition of sensation seeking and includes both physical risk-taking and a broader concept of legal, social, and financial risk-taking. High scorers on TPQ NS are exploratory and curious, impulsive, extravagant, and enthusiastic as well as disorderly. The NS personality trait is defined by such statements as, "I often try new things just for fun or thrills, even if most people think it is a waste of time," or "When nothing new is happening, I usually start looking for something that is thrilling or exciting."

GENES AND PERSONALITY

Many twin studies demonstrate that 1) personality traits measured by self-report questionnaires show moderate heritability and 2) almost all environmental variance is nonshared, although environmental influence is also important (Loehlin, 1992). Heritabilities in the 30–50% range are typical. Extroversion, a trait akin to sensation seeking, is one of the most highly heritable categories (~50%), closely followed by neuroticism, akin to harm avoidance or emotional stability (~40%).

DOPAMINE D4 RECEPTOR AND NOVELTY SEEKING

Only recently has an association between a specific genetic polymorphism and a specific personality trait, NS, been reported (Benjamin et al., 1996; Ebstein et al., 1996). Our seminal study catalyzed many investigations by others, and we aimed to validate these first reports and identify other genes that contribute to personality factors.

The two initial studies reported simultaneously by Benjamin et al. (1996) and Ebstein et al. (1996) examined the role of the exon III 48 base pair repeat dopamine D4 receptor (DRD4) polymorphism (Lichter et al., 1993; Van Tol et al., 1992) in personality. This gene has a highly polymorphic 16 amino acid repeat region in the putative third cytoplasmic loop that varies between 2 and 10 repeats in most populations and changes the length of the receptor protein. There is some evidence that the long and short forms of this protein have a moderate functional significance (Asghari et al., 1994, 1995). Two designs were used. The Israeli study (Epstein et al., 1996) was a case-control design, whereas the group's sample of Benjamin et al. (1996) also included many sib pairs allowing for both a between- and within-families design. Both studies suggested an association between NS and the long alleles of the DRD4. Although some subsequent studies confirmed our initial findings (Kuhn et al., 1999; Noble et al., 1997; Ono et al., 1997; Strobel et al., 1999), others did not (Gelernter et al., 1997; Jonsson et al., 1997; Malhotra et al., 1996; Vanderbergh et al., 1997).

Note, however, that three recent studies appear to confirm the relevancy of the DRD4 gene to NS. A Japanese group has characterized several polymorphisms in the upstream promoter region of the DRD4 gene, and one of these was associated with higher NS scores in a group of Japanese subjects (Okuyama et al., 2000). This particular promoter region polymorphism is functionally significant, and the T variant of the C-521T polymorphism reduces transcriptional efficiency. In a second study, a Finnish group has shown an association between the DRD4 exon III 2 and 5 repeat alleles and high NS scores in a large and homogeneous Finnish birth cohort of more than 4,700 subjects (Ekelund et al., in press). Both these studies suggest that our original observation of an association between the DRD4 48 base pair repeat region and TPQ NS (Ebstein et al, 1996) may have been due to linkage disequilibrium between this polymorphism and another polymorphism within the DRD4 gene (the promoter region?) or in a neighboring gene. Finally, the first genome-wide scan in personality genetics in a group of alcoholic families discussed above (Cloninger et al., 1998), which reported a linkage between anxiety-related traits and a region on chr 8p, also observed a linkage between NS and the region on chr 11 where the DRD4 gene is located. This finding is being replicated in the second panel from this cohort (C.R. Cloninger, personal communication).

SEROTONIN TRANSPORTER PROMOTER REGION POLYMORPHISM AND NEUROTICISM

After our report of an association between DRD4 and NS, Heils et al. (1996) showed an association between a newly discovered 44 base pair deletion in the promoter region of the serotonin transporter promoter region (5-HTTLPR) affecting transcription of the gene (Heils et al., 1996, 1997) and the personality trait of neuroticism or harm avoidance. Three subsequent reports replicated the initial association (Murakami et al., 1999; Ricketts et al., 1998), whereas two studies rendered somewhat ambiguous results (Gelernter et al., 1998; Mazzanti et al., 1998). Other studies failed to show an association (Ball et al., 1997; Ebstein et al., 1997a; Gustaysson et al., 1999; Hamilton et al., 1999; Kumakiri et al., 1999; Sander et al., 1997a).

DOPAMINE D4 RECEPTOR AND PSYCHOPATHOLOGY

A complementary strategy for examining the role of polymorphic genes such as DRD4 in contributing to particular personality traits such as NS is to study these genes in disorders characterized by extremes of such behaviors. Two DSM disorders, in particular, substance abuse and attention deficit hyperactivity disorder (ADHD), show exaggerated elements of impulsive and excitable behavior somewhat akin to TPQ NS. Most interesting is that adult ADHD subjects score higher on and are comorbid for substance abuse, antisocial personality disorder, and depressive disorders (Downey et al., 1996, 1997). NS is pronounced in substance abusers, who score higher in this dimension than control subjects (Cloninger et al., 1995; Mel et al., 1998; Pomerleau et al., 1992).

SUBSTANCE ABUSE AND DOPAMINE D4 RECEPTOR

The role of dopamine in mediating TPQ NS in humans and this neurotransmitter's importance in mediating drug reinforcement and reward mechanisms in many animal studies (Koob et al., 1997) prompted us to examine a group of Israeli heroin addicts for prevalence of the DRD4 repeat polymorphism. We demonstrated that the 7-repeat allele is significantly overrepresented in the opioid-dependent cohort and confers a relative risk of 2.46 (Kotler et al., 1997). To our knowledge this was the first report of an association between a specific genetic polymorphism and opioid addiction. A subsequent study we conducted confirmed an excess of the 7-repeat allele in another group of heroin addicts (Mel et al., 1998). Similar results showing an excess of the long alleles (>5) of the DRD4 were obtained in a group of Chinese heroin addicts (Li et al., 1997). Although the 7-repeat is rare in Asian populations, the only two 7-repeats observed were among the addicts.

The DRD4 polymorphism has also been examined in a study of alcoholism that illustrated the importance of gene interactions in determining such phenotypes. A point mutation in the aldehyde dehydrogenase 2 gene (ALDH2) allele is considered a genetic deterrent for alcoholism. Nevertheless 80 of 655 Japanese alcoholics had the protective ALDH2 allele (Muramatsu et al., 1996). Genotype factors that might increase susceptibility by overriding the deterrent included a higher frequency of a five repeat allele of the DRD4 polymorphism in alcoholics with ALDH2 than in 100 other alcoholics and 144 controls. Alcoholics with the 5 repeat allele also abused other drugs more often than those without this polymorphism.

Shields et al. (1998) examined the DRD4 genotype for an association with smoking in subjects after a single minimal-contact session of smoking cessation counseling who were then followed for up to 1 year. African-Americans (n = 72) who had at least one DRD4 long allele had a higher risk of smoking (odds ratio 7.7; P = 0.006), waited less time for the first cigarette in the morning (P = 0.03), and started smoking younger (P = 0.09) than homozygote genotypes for the short-short alleles. After smoking cessation counseling, no African-American smoker with a long DRD4 allele was abstinent at 2 months, compared with 35% of the smokers homozygote for the short genotype (P = 0.02).

The analysis of Caucasians did not suggest a similar smoking risk for the DRD4 genotypes. If replicated, the data indicate that a single minimal-contact session of cessation counseling, similar to what is typically provided in primary care physician offices, is ineffective for African-American smokers with at least one long DRD4 allele. These results are consistent with a study in a DRD4 knockout mouse that was characterized as supersensitive to ethanol, cocaine, and methamphetamine (Rubenstein et al., 1997). However, in three studies with Caucasian populations (Geijer et al., 1997; Malhotra et al., 1996; Sander et al., 1997b) and one in Taiwan (Chang et al., 1997), no evidence was found for an association between DRD4 and alcoholism.

SUBSTANCE ABUSE AND 5-HTTLPR AND DOPAMINE D3 RECEPTOR *BalI* POLYMORPHISM

We have examined two other polymorphisms, 5-HTTLPR and dopamine D3 receptor Bal I receptor [linked to personality traits of harm avoidance or neuroticism (Lesch et al., 1996) and reward, respectively)], in a group of Israeli heroin addicts (Kotler et al., 1999). The dopamine D3 receptor has also been linked to NS in a small group of bipolar patients (Staner et al., 1998) and to substance abuse in schizophrenia (Duaux et al., 1998; Krebs et al., 1998). We failed to replicate the relationship between the DRD3 receptor and substance abuse in our sample of 186 heroin addicts and 217 gender and ethnically matched controls. DRD3 has also been examined in alcoholism, again with conflicting results (Dobashi et al., 1997; Higuchi et al., 1996; Parsian et al., 1997). Nor did we observe an association between the 5-HTTLPR promoter-region polymorphism and heroin addiction (Kotler et al., 1999).

DRD4 AND ADHD

Several studies have examined the DRD4 polymorphism in ADHD (Castellanos et al., 1998; Eisenberg et al., 2000; LaHoste et al., 1996; Rowe et al., 1998; Smalley et al., 1998; Swanson et al., 1998). Except for a family-based study from our own group (Eisenberg et al., 2000) and a single case-control report (Castellanos et al., 1998), these investigations show an excess of the 7-repeat allele in ADHD. Overall, these results strengthen the notion that the DRD4 contributes modestly to impulsive and NS behaviors presenting in children as ADHD and in adults as substance abuse. The dopamine transporter polymorphism has also been examined in ADHD, and a positive association has been reported (Comings et al., 1996; Cook et al., 1995; Gill et al., 1997). Recently the dopamine transporter has also been shown to be associated with NS and cigarette addiction (Saboz et al., 1999).

CATECHOL-*O*-METHYLTRANSFERASE

Another polymorphism examined in ADHD (Eisenberg et al., 1999), schizophrenia (Kotler et al., in press), personality (Benjamin et al., 2000a,b), executive function (hypnotizability) (P. Lichtenberg et al., unpublished data), and heroin addiction (R. Horowitz et al., unpublished data) is catechol-*O*-methyltransferase (COMT). A common COMT polymorphism coding for a thermolabile low activity enzyme has been recognized for two decades (Lotta et al., 1997; Weinshilboum et al., 1981). Lachman et al. (1996) found a common biallelic polymorphism (val/met) that results in high (val/val), low (met/met), and intermediate levels of enzyme activity (val/met). COMT contributes to the clearance of dopamine and norepinephrine but not serotonin.

The high enzyme activity COMT *val* allele has recently been linked, in a case-control study, to substance abuse (Vandenbergh et al., 1997), which is often an adult developmental outcome of childhood ADHD (Biederman et al., 1997; Milberger et al., 1997a,b). We have recently confirmed this finding using a haplotype relative risk family-based design in a group of Israeli heroin addicts and their parents (R. Horowitz et al., unpublished data).

Using a family-based design and a parent to proband allele transmission test with 48 ADHD triads, we also found an association between COMT val allele and ADHD ($\chi^2 = 4.72$, $P = 0.03$, df = 1) (Eisenberg et al., 1999). In particular, the impulsive-hyperactive type of ADHD (excluding inattention) ascertained by DSM-IV criteria ($\chi^2 = 8.34$, $P = 0.004$, df = 1), Conners Teaching Rating Hyperactivity Scale (Pearson $\chi^2 = 5.32$, $P = 0.02$, df = 1), and Continuous Performance Test False Alarm scale ($\chi^2 = 2.78$, $P = 0.096$, df = 1) was associated with the high enzyme activity COMT val allele. Similar results were obtained when genotype frequencies were compared. Note that the association between the high-enzyme activity COMT val allele that increases CNS dopamine (and norepinephrine) clearance is consistent with the use of methylphenidate, an agent that increases dopamine (and norepinephrine) turnover in the treatment of ADHD.

COMT AND AGGRESSION

Lachman et al. (1998) and Strous et al. (1997) reported an association of the COMT polymorphism and aggressive behavior in schizophrenia that prompted us to also examine the role of this gene in a group of 30 male schizophrenic patients who displayed extreme aggressiveness by committing homicide (Kotler et al., in press). Subjects were also inventoried for two additional polymorphisms that have likewise been linked to both normal and abnormal personality traits, DRD4 and 5-HTTLPR. Significant excess (46.7% versus 21.0%) homozygosity of the low activity COMT met/met genotype was observed in 30 mostly male (28/30) homicidal schizophrenic patients compared with 415 control subjects (Pearson $\chi^2 = 10.53$, $P = 0.005$, df = 2).

No difference in COMT genotype was found between 62 nonviolent schizophrenic patients and the 415 control subjects ($\chi^2 = 0.963$, $P > 0.1$, df = 2). A nonsignificant trend for excess (46.7% versus 25.8%) homozygosity of the low activity COMT met/met genotype was also observed when the homicidal schizophrenic subjects were compared directly with the nonviolent schizophrenic patients ($\chi^2 = 4.03$, $P = 0.1$, df = 2). Similarly, an excess of the low activity COMT met allele was observed in homicidal versus nonviolent schizophrenic patients (likelihood ratio ($^2 = 2.92$, $P = 0.087$, df = 2). Finally, no association was observed between homicidal behavior in schizophrenic patients and the dopamine D4 exon III repeat length polymorphism (D4DR) or the serotonin transporter promoter-region polymorphism (5-HTTLPR).

In summary, both the COMT and DRD4 polymorphisms appear to contribute to psychopathological behaviors that share common features with the TPQ personality trait of NS. These effects have been observed in ADHD, substance abuse, and violent behavior in schizophrenia. Indeed, the most robust finding to date in genetic studies of ADHD is the association of the 7-repeat allele of the DRD4 gene with this illness.

MULTIPLE GENE INTERACTIONS

The small effect of these polymorphisms, the failure to observe these relationships in some studies (especially across ethnic and cultural categories), and the complex nature of behavioral and personality prompted us to examine three of these polymorphisms (COMT, DRD4, and 5-HTTLPR) in our extended group of subjects administered the TPQ (Benjamin et al., 2000a,b). We hypothesized that a simultaneous analysis of all three polymorphisms would help us to better understand the complex interactions that undoubtedly underlie the genetic architecture of NS and perhaps to clarify some reasons behind the failure to replicate initial findings in molecular personality genetics.

DRD4, COMT, and 5-HTTLPR polymorphisms were therefore examined for an association with TPQ personality factors in a large group of 455 subjects (Benjamin et al., 2000b). Significant interactions were observed by multivariate analysis and by subsequent univariate three-way way analysis of variance with NS as the dependent variable. In the absence of the short 5-HTTLPR allele and the presence of the high-enzyme activity COMT val/val genotype, NS scores are higher in the presence of the DRD4 7-repeat allele (Fig. 13-1).

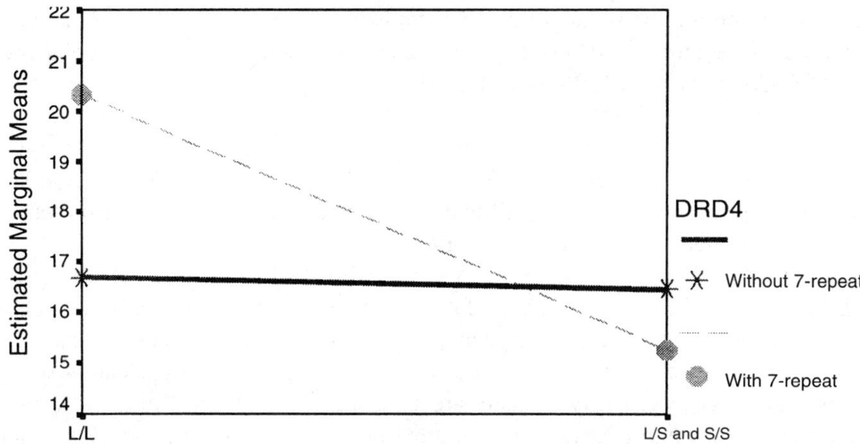

FIG. 13-1. Marginal mean value of TPQ novelty seeking scores (adjusted for age and sex covariates) grouped by three polymorphisms: COMT, DRD4, and 5-HTTLPR. Left Y-axis groups subjects with long/long 5-HTTLPR; right Y-axis groups subjects with short genotypes associated in some studies with harm avoidance or neuroticism. Connecting lines group subjects with and without the DRD4 7-repeat allele (solid line, subjects without 7-repeat; dashed line, subjects with 7-repeat). All subjects carry val/val COMT genotype (high enzyme activity). In absence of 5-HTTLPR neuroticism short allele, the presence of the DRD4 7-repeat allele significantly raises NS scores. L/L, long/long; L/S, long/short; S/S, short/short.

About 70% of these subjects were independently recruited sib pairs, allowing us to examine the effect of these three polymorphisms on NS using within-families strategy. First, intraclass correlation coefficients for NS were calculated for sib pairs who shared identical genotype groupings for each of the three polymorphisms. A significant intraclass correlation was observed for NS scores within sib pairs (coefficient = 0.39, $F = 2.26$, $P = 0.008$, $N = 49$). However, sib pairs who shared at least one dissimilar genotype of the three showed no significant correlation for NS scores (coefficient = 0. 177, $F = 1.43$, $P = 0.09$, $N = 110$). When we examined siblings sharing either of the two homozygous (val/val versus met/met) COMT genotypes (and who were identical for 5-TTLPR and DRD4), sib pairs with the val/val genotype were found to have significantly correlated NS scores (coefficient = 0.67, $F = 5.11$, $P = 0.009$, $N = 13$). However, no significant difference in mean NS scores was observed using a paired t test ($t = 0.07$, $P > 0.1$). Conversely, sib pairs with the COMT met/met genotype (and identical for 5-HTTLPR and DRD4) showed no correlation in NS scores (coefficient = 0.16, $F = 1.36$, $P = 0.9$, $N = 10$) but displayed a marginally significant difference in mean NS scores by paired t test [15.00 ± 1.49 versus 18.70 ± 4.62 (±SD), $t = 2.55$, $P = 0.09$]. Similar results regarding the permissive role of the val/val COMT genotype were also observed by using a between-families analysis. We note that similar interactions were also observed between these three polymorphisms and NS when the 150 independently recruited and nonrelated subjects were analyzed.

Our results showing modulation of D4DR on NS by at least two other functional polymorphisms, COMT and 5-HTTLPR, suggest the importance of epistatic interactions in determining personality traits. Others have also recently addressed the issue of multiple gene effects and how they mediate complex behavioral traits (Cloninger et al., 1998; Comings et al., 1996; Weinshilboum et al., 1981). These considerations suggest to us that in the absence of additional genetic information, first results showing association between particular polymorphisms may be difficult to replicate. The presence of modifying genes confounds the interpretation of genetic studies of complex traits, and replication is especially difficult across ethnic categories or in mixed populations when allele frequencies often differ. In a population with an increased frequency of COMT val/val genotype and the 5-HTTLPR short allele, the lack of effect of DRD4 on NS might be reported as a false-negative. We believe these considerations have often been overlooked to explain inconsistent findings in human behavioral genetics. Even family-based designs are of doubtful usefulness in preventing type I errors when unknown modifying genes are present in the sib pairs. Failure to account for such modifiers introduces a source of error, depending on the strength of the main gene effect and that of the epistatic interactions.

TPQ REWARD-DIRECTED BEHAVIOR

The first demonstration of polygenic interactions in molecular personality genetics is illustrated in a study in which we examined two additional coding region polymorphisms, a glycine to serine substitution in the dopamine D3 receptor (*Bal* I) and a cysteine to serine substitution in the 5-HT2C serotonin receptor (HTR2C) (Ebstein et al., 1997b). A three-way analysis of variance (TPQ score grouped by D4DR, dopamine D3 receptor, and 5-HT2C) demonstrated that TPQ reward-directed behavior and TPQ persistence scores were significantly reduced by the presence of the less common 5-HT2Cser polymorphism. The effect of the serine substitution in this X-linked serotonin receptor polymorphism on reward was also observed when males and females were separately analyzed. There was also a significant interaction between the two dopamine receptor polymorphisms and the serotonin polymorphism on reward. In particular, the effect of the 5-HT2C polymorphism on reward was markedly accentuated in individuals who had the long version of the D4DR exon III repeat polymorphism. When present in the same individual, the 5-HT2C and dopamine receptor polymorphisms account for 30% of the observed variance for persistence and 13% of the variance for reward scores. However, the number of subjects with both less common D4DR and 5-HT2C polymorphisms is small, underscoring the importance of verifying this interaction in a larger cohort. Kuhn et al. (1999) have reported a replication of this study.

NEONATAL BEHAVIOR

In addition to our studies of candidate genes in adults using self-report questionnaires, we have examined the effect of two of these well-studied candidates (5-HTTLPR and DRD4) for their role in neonate and infant behavior (Auerbach et al., 1999; Ebstein et al., 1998). Extending our examination of candidate genes purportedly affecting adult personality to neonate and child temperament offers the opportunity to further probe the validity of adult findings and examine how the expression of genetically determined behavioral phenotypes may vary during development. We also theorized that in neonates and infants genetic effects might be maximized, because environmental influences exerted by the caregivers and home environment are minimal. Moreover, measurement of neonate, infant, and child temperaments and behaviors are based on observer-based inventories (by caregivers, psychologists, teachers, etc.) in "laboratory" settings.

We demonstrated an interaction between the 5-HTTLPR and DRD4 7-repeat on Brazelton Orientation scores (a putative antecedent temperament of adult NS?) in 2-week-old neonates (Ebstein et al., 1998). At age 2 months these children were again assessed using the infant behavioral questionnaire, and a significant interaction between the DRD4 7-repeat × 5-HTTLPR promoter region polymorphisms on negative emotionality and distress to limitations was observed (Auerbach et al., 1999). In those infants lacking the DRD4 7-repeat, the effect of 5-HTTLPR s/s genotype was to significantly raise scores for negative emotionality and distress to limitations. These infants also reacted more negatively when presented with sudden or novel stimuli. In both infants and adults, short alleles of 5-HTTLPR and long alleles of DRD4 appear to oppose each other's effects; approach or arousal behaviors (orientation to environmental stimuli in infants and NS in adults) are promoted by long DRD4 alleles, whereas short alleles of 5-HTTLPR increase avoidance behaviors. These results are intuitive because commonsense dictates that individuals characterized by a drive for new experiences and sensations are not likely to be characterized by high harm avoidance (fearful, shy, fatigable).

CONCLUSIONS

Studies of brain imaging (Maas et al., 1998; Pidoplichko et al., 1997; Stein et al., 1998; Volkow et al., 1997a,b) after administration of addictive drugs such as cocaine and nicotine suggest that the motive circuit described overall in rats is involved in humans. For example, the same concentration of nicotine achieved by smokers activates and desensitizes multiple nicotinic receptors, thereby regulating the activity of mesolimbic dopamine neurons (Pidoplichko et al., 1997).

Rat psychologists do not distinguish among individual animals, whereas people psychologists make their living from such individual differences. Personality traits reflect these individual differences, and we now know that genes account for a substantial percentage of the variance in personality dimensions measured by self-report questionnaires. People differ in how they respond to environmental stimuli, and the motivational value attached to appetitive events (e.g., sex and food) varies markedly among individuals.

Why is this so? We have discussed recent genetics studies, including many from our laboratory, suggesting that common dopaminergic polymorphisms account for some variance in personality traits such as NS or sensation seeking and harm avoidance or neuroticism. NS is a personality trait that apparently reflects how much stimulation is needed from environmental events to reach each individual's optimal level of arousal. Thrill seekers need more stimulation than the average; some obtain stimulation by bungee jumping and others in less socially acceptable ways such as substance abuse.

These genetics studies illuminate the neural basis of individual differences in human motivational states. Common polymorphisms in the DRD4, the dopamine transporter, the serotonin transporter promoter region, and the COMT enzyme may partially determine individual differences in personality traits by contributing to brain dopaminergic tone. Personality traits such as NS reflect individual differences in the mesolimbic motive circuit and determine the motivational value that people give to environmental reward cues. Dopamine neurons in the motive circuit are tuned to change and novelty, and it is therefore not surprising that genes modulating brain dopamine levels or receptor response have also been shown to contribute to higher level expressions of these molecular events, i.e., extroverted versus introverted personality traits.

REFERENCES

Asghari V, et al. (1994). Dopamine D4 receptor repeat: analysis of different native and mutant forms of the human and rat genes. *Mol Pharmacol* 46,364–373.

Asghari V, et al. (1995). Modulation of intracellular cyclic AMP levels by different human dopamine D4 receptor variants. *J Neurochem* 65,1157–1165.

Auerbach J, et al. (1999). Dopamine D4 receptor (D4DR) and serotonin transporter promoter (5-HTTLPR) polymorphisms in the determination of temperament in two month old infants. *Mol Psychiatry* 4,369–373.

Ball D, et al. (1997). The serotonin transporter gene and peer-rated neuroticism. *Neuroreport* 8,1301–1304.

Benjamin J, et al. (2000a). Association between tridimensional personality questionnaire (TPQ) traits and three functional polymorphisms: dopamine receptor D4 (DRD4), serotonin transporter promoter region (5-HTTLPR) and catechol O-methyltransferase (COMT). *Mol Psychiatry* 5,96–100 (2000.

Benjamin J, et al. (2000b). An interaction between the catechol-*O*-methyltransferase (COMT) and serotonin promoter region (5-HTTLPR) polymorphisms contributes to tridimensional personality questionnaire (TPQ) persistence scores in normal subjects. *Neuropsychobiology* 41,48–53.

Benjamin J, et al. (1996). Population and familial association between the D4 dopamine receptor gene and measures of novelty seeking. *Nat Genet* 12,81–84.

Biederman J, et al. (1997). Is ADHD a risk factor for psychoactive substance use disorders? Findings from a four-year prospective follow-up study. *J Am Acad Child Adolesc Psychiatry* 36,21–29.

Blum K, et al. (1997). Association of polymorphisms of dopamine D2 receptor (DRD2) and dopamine transporter (DAT1) genes with schizoid/avoidant behaviors (SAB). *Mol Psychiatry* 2,239–246.

Castellanos FX, et al. (1998). Lack of an association between a dopamine-4 receptor polymorphism and attention-deficit/hyperactivity disorder: genetic and brain morphometric analyses. *Mol Psychiatry* 3,431–434.

Chang FM, Ko HC, Lu RB, et al. (1997). The dopamine D4 receptor gene (DRD4) is not associated with alcoholism in three Taiwanese populations: six polymorphisms tested separately and as haplotypes. *Biol Psychiatry* 41,394–405.

Cloninger CR (1987). A systematic method for clinical description and classification of personality variants. A proposal. *Arch Gen Psychiatry* 44,573–588.

Cloninger CR, et al. (1998). Anxiety proneness linked to epistatic loci in genome scan of human personality traits. *Am J Med Genet* 81,313–317.

Cloninger CR, Sigvardsson S, Przybeck TR, et al. (1995). Personality antecedents of alcoholism in a national area probability sample. *Eur Arch Psychiatry Clin Neurosci* 245,239–244.

Comings DE, et al. (1996). Polygenic inheritance of Tourette syndrome, stuttering, attention deficit hyperactivity, conduct, and oppositional defiant disorder: the additive and subtractive effect of the three dopaminergic genes—DRD2, D beta H, and DAT1. *Am J Med Genet* 67,264–288.

Cook EH Jr., et al. (1995). Association of attention-deficit disorder and the dopamine transporter gene. *Am J Hum Genet* 56,993–998.

Dobashi I, Inada T, Hadano K (1997). Alcoholism and gene polymorphisms related to central dopaminergic transmission in the Japanese population. *Psychiatr Genet* 7,87–91.

Downey KK, Pomerleau CS, Pomerleau OF (1996). Personality differences related to smoking and adult attention deficit hyperactivity disorder. *J Subst Abuse* 8,129–135.

Downey KK, Stelson FW, Pomerleau OF, et al. (1997). Adult attention deficit hyperactivity disorder: psychological test profiles in a clinical population. *J Nerv Ment Dis* 185,32–38.

Duaux, E. et al. (1998). Homozygosity at the dopamine D3 receptor gene is associated with opiate dependence. *Mol Psychiatry* 3,333–336.

Ebstein RP, et al. (1996). Dopamine D4 receptor (D4DR) exon III polymorphism associated with the human personality trait of novelty seeking. *Nat Genet* 12,78–80.

Ebstein RP, et al. (1997a). No association between the serotonin transporter gene regulatory region polymorphism and the tridimensional personality questionnaire (TPQ) temperament of harm avoidance. *Mol Psychiatry* 2,224–226.

Ebstein RP, et al. (1997b). 5-HT2C (HTR2C) serotonin receptor gene polymorphism associated with the human personality trait of reward dependence: interaction with dopamine D4 receptor (D4DR) and dopamine D3 receptor (D3DR) polymorphisms. *Am J Med Genet* 74,65–72.

Ebstein RP, et al. (1998). Dopamine D4 receptor and serotonin transporter promoter in the determination of neonatal temperament. *Mol Psychiatry* 3,238–246.

Eisenberg J, et al. (1999). Haplotype relative risk study of catechol-O-methyltransferase (COMT) and attention deficit hyperactivity disorder (ADHD): association of the high-enzyme activity Val allele with ADHD impulsive-hyperactive phenotype. *Am J Med Genet (Neuropsychiatr Genet)* 88,497–502.

Eisenberg J, et al. (2000). A haplotype relative risk study of the dopamine D4 receptor (DRD4) exon III repeat polymorphism and attention deficit hyperactivity disorder (ADHD). *Am J Med Genet (Neuropsychiatr Genet)* 96,258–261.

Ekelund J, Lichtermann D, Jarvelin MR, et al. Association between novelty seeking and the type 4 dopamine receptor gene in a large Finnish cohort sample. *Am J Psychiatry*, in press.

Eysenck SB, Eysenck HJ (1967). Physiological reactivity to sensory stimulation as a measure of personality. *Psychol Rep* 20,45–46.

Geijer T, et al. (1997). Tyrosine hydroxylase and dopamine D4 receptor allelic distribution in Scandinavian chronic alcoholics. *Alcohol Clin Exp Res* 21,35–39.

Gelernter J, et al. (1997). D4 dopamine-receptor (DRD4) alleles and novelty seeking in substance-dependent, personality-disorder, and control subjects. *Am J Hum Genet* 61,1144–1152.

Gelernter J, Kranzler H, Coccaro EF, et al. (1998). Serotonin transporter protein gene polymorphism and personality measures in African American and European American subjects. *Am J Psychiatry* 155,1332–1338.

Gill M, Daly G, Heron S, et al. (1997). Confirmation of association between attention deficit hyperactivity disorder and a dopamine transporter polymorphism. *Mol Psychiatry* 2,311–313.

Gray JA (1981). A critique of Eysenck's theory of personality. In: *A Model for Personality*, Eysenck HJ, ed. Berlin: Springer-Verlag.

Hamilton SP, et al. (1999). Lack of genetic linkage or association between a functional serotonin transporter polymorphism and panic disorder. *Psychiatr Genet* 9,1–6.

Heils A, et al. (1996). Allelic variation of human serotonin transporter gene expression. *J Neurochem* 66,2621–2624.

Heils A, Mossner R, Lesch KP (1997). The human serotonin transporter gene polymorphism—basic research and clinical implications. *J Neural Transm* 104,1005–1014.

Higuchi S, Muramatsu T, Matsushita S, et al. (1996). No evidence of association between structural polymorphism at the dopamine D3 receptor locus and alcoholism in the Japanese. *Am J Med Genet* 67,412–414 .

Jonsson EG, et al. (1997). Lack of evidence for allelic association between personality traits and the dopamine D4 receptor gene polymorphisms. *Am J Psychiatry* 154,697–699.

Kalivas PW, Nakamura M (1999). Neural systems for behavioral activation and reward. *Curr Opin Neurobiol* 9,223–227.

Koob GF, Nestler EJ (1997). The neurobiology of drug addiction. *J Neuropsychiatry Clin Neurosci* 9,482–497.

Kotler M, et al. (1997). Excess dopamine D4 receptor (D4DR) exon III seven repeat allele in opioid-dependent subjects. *Mol Psychiatry* 2,251–254.

Kotler M, et al. (1999). No association between the serotonin transporter promoter region (5-HTTLPR) and the dopamine D3 receptor (Bal I D3DR) polymorphisms and heroin addiction. *Mol Psychiatry* 4,313–316.

Kotler M, et al. Homicidal behavior in schizophrenia associated with a genetic polymorphism determining low catechol-*O*-methyltransferase (COMT) activity. *Am J Med Genet (Neuropsychiatr Genet)*, in press.

Krebs MO, et al. (1998). Dopamine D3 receptor gene variants and substance abuse in schizophrenia. *Mol Psychiatry* 3,337–341.

Kuhn KU, et al. (1999). Allelic variants of dopamine receptor D4 (DRD4) and serotonin receptor 5HT2c (HTR2c) and temperament factors: replication tests. *Am J Med Genet* 88,168–172.

Kumakiri C, et al. (1999). Study of the association between the serotonin transporter gene regulatory region polymorphism and personality traits in a Japanese population. *Neurosci Lett* 263,205–207.

Lachman HM, et al. (1996). Human catechol-*O*-methyltransferase pharmacogenetics: description of a functional polymorphism and its potential application to neuropsychiatric disorders. *Pharmacogenetics* 6,243–250.

Lachman HM, Nolan KA, Mohr P, et al. (1998). Association between catechol-*O*-methyltransferase genotype and violence in schizophrenia and schizoaffective disorder. *Am J Psychiatry* 155,835–837.

LaHoste GJ, et al. (1996). Dopamine D4 receptor gene polymorphism is associated with attention deficit hyperactivity disorder. *Mol Psychiatry* 1,121–124.

Lesch KP, et al. (1996). Association of anxiety-related traits with a polymorphism in the serotonin transporter gene regulatory region. *Science* 274,1527–1531.

Li T, et al. (1997). Association analysis of the dopamine D4 gene exon III VNTR and heroin abuse in Chinese subjects. *Mol Psychiatry* 2,413–416.

Lichter JB, et al. (1993). A hypervariable segment in the human dopamine receptor D4 (DRD4) gene. *Hum Mol Genet* 2,767–773.

Loehlin JC (1992). *Genes and Environment in Personality Development*. Newbury Park: Sage Publications.

Lotta T, et al. (1995). Kinetics of human soluble and membrane-bound catechol-*O*-methyltransferase: a revised mechanism and description of the thermolabile variant of the enzyme. *Biochemistry* 34,4202–4210.

Maas LC, et al. (1998). Functional magnetic resonance imaging of human brain activation during cue-induced cocaine craving. *Am J Psychiatry* 155,124–126.

Malhotra AK. et al. (1996). The association between the dopamine D4 receptor (D4DR) 16 amino acid repeat polymorphism and novelty seeking. *Mol Psychiatry* 1,388–391.

Mazzanti CM, et al. (1998). Role of the serotonin transporter promoter polymorphism in anxiety-related traits. *Arch Gen Psychiatry* 55,936–940.

Mel H, et al. (1998). Additional evidence for an association between the dopamine D4 receptor (D4DR) exon III seven-repeat allele and substance abuse in opioid dependent subjects: relationship of treatment retention to genotype and personality. *Addict Biol* 3,473–481.

Milberger S, Biederman J, Faraone SV, et al. (1997a). Associations between ADHD and psychoactive substance use disorders. Findings from a longitudinal study of high-risk siblings of ADHD children. *Am J Addict* 6,318–329.

Milberger S, Biederman J, Faraone SV, et al. (1997b). Further evidence of an association between attention-deficit/hyperactivity disorder and cigarette smoking. Findings from a high-risk sample of siblings. *Am J Addict* 6,205–217.

Murakami F, et al. (1999). Anxiety traits associated with a polymorphism in the serotonin transporter gene regulatory region in the Japanese. *J Hum Genet* 44,15–17.

Muramatsu T, Higuchi S, Murayama M, et al. (1996). Association between alcoholism and the dopamine D4 receptor gene. *J Med Genet* 33,113–115.

Noble EP, et al. (1998). D2 and D4 dopamine receptor polymorphisms and personality. *Am J Med Genet* 81,257–267.

Okuyama Y, et al. (2000). Identification of a polymorphism in the promoter region of DRD4 associated with the human novelty seeking personality trait. *Mol Psychiatry* 5,64–69.

Ono Y, et al. (1997). Association between dopamine D4 receptor (D4DR) exon III polymorphism and novelty seeking in Japanese subjects. *Am J Med Genet* 74,501–503.

Parsian A, Chakraverty S, Fisher L, et al. (1997). No association between polymorphisms in the human dopamine D3 and D4 receptor genes and alcoholism. *Am J Med Genet* 74,281–285.

Pidoplichko VI, DeBiasi M, Williams JT, et al. (1997). Nicotine activates and desensitizes midbrain dopamine neurons. *Nature* 390,401–404.

Pomerleau CS, Pomerleau OF, Flessland KA, et al. (1992). Relationship of tridimensional personality questionnaire scores and smoking variables in female and male smokers. *J Subst Abuse* 4,143–154.

Revelle W (1989). Personality, motivation, and cognitive performance. In: *Learning and Individual Differences: Abilities, Motivation, and Methodology*, Ackerman P, Kanfer R, Cudeck, R, eds. Erlbaum, pp. 297–341.

Ricketts MH, et al. (1998). Association of a serotonin transporter gene promoter polymorphism with harm avoidance behaviour in an elderly population. *Psychiatr Genet* 8,41–44.

Robbins TW, Everitt BJ (1996). Neurobehavioural mechanisms of reward and motivation. *Curr Opin Neurobiol* 6,228–236.

Rowe DC, et al. (1998). Dopamine DRD4 receptor polymorphism and attention deficit hyperactivity disorder. *Mol Psychiatry* 3,419–426.

Rubinstein M, et al. (1997). Mice lacking dopamine D4 receptors are supersensitive to ethanol, cocaine, and methamphetamine. *Cell* 90,991–1001.

Sabol SZ, et al. (1999). A genetic association for cigarette smoking behavior. *Health Psychol* 18,7–13.

Sander T, et al. (1997a). Association analysis of a regulatory variation of the serotonin transporter gene with severe alcohol dependence. *Alcohol Clin Exp Res* 21,1356–1359.

Sander T, et al. (1997b). Dopamine D4 receptor exon III alleles and variation of novelty seeking in alcoholics. *Am J Med Genet* 74,483–487.

Schultz W (1997). Dopamine neurons and their role in reward mechanisms. *Curr Opin Neurobiol* 7,191–197.

Shields PG, et al. (1998). Dopamine D4 receptors and the risk of cigarette smoking in African-Americans and Caucasians. *Cancer Epidemiol Biomarkers Prev* 7,453–458.

Smalley SL, et al. (1998). Evidence that the dopamine D4 receptor is a susceptibility gene in attention deficit hyperactivity disorder. *Mol Psychiatry* 3,427–430.

Staner L, et al. (1998). Association between novelty-seeking and the dopamine D3 receptor gene in bipolar patients: a preliminary report. *Am J Med Genet* 81,192–194.

Stein EA, et al. (1998). Nicotine-induced limbic cortical activation in the human brain: a functional MRI study. *Am J Psychiatry* 155,1009–1015.

Strobel A, Wehr A, Michel A, et al. (1999). Association between the dopamine D4 receptor (DRD4) exon III polymorphism and measures of novelty seeking in a German population. *Mol Psychiatry* 4,378–384.

Strous RD, Bark N, Parsia SS, et al. (1997). Analysis of a functional catechol-*O*-methyltransferase gene polymorphism in schizophrenia: evidence for association with aggressive and antisocial behavior. *Psychiatry Res* 69,71–77.

Swanson JM, et al. (1998). Association of the dopamine receptor D4 (DRD4) gene with a refined phenotype of attention deficit hyperactivity disorder (ADHD): a family-based approach. *Mol Psychiatry* 3,38–41.

Van Tol HH, et al. (1992). Multiple dopamine D4 receptor variants in the human population. *Nature* 358,149–152.

Vandenbergh DJ, Rodriguez LA, Miller IT, et al. (1997). High-activity catechol-*O*-methyltransferase allele is more prevalent in polysubstance abusers. *Am J Med Genet* 74,439–442.

Vandenbergh DJ, Zonderman AB, Wang J, et al. (1997). No association between novelty seeking and dopamine D4 receptor (D4DR) exon III seven repeat alleles in Baltimore longitudinal study of aging participants. *Mol Psychiatry* 2,417–419.

Volkow ND, et al. (1997a). Relationship between subjective effects of cocaine and dopamine transporter occupancy. *Nature* 386,827–830.

Volkow ND, et al. (1997b). Decreased striatal dopaminergic responsiveness in detoxified cocaine-dependent subjects. *Nature* 386,830–833.

Weinshilboum R, Dunnette J (1981). Thermal stability and the biochemical genetics of erythrocyte catechol-*O*-methyl-transferase and plasma dopamine-beta-hydroxylase. *Clin Genet* 19,426–437.

Wise RA (1996a). Neurobiology of addiction. *Curr Opin Neurobiol* 6,243–251.

Wise RA (1996b). Addictive drugs and brain stimulation reward. *Annu Rev Neurosci* 19,319–340.

Zuckerman M (1994). *Behavioral Expressions and Biosocial Bases of Sensation Seeking*. New York: Cambridge University Press.

14.

Dopamine Genes and Neuropsychiatric Disease

Livia Martucci and James L. Kennedy

ABSTRACT

The dopamine system is strongly implicated in the pathophysiology of several neuropsychiatric diseases, such as schizophrenia, bipolar disorder, obsessive compulsive disorder, and Parkinson's disease, suggesting a role for dopamine in the etiology of these disorders. Candidate gene studies between the D2 dopamine receptor (DRD2) gene and schizophrenia and bipolar disorder have been mostly negative, whereas a recent study has shown an association between a DRD2 polymorphism and obsessive compulsive disorder. An association between schizophrenia and the amino acid substitution on dopamine D3 receptor gene has been found, as well as an association with tardive dyskinesia. Genetics studies have failed to find conclusive evidence of linkage between the dopamine D4 receptor gene and schizophrenia and bipolar disorder. An increase in the 7-repeat allele of the dopamine D4 receptor gene 48 base pair repeat polymorphism has been found in obsessive compulsive disorder patients with tics compared with those without tics. The other two known dopamine receptor genes, D1 and D5 ("D1-like"), have not been studied as extensively as the D2-like receptor genes. Association studies between a polymorphism in the dopamine transporter DAT1 gene and bipolar disorder have produced both positive and negative results, whereas no association was found between DAT1 and obsessive compulsive disorder, schizophrenia, and tardive dyskinesia. Results of the studies on Parkinson's disease and dopamine system genes are showing a lack of association thus far, but more studies are needed. Overall, the use of molecular genetics strategies to study the dopamine system in neuropsychiatric disease is a powerful new approach and will undoubtedly lead to findings relevant to clinical care. This chapter reviews recent developments in the use of dopamine system genes to investigate neuropsychiatric disorders.

SCHIZOPHRENIA

Schizophrenia is a severe illness characterized by peculiar anomalies of thought, perception, and emotion that produces a severe deterioration of social and occupational functioning. The lifetime prevalence of schizophrenia worldwide is estimated to be 1%. The disease onset is most often observed in young adults, with men typically having a peak age of onset in their early 20s and women in their late 20s (Hefner et al., 1998). It is now clearly established, on the basis of results from family, twin, and adoption studies, that genetic factors are a major factor in the etiology of schizophrenia (McGuffin et al., 1995).

Studying the recurrence risk in relatives of schizophrenic patients has allowed us to largely exclude the possibility that schizophrenia is either a single gene disorder or a collection of single gene disorders, even when incomplete penetrance is considered. Rather, in schizophrenia, the mode of transmission, like other common disorders, is complex and non-Mendelian (McGue and Gottesman, 1989). The most common mode of transmission probably involves multiple susceptibility loci (McGuffin et al., 1994), but the number of such loci, the risk for disease conferred by each locus, and the degree of interaction between loci remain unknown. The basis for candidate gene selection has originated from neuropharmacological studies suggesting that abnormalities in monoamine neurotransmission are involved in the pathophysiology of schizophrenia. Given the importance of the dopaminergic hypothesis, dopamine system genes may be vital in the etiology and treatment of schizophrenia.

Despite many studies, the etiology of schizophrenia still remains unclear. However, a strong link to the dopamine system has been developed from the observation that high doses or chronic use of drugs that induce dopamine release can create psychotic episodes indistinguishable from those experienced by a paranoid schizophrenia patient (Randrup and Munkvad, 1965).

The longstanding dopamine hypothesis for schizophrenia has proposed that the psychotic thoughts result from excess dopamine affecting the brain areas responsible for cognition. Dopaminergic overactivity could result from either excess neurotransmitter or oversensitivity to dopamine, perhaps from an increased number of dopamine receptors. For more than three decades, the hypothesis that schizophrenia is caused by excessive dopaminergic neurotransmission has dominated biological thinking.

Our present knowledge, derived mostly from the pharmacology of neuroleptics, has favored disordered transmission at the dopamine D2 receptor gene (DRD2); however, with few exceptions, the results of candidate gene studies of an association between DRD2 and schizophrenia have been negative (O'Donovan and Owen, 1999). However, the single nucleotide polymorphism at position –141 in the D2 receptor upstream putative regulatory region has been implicated. The dopamine receptor D3 (DRD3) gene has been tested extensively in schizophrenia, partly because of its similarity to DRD2 and because of its neuroanatomical location in the limbic system, which is consistent with circuits that might be involved in psychotic symptomatology.

DRD3 maps to chromosome 3 at q13.3. A serine to glycine polymorphism is at position 9 in the N-terminal extracellular domain of the D3 receptor coded by an MscI restriction site in exon I of the DRD3 gene (Lannfelt et al., 1992). Evidence of an association between schizophrenia and homozygosity for the serine/glycine variant was reported by Croq et al. (1992). These results were independently replicated by Williams et al. (1998), and other studies have also indicated an association between the Gly-Gly genotype as well as an allele-wise association for the Gly variant and schizophrenia (Ebstein et al., 1997; Kennedy et al., 1995). The substitution of a polar serine residue to a nonpolar glycine residue may alter the tertiary structure of the D3 receptor. Lundstrom and Turpin (1996) reported significantly higher affinity for the glycine homozygote cells compared with both heterozygote binding and serine/serine homozygotes.

The dopamine D4 receptor (DRD4) gene has also been investigated in the etiology of schizophrenia because different polymorphic variants exist in the human population, and these vary in the number of repeats of a 16 amino acid sequence within the functionally critical third cytoplasmic loop. There can be from 2 to 11 repeats, with 2, 4, and 7 being common in Caucasians. The anatomical distribution of D4 receptors appears to be primarily cortical and has far less density than that of D2 in the basal ganglia. Genetics studies have failed to find conclusive evidence of linkage between the DRD4 gene and schizophrenia (Macciardi et al., 1994). DRD4 was cloned in 1991, and the variation in the third exon was documented in 1992 (Van Tol et al., 1992). This 48 base pair repeat variant created a great deal of interest because of the fact that the atypical neuroleptic clozapine has the highest affinity for D4 among all the dopamine receptors. However, extensive testing of this 48 base pair polymorphism, as well as markers in other regions of the gene (Paterson et al., 1996; Petronis et al., 1994), have revealed mostly negative results when the phenotype of schizophrenia was the target.

Based on the high affinity of clozapine for the D4 receptor, the role of polymorphisms in DRD4 was examined in predicting response of schizophrenic patients to clozapine treatment. Although the D4 exon III 48 base pair polymorphism did not predict overall response, it showed some evidence of prediction of change in positive symptoms (e.g., hallucinations, disorganization, bizarre behavior) (Ozdemir et al., 1999). As is the case in general for the other dopamine system genes, the regulatory region of DRD4 has not been investigated adequately, although additional polymorphisms in the upstream region have been discovered (Paterson et al., 1999).

The other two known dopamine receptor genes, DRD1 and DRD5 ("D1-like"), have not been studied as extensively in schizophrenia as the D2-like receptor genes. Part of the reason is that because the D1-like genes have no introns, there is less polymorphic information at the DNA level. Association studies examining dopamine D1 receptor and schizophrenia have mostly revealed nonsignificant results (Cichon et al., 1996; Fang et al., 1998; Kojima et al., 1999). Molecular genetics studies have found only a weak association between DRD5 and schizophrenia: positive results were reported for the nearby anonymous markers D4S394 and D4S2917 (Kennedy et al., 1998, 1999).

BIPOLAR DISORDER

Bipolar affective disorder is common and affects roughly 0.8% of the general population. This mood disorder presents with episodes of mania and depression, although an episode of mania alone is sufficient for the diagnosis. The major genetic contribution to bipolar disorder has been shown by family, twin, and adoption studies. However, the mode of inheritance, like that of other common disorders, is complex and non-Mendelian. Transmission in most cases probably involves the interaction of several genes together with environmental factors (Craddock et al., 1995). Several lines of evidence implicate the dopaminergic system in the pathogenesis of both manic and depressive episodes. Dopaminergic drugs such as amphetamines and L-DOPA can provoke manic episodes in susceptible individuals (Goodwin and Jamison, 1990; Murphy et al., 1971). Antipsychotic drugs that are dopamine antagonists are effective in the treatment of mania; however, they can also induce depression (Diehl and Gershon, 1992; Willner 1995). This leads to the hypothesis that genes encoding dopamine receptors and also the dopamine transporter DAT1 (which acts to move released dopamine back into presynaptic terminals) are important candidates for investigation in bipolar disorder.

Association studies between a variable number of tandem repeat (VNTR) polymorphisms consisting of a 40 base pair repeat in the 3′ untranslated region of the DAT1 gene and bipolar disorder have been positive (Gomez-Casero et al., 1996; Waldman et al., 1997) and negative (Manki et al., 1996; Souery et al., 1996). Linkage of bipolar disorder to markers in the vicinity of DRD2 has been excluded in several studies (Byerley et al., 1990; De Bruyn et al., 1996; Ewald et al., 1995; Holmes et al., 1991; Mitchell et al., 1992; Nothen et al., 1992). DRD2 maps to chromosome 11q22.3-q23 and previous intensive searches for nucleotide variants causing alterations in the amino acid sequence have identified only a few variants. Of interest, a recently identified polymorphism in the promoter region of DRD2 (the –141 insertion/deletion) has been shown to alter gene expression in vitro (Arinami et al., 1997). Because this functional variant is in the regulatory region, a dysregulation of dopaminergic neurotransmission has been implicated in the manic episodes of bipolar disorder. Two studies investigated the association between the –141 insertion/deletion polymorphism and bipolar disorder with negative results (Furlong et al., 1998; Stober et al., 1998). These results do not support a major role for DRD2 in the etiology of bipolar disorder.

Linkage between bipolar disorder and the serine/glycine variant of DRD3 was excluded in two studies (De Bruyn et al., 1996; Mitchell et al., 1993). An increased transmission of the serine allele in bipolar families has been reported (Parsian et al., 1995) but not in another study (Piccardi et al., 1997). Association with the DRD3 gene was not found in several case-control samples (Gomez-Casero et al., 1996; Manki et al., 1996; Mitchell et al., 1993; Oruc et al., 1996; Rietschel et al., 1993; Shaikh et al., 1993; Suoery et al., 1996).

Genetic linkage studies of DRD4 and bipolar disorder have been mostly negative, apart from a weak positive cosegregation of a haplotype containing the DRD4 and tyrosine hydroxylase gene markers in a core section of Old Order Amish kindred (Sidenberg et al., 1993). Association studies between DRD4 and bipolar disorder have had both positive and negative (Serretti et al., 1998b) results: in a study by Serretti et al. (1998a), the DRD4 7-repeat allele was significantly associated with delusional symptoms in bipolar disorder and could therefore be considered a liability factor for delusional symptoms in mood disorder, if this finding can be replicated.

DRD5 maps to the area of chromosome 4q15.1–16.1 where relatively strong linkage to bipolar disorder was reported in a large multiply affected pedigree (Blackwood et al., 1996). The DRD5 locus shows a highly polymorphic dinucleotide repeat (CT/GT/GA)n, and there was a trend for the most common allele

(allele 8) to be preferentially transmitted in one study (Asherson et al., 1998). There have been three positive linkage results involving the area of DRD5 on chromosome 4p (Asherson et al., 1998; Blackwood et al., 1996; Ewald et al., 1998). Absence of linkage to this region has also been reported (Asherson et al., 1998; De Bruyn et al., 1996).

TARDIVE DYSKINESIA

Neuroleptic medications are frequently used to alleviate psychotic symptoms in schizophrenia and bipolar patients and can be used as an addition in therapy of treatment resistant obsessive compulsive patients. One major drawback to chronic treatment with typical neuroleptic drugs is the potential for development of severe extrapyramidal side effects, such as tardive dyskinesia (TD). TD occurs in predisposed individuals during or after cessation of prolonged typical neuroleptic treatment (Gerlach and Casey, 1984). Although the mechanism of TD remains unknown, it has been postulated that an overactivity of dopaminergic neurotransmission in the basal ganglia may be involved in its manifestation (Tarsy and Baldessarini, 1977). The hypothesis speculates that TD results from chronic neuroleptic blockade of dopamine D2-like receptors in the basal ganglia and states that long-term blockade results in an up-regulation of dopamine receptors residing on postsynaptic membranes (Casey et al., 1982; Gerlach and Casey 1984; Meshul and Casey 1989). It has been suggested that the neuroleptic-induced increase in dopamine receptor density eventually results in an overactivity of the nigrostriatal dopaminergic tract, a brain region involved in regulation of motor behavior (Gordon and Fields, 1989).

In the treatment of schizophrenia with typical neuroleptics, approximately 20–30% of patients suffer from TD (Awouters et al. 1990; Casey 1991; Hoffman et al., 1987; Jeste and Caligiuri 1993; Lieberman et al., 1988), and neuroleptic-treated patients with bipolar disorder have been reported to have rates of TD as high as or higher than patients with schizophrenia, thus implying variable susceptibility to the disorder. Epidemiological data suggest that the occurrence of TD may be based on a genetic predisposition, the effect of which may become expressed in conjunction with other variables, in particular age, ethnicity, sex, and neuroleptic history (Cavallaro and Smeraldi, 1995).

In terms of candidate genes, the D2 receptor gene was initially thought to be the most likely candidate involved in TD. Chen et al. (1997) reported a significant association between the DRD2 gene and TD; however, Inada et al., (1997) did not find any association between the DRD2 gene and TD. An analysis by Badri et al. (1996) of DRD2 and TD revealed no significant effect. One candidate from the D2-like receptor family is the dopamine D3 receptor. Autoradiographic studies, as well histochemical studies, have localized dopamine D3 mRNA and protein to the ventral side of the striatum and the ventral putamen in the basal ganglia, a brain region implicated in motor control (Joyce et al., 1997; Suzuki et al., 1998). Several studies have demonstrated that dopamine D3 preferring agonists inhibit locomotor activity, whereas dopamine D3 antagonists increase locomotor activity (Fink-Jensen 1998; Gendreau et al., 1997; Van Hartesveldt 1997). Thus, evidence suggests that the dopamine D3 receptor may be involved in motor control.

Several studies have investigated the putative role of the serine to glycine polymorphism at amino acid position 9 as a predisposing factor to neuroleptic induced TD. A preliminary report by Macciardi et al. (1996) demonstrated an association between DRD3 and TD. However, Inada et al. (1997) and Gaitonde et al. (1996) did not find any association between DRD3 and TD. Basile et al. (1999) found a statistically significant association between the glycine variant of DRD3 and TD, suggesting the involvement of this polymorphism as a predisposing risk factor for TD. Perhaps the functional differences of the serine versus glycine variants described by Lundstrom and Turpin (1996) may contribute to the TD phenotype, although it is difficult to speculate further on the precise mechanism involved.

OBSESSIVE COMPULSIVE DISORDER

Obsessive compulsive disorder (OCD) is characterized by recurrent unwanted thoughts (obsessions), usually accompanied by repetitive behaviors (compulsions). Insight is generally preserved into the senseless nature of the symptoms. Several studies have shown OCD to be relatively common, with a lifetime prevalence of 2–3%. There is solid evidence for the involvement of a genetic factor in the etiology of OCD, derived from family and twin studies (Rasmussen, 1993).

Although the serotonin hypothesis has been given more attention because of the successful treatment of OCD patients with selective serotonin reuptake inhibitors (SSRI), several observations have been made providing evidence for an involvement of dopamine in the pathogenesis. Both clomipramine and fluoxetine, successful drugs in the treatment of OCD, display antidopaminergic activity (Austin et al., 1991; Lipinski et al., 1989). Furthermore, there is a connection between OCD and the basal ganglia, where the neurotransmitter dopamine and serotonin interact (Baxter et al., 1991; Insel 1992; Rapoport 1991; Schilder et al., 1938; Swedo et al., 1989). In addition, some patients with OCD never respond to SSRIs, and for those that do respond, the symptoms are never eradicated. Several clinical trials have shown that SSRI-resistant patients benefit from the addition of a neuroleptic to their treatment (McDougle et al., 1994; Riddle et al., 1988), especially in OCD patients with comorbid tic disorder.

Preliminary studies of dopamine receptor genes and OCD have been controversial: Novelli et al. (1994) found no relationship between OCD and the dopamine D2 receptor; Billet et al. (1998) genotyped a sample of OCD patients and matched controls for the TaqIA polymorphism and the serine-cysteine variation in the DRD2 gene with negative results; and a study by Catalano et al. (1994) failed to demonstrate an association between OCD and the dopamine D3 receptor serine/glycine polymorphism. This lack of association has been confirmed by Billet et al. (1998). It has also been confirmed by autoradiographic studies that the D3 receptor is expressed to a significant degree in the nucleus accumbens (Lathi et al., 1995; Tarazi et al., 1995), which is a convergence site for inputs from brain regions that have been associated with OCD, such as hippocampus, cingulate, temporal lobe, and other parts of the limbic system. Recently, Cruz et al. (1997) have reported an increase in the 7-repeat allele of the D4 receptor gene 48 base pair repeat polymorphism in OCD patients with tics. Significant differences in allele frequencies were also found between patients and controls for the D4 receptor gene by Billet et al. (1998).

A study by Nicolini et al. (1998) confirmed these results and showed an association between the DRD2 cysteine/serine polymorphism and OCD patients with tics. Similarly, when both DRD4 7-repeat allele and DRD2 cysteine/cysteine allele are combined (at least one copy of both), patients with tics show a higher frequency of this genotype compared with OCD patients without tics. Tic-positive OCD patients may therefore represent a different clinical and genetic subtype of the disorder.

Furthermore, there have been numerous reports of clozapine-induced OCD in schizophrenic patients (Gahemi et al., 1995). Unlike many traditional antipsychotic drugs, atypical neuroleptics are not only antagonists of the dopamine receptors but also potent antagonists of serotonin-2 receptors. These findings suggest a more complex biological basis of OCD, based on the functional overlapping between serotonergic and dopaminergic systems and not just serotonin system deficiency.

Another dopamine system polymorphism that has been studied is the 40 base pair VNTR of the dopamine transporter gene DAT1. Cocaine exacerbates obsessive compulsive behavior in OCD patients (McDougle et al., 1989), and cocaine binds to the dopamine transporter in the CNS, inhibiting dopamine reuptake (Gawin and Ellinwood, 1988). Billet et al. (1998) genotyped a sample of OCD patients and matched controls for the 40 base pair repeat VNTR and found nonsignificant results.

PARKINSON'S DISEASE

Parkinson's disease is an age-related neurodegenerative disorder. It is characterized by resting tremor, rigidity, bradykinesia, gait disturbance, and postural instability. Pathological features include degeneration of dopaminergic neurons in the substantia nigra pars compacta coupled with intracytoplasmic inclusions known as Lewi bodies. The pathogenesis of idiopathic Parkinson's disease is unknown but is thought to be multifactorial, deriving from environmental factors acting on genetically predisposed individuals with aging. Recently it has been shown that α-synuclein is accumulated in Lewi bodies of sporadic Parkinson's disease and mutated in some rare families with an autosomal dominant trait of the disease (Riess and Kruger, 1999). Evidence from necropsy brain samples and pharmacokinetics suggests involvement of dopamine receptors in the pathophysiology.

Genetic association studies between Parkinson's disease and dopamine D2, D3, and D4 receptor gene polymorphisms have been conducted, mostly with negative results (Nanko et al., 1994). However, Nagay et al. (1996) investigated the dopamine receptor mRNA expression in peripheral blood lymphocytes and found a statistically significant decrease of the dopamine D3 receptor mRNA expression in Parkinson's disease patients compared with that in controls. A further binding study showed reduction of D3 receptor binding sites in Parkinson's disease lymphocytes. The decrease of the DRD3 mRNA expression correlated with the degree of clinical severity.

Although results of the studies on Parkinson's disease and dopamine system genes seem to show a lack of association thus far, the sample sizes have been relatively small, and the full set of DNA markers at each dopamine system gene has not been fully examined. The major role of the dopamine system in the pathophysiology suggests a rationale for further investigation regarding the role of genetic variants in the etiology.

FUTURE DIRECTION

We anticipate a scenario in the not-so-distant future wherein a patient will arrive at his or her doctor's office and give a small blood sample to the receptionist. The receptionist will then feed the DNA from the sample into a computerized polymerase chain reaction and gene sequencing machine. In about 30 minutes, the patient will meet with the doctor, who will hold the results from the disease gene risk assessment just completed. The patient and doctor will then discuss the probabilities and risk factors arising from the "DNA printout," particularly those genetic findings that relate to the presenting complaint. The doctor may then choose a medication that is highly likely to be effective as predicted by the patient's genetic makeup, and the chosen medication will also avoid the major side effects to which the patient is genetically predisposed. In this way, findings of current research in the genetics of psychiatric disease (and most other medical disorders) will be applied at the clinical level, eventually in the primary care setting. If the results reviewed in this chapter replicate and are further validated, then this scenario for a revolution in medical care is not far off.

REFERENCES

Arinami T, Gao M, Hamaguchi H, et al. (1997). A functional polymorphism in the promoter region of the dopamine D2 receptor gene is associated with schizophrenia. *Hum Mol Genet* 6,577–582.

Asherson P, Mant R, Williams N, et al. (1998). A study of chromosome 4p markers and dopamine D5 receptor gene in schizophrenia and bipolar disorder. *Mol Psychiatry* 3,310–320.

Austin LS, Lydiard RB, Ballenger JC, et al. (1991). Dopamine blocking activity of clomipramine in patients with obsessive-compulsive disorder. *Biol Psychiatry* 30,225–232.

Awouters F, Niemegeers CJ, Janssen PA (1990). "Tardive" dyskinesia: etiological and therapeutic aspects. *Pharmacopsychiatry* 23,33–37.

Badri F, Masellis M, Petronis A, et al. (1996). Dopamine and serotonin system genes may predict clinical response to clozapine, *Am J Hum Genet* 59(suppl),A247.

Basile VS, Masellis M, Badri F, et al. (1999). Association of the MscI polymorphism of the dopamine D3 receptor gene with tardive dyskinesia in schizophrenia. *Neuropsychopharmacology* 21,17–27.

Baxter LR, Schwartz JM, Guze BH (1991). Brain imaging: toward a neuroanatomy of OCD. In: *The Psychobiology of Obsessive Compulsive Disorder*, Zohar J, Insel TR, Rasmussen S, eds. New York: Springer.

Billett EA, Richter MA, King N, et al. (1997). Obsessive compulsive disorder, response to serotonin reuptake inhibitors and the serotonin transporter gene. *Mol Psychiatry* 2,403–406.

Billett EA, Richter MA, Swinson RP, et al. (1998). Investigation of dopamine system genes in obsessive compulsive disorder. *Psychiatr Genet* 8,163–169.

Blackwood DH, He L, Morris SW, et al. (1996). A locus for bipolar affective disorder on chromosome 4p. *Nat Genet* 12,427–430.

Byerley W, Leppert M, O'Connell P, et al. (1990). D2 dopamine receptor not linked to manic-depression in three families. *Psychiatr Genet* 1,55–62.

Caligiuri MP, Harris MJ, Jeste DV (1988). Quantitative analyses of voluntary orofacial motor control in schizophrenia and tardive dyskinesia. *Biol Psychiatry* 24,787–800.

Casey DE (1991). Neuroleptic drug-induced extrapyramidal syndromes and tardive dyskinesia. *Schizophr Res* 4,109–120.

Casey DE, Gerlach J, Bjorndal N (1982). Levodopa and receptor sensitivity modification in tardive dyskinesia. *Psychopharmacology* 78,89–92.

Catalano M, Sciuto G, Di Bella D, et al. (1994). Lack of association between obsessive-compulsive disorder and the dopamine D3 receptor gene: some preliminary considerations. *Am J Med Genet* 54,253–255.

Cavallaro R, Smeraldi E (1995). Recognition, avoidance and management of antipsychotic-induced tardive dyskinesia. *CNS Drugs* 4,278–293.

Chen CH, Wei FC, Koong FJ, et al. (1997). Association of TaqI a polymorphism of dopamine D-2 receptor gene and tardive dyskinesia in schizophrenia. *Biol Psychiatry* 41,827–829.

Cichon S, Nothen MM, Stober G, et al. (1996). Systematic screening for mutations in the 5′ regulatory region of the human dopamine D1 receptor (DRD1) gene in patients with schizophrenia and bipolar affective disorder. *Am J Med Genet* 26,424–428.

Craddock N, Khodel V, Van Eerdewegh P, et al. (1995). Mathematical limits of multilocus models: the genetic transmission of bipolar disorder. *Am J Hum Genet* 57,690–702.

Crocq MA, Mant R, Asherson P, et al. (1992). Association between schizophrenia and homozygosity at the dopamine D3 receptor gene. *J Med Genet* 29,858–860.

Cruz C, Camarena B, King N, et al. (1997). Increased prevalence of the seven-repeat variant of the dopamine D4 receptor gene in patients with obsessive-compulsive disorder with tics. *Neurosci Lett* 231,1–4.

De Bruyn A, Souery D, Mendelbaum K, et al. (1996). A linkage study between bipolar disorder and genes involved in dopaminergic and GABAergic neurotransmission. *Psychiatr Genet* 6,67–73.

Diehl DJ, Gershon S (1992). The role of dopamine in mood disorders. *Compr Psychiatry* 33,115–120.

Ebstein RP, Macciardi F, Heresco-Levi U, et al. (1997). Evidence for an association between the dopamine D3 receptor gene DRD3 and schizophrenia. *Hum Hered* 47,6–16.

Ewald H, Degn B, Mors O, et al. (1998). Support for the possible locus on chromosome 4p16 for bipolar affective disorder. *Mol Psychiatry* 3,442–448.

Ewald H, Mors O, Flint T, et al. (1995). Linkage analysis between manic-depressive illness and markers on the long arm of chromosome 11. *Am J Med Genet* 60,386–392.

Feng J, Sobell JL, Heston LL, et al. (1998). Scanning of the dopamine D1 and D5 receptor genes by REF in neuropsychiatric patients reveals a novel missense change at a highly conserved amino acid. *Am J Med Genet* 28,172–178.

Fink-Jensen A, Nielsen EB, Hansen L, et al. (1998). Behavioral and neurochemical effects of the preferential dopamine D3 receptor agonist cis-8-OH-PBZI. *Eur J Pharmacol* 342,153–161.

Furlong RA, Coleman TA, Ho L, et al. (1998). No association of a functional polymorphism in the dopamine D2 receptor promoter region with bipolar or unipolar affective disorders. *Am J Med Genet* 81,385–387.

Gaitonde EJ, Morris A, Sivagnanasundaram S, et al. (1996). Assessment of association of D3 dopamine receptor MscI polymorphism with schizophrenia: analysis of symptom ratings, family history, age at onset, and movement disorders. *Am J Med Genet* 67,455–458.

Gawin FH, Ellinwood EH Jr. (1988). Cocaine and other stimulants. Actions, abuse, and treatment. *N Engl J Med* 318,1173–1182.

Gendreau PL, Petitto JM, Schnauss R, et al. (1997). Effects of the putative dopamine D3 receptor antagonist PNU 99194A on motor behavior and emotional reactivity in C57BL/6J mice. *Eur J Pharmacol* 337,147–155.

Gerlach J, Casey DE (1984). Sulpiride in tardive dyskinesia. *Acta Psychiatr Scand Suppl* 311,93–102.

Ghaemi SN, Zarate CA Jr, Popli AP, et al. (1995). Is there a relationship between clozapine and obsessive-compulsive disorder? A retrospective chart review. *Compr Psychiatry* 36,267–270.

Gomez-Casero E, Perez de Castro I, Saiz-Ruiz J, et al. (1996). No association between particular DRD3 and DAT gene polymorphisms and manic-depressive illness in a Spanish sample. *Psychiatr Genet* 6,209–212.

Goodwin FK, Jamison KR. *Manic-depressive Illness*. New York: Oxford University Press, 1990

Gordon JH, Fields JZ (1989). A permanent dopamine receptor up-regulation in the ovariectomized rat. *Pharmacol Biochem Behav* 33,123–125.

Guala A, Mittino D, Ghini T, et al. (1992). Are metoclopramide dystonias familial? *Pediatr Med Chir* 14,617–618.

Hafner H, Van der Heiden W, Behrens S, et al. (1998). Causes and consequences of the gender difference in age at onset of schizophrenia. *Schizophr Bull* 24,99–113.

Hoffman WF, Labs SM, Casey DE (1987). Neuroleptic-induced parkinsonism in older schizophrenics. *Biol Psychiatry* 22,427–439.

Holmes D, Brynjolfsson J, Brett P, et al. (1991). No evidence for a susceptibility locus predisposing to manic depression in the region of the dopamine (D2) receptor gene. *Br J Psychiatry* 158,635–641.

Inada T, Dobashi I, Sugita T, et al. (1997). Search for a susceptibility locus to tardive dyskinesia. *Hum Psychopharmacol Clin Exp Med* 12,35–39.

Insel TR (1992). Toward a neuroanatomy of obsessive-compulsive disorder. *Arch Gen Psychiatry* 49,739–744.

Jeste DV, Caligiuri MP (1993). Tardive dyskinesia. *Schizophr Bull* 19,303–315.

Joyce JN, Meador Woodruff JH (1997). Linking the family of D-2 receptors to neuronal circuits in human brain: insights into schizophrenia. *Neuropsychopharmacology* 16,375–384.

Kennedy JL, Basile VS, Macciardi F (1999). Chromosome 4 workshop summary. *Sixth World Congress on Psychiatric Genetics*, Bonn, Germany, Oct 6–10.

Kennedy JL, Billet EA, Macciardi FM, et al. (1995) Association study of dopamine D3 receptor gene and schizophrenia. *Am J Med Genet* 60,558–562.

Kennedy JL, Macciardi FM (1998). Chromosome 4 workshop. *Psychiatr Genet* 8,67–71.

Kojima H, Ohmori O, Shinkai T, et al. (1999). Dopamine D1 receptor gene polymorphism and schizophrenia in Japan. *Am J Med Genet* 16,116–119.

Lannfelt L, Sokoloff P, Martres MP, et al. (1992). Amino acid substitution in the dopamine D3 receptor as a useful polymorphism for investigating psychiatric disorders. *Psychiatr Genet* 2,249–256.

Lathi RA, Conley R, Grubowski L, et al. (1995). Distribution of dopamine D2, D3 and D4 receptors in human post-mortem brain section. *Schizophr Res* 15,63.

Lieberman J, Pollack S, Lesser M, et al. (1988). Pharmacologic characterization of tardive dyskinesia. *J Clin Psychopharmacol* 8,254–260.

Lipinski JF Jr, Mallya G, Zimmerman P, et al. (1989). Fluoxetine-induced akathisia: clinical and theoretical implications. *J Clin Psychiatry* 50,339–342.

Lundstrom K, Turpin MP (1996). Proposed schizophrenia-related gene polymorphism: expression of the Ser9Gly mutant human dopamine D3 receptor with the Semliki Forest virus system. *Biochem Biophys Res Commun* 225,1068–1072.

Macciardi F, Verga M, Cavallaro R, et al. (1996). A genetic study of tardive dyskinesia in and Italian population of chronic schizophrenics. *Fifth World Congress on Psychiatric Genetics*. San Francisco, Oct 27–28.

Macciardi F, Verga M, Kennedy J, et al. (1994). An association study between schizophrenia and the dopamine receptor genes DRD3 and DRD4 using haplotype relative risk. *Hum Hered* 44,328–336.

Manki H, Kanba S, Muramatsu T, et al. (1996). Dopamine D2, D3 and D4 receptor and transporter gene polymorphisms and mood disorders. *J Affect Disord* 40,7–13.

McDougle CJ, Goodman WK, Delgado PL, et al. (1989). Pathophysiology of obsessive-compulsive disorder. *Am J Psychiatry* 146,1350–1351 (letter).

McDougle CJ, Goodman WK, Leckman JF, et al. (1994). Haloperidol addition in fluvoxamine-refractory obsessive-compulsive disorder. A double-blind, placebo-controlled study in patients with and without tics. *Arch Gen Psychiatry* 51,302–308.

McGue M, Gottesman II. (1989). A single dominant gene still cannot account for the transmission of schizophrenia. *Arch Gen Psychiatry* 46,478–480.

McGuffin P, Owen MJ, Farmer AE (1995). The genetic basis of schizophrenia. *Lancet* 346,678–682.

McGuffin P, Owen MJ, O'Donovan MC, et al. (1994).*Seminars in Psychiatric Genetics*. London: Gaskell.

Meshul CK, Casey DE (1989). Regional, reversible ultrastructural changes in rat brain with chronic neuroleptic treatment. *Brain Res* 489,338–346.

Mitchell P, Selbie L, Waters B, et al. (1992). Exclusion of close linkage of bipolar disorder to dopamine D1 and D2 receptor gene markers. *J Affect Disord* 25,1–11.

Mitchell P, Waters B, Vivero C, et al. (1993). Exclusion of close linkage of bipolar disorder to the dopamine D3 receptor gene in nine Australian pedigrees. *J Affect Disord* 27,213–224.

Murphy DL, Brodie HK, Goodwin FK, et al. (1971). Regular induction of hypomania by L-dopa in manic-depressive patients. *Nature* 229,135–136.

Nagai Y, Ueno S, Saeki Y, et al. (1996). Decrease of the D3 dopamine receptor mRNA expression in lymphocytes from patients with Parkinson's disease. *Neurology* 46,791–795.

Nanko S, Ueki A, Hattori M, et al. (1994). No allelic association between Parkinson's disease and dopamine D2, D3, and D4 receptor gene polymorphisms. *Am J Med Genet* 54,361–364.

Nicolini H, Cruz C, Paez F, et al. (1998). Dopamine D2 and D4 receptor genes distinguish the clinical presence of tics in obsessive-compulsive disorder. *Gac Med Mex* 134,521–527.

Nothen MM, Erdmann J, Korner J, et al. (1992). Lack of association between dopamine D1 and D2 receptor genes and bipolar affective disorder. *Am J Psychiatry* 149,199–201.

Novelli E, Nobile M, Diaferia G, et al. (1994). A molecular investigation suggests no relationship between obsessive-compulsive disorder and the dopamine D2 receptor. *Neuropsychobiology* 29,61–63.

O' Callaghan E, Larkin C, Kinsella A, et al. (1990). Obstetric complications, the putative familial-sporadic distinction, and tardive dyskinesia in schizophrenia. *Br J Psychiatry* 157,578–584.

O'Donovan MC, Owen MJ (1999). Candidate gene association studies of schizophrenia. *Am J Hum Genet* 65,587–592.

Oruc L, Furac I, Croux C, et al. (1996). Association study between bipolar disorder and candidate genes involved in dopamine-serotonin metabolism and GABAergic neurotransmission: a preliminary report. *Psychiatr Genet* 6,213–217 (letter).

Özdemir V, Masellis M, Basile VS, et al. (1999). Variability in response to clozapine: potential role of cytochrome-P450 1A2 and the dopamine D_4 receptor gene. *CNS Spectrums* 4,30–56.

Parsian A, Chakraverty S, Todd RD (1995). Possible association between the dopamine D3 receptor gene and bipolar affective disorder. *Am J Med Genet* 60,234–237.

Paterson AD, Sunohara GA, Kennedy JL (1999) The dopamine D4 receptor gene: novelty or nonsense? *Neuropsychopharmacology* 21,3–16.

Paterson AD, Ying D-J, Petronis A, et al. (1996). A Pstl restriction fragment length polymorphism in the 5′ untranslated region of DRD4 is not associated with schizophrenia. *Psychiatr Genet* 6,191–193.

Petronis A, Macciardi F, Athanassiades A, et al. (1995). Association study between the dopamine D4 receptor gene and schizophrenia. *Am J Med Genet* 60,452–455.

Piccardi MP, Severino G, Bocchetta A, et al. (1997). No evidence of association between dopamine D3 receptor gene and bipolar affective disorder. *Am J Med Genet* 74,137–139.

Randrup A, Munkvad I (1965). Special antagonism of amphetamine-induced abnormal behaviour. Inhibition of stereotyped activity with increase of some normal activities. *Psychopharmacologia* 7,416–422.

Rapoport JL (1991). Recent advances in obsessive-compulsive disorder. *Neuropsychopharmacology* 5,1–10.

Rasmussen SA (1993). Genetic studies of obsessive-compulsive disorder. *Ann Clin Psychiatry* 5,241–247.

Riddle MA, Scahill L, King R, et al. (1990). Obsessive compulsive disorder in children and adolescents: phenomenology and family history. *J Am Acad Child Adolesc Psychiatry* 29,766–772.

Riess O, Kruger (1999). Parkinson's disease—a multifactorial neurodegenerative disorder. *J Neural Transm Suppl* 56,113–125.

Rietschel M, Nothen MM, Lannfelt L, et al. (1993). A serine to glycine substitution at position 9 in the extracellular N-terminal part of the dopamine D3 receptor protein: no role in the genetic predisposition to bipolar affective disorder. *Psychiatry Res* 46,253–259.

Rosengarten H, Schweitzer JW, Friedhoff AJ (1993a). A mechanism underlying neuroleptic induced oral dyskinesias in rats. *Pol J Pharmacol* 45,391–398.

Schilder P (1938). The organic background of obsessions and compulsions. *Am J Psychiatry* 94,1397–1414.

Serretti A, Lattuada E, Cusin C, et al. (1999). Factor analysis of delusional disorder symptomatology. *Compr Psychiatry* 40,143–147.

Serretti A, Macciardi F, Cusin C, et al. (1998a). Dopamine receptor D4 gene is associated with delusional symptomatology in mood disorders. *Psychiatry Res* 80,129–136.

Serretti A, Macciardi F, Di Bella D, et al. (1998b). Self-esteem in remitted patients with mood disorders is not associated with the dopamine receptor D4 and the serotonin transporter genes. *Psychiatry Res* 80,137–144.

Shaikh S, Ball D, Craddock N, et al. (1993). The dopamine D3 receptor gene: no association with bipolar affective disorder. *J Med Genet* 30,308–309.

Sidenberg DG, Bassett AS, Demchyshyn L, et al. (1993). New polymorphism for the human serotonin 1D receptor variant (5-$HT_{1D\text{-}[gb]}$) not linked to schizophrenia in five Canadian pedigrees. *Hum Hered* 43,315–318.

Souery D, Lipp O, Mahieu B, et al. (1996). Association study of bipolar disorder with candidate genes involved in catecholamine neurotransmission: DRD2, DRD3, DAT1, and TH genes. *Am J Med Genet* 67,551–555.

Staner L, Hilger C, Hentges F, et al. (1998). Association between novelty-seeking and the dopamine D3 receptor gene in bipolar patients: a preliminary report. *Am J Med Genet* 81,192–194.

Stober G, Jatzke S, Heils A, et al. (1998). Insertion/deletion variant (–141C Ins/Del) in the 5′ regulatory region of the dopamine D2 receptor gene: lack of association with schizophrenia and bipolar affective disorder. Short communication. *J Neural Transm* 105,101–109.

Suzuki M, Hurd YL, Sokoloff P, et al. (1998). D3 dopamine receptor mRNA is widely expressed in the human brain. *Brain Res* 779,58–74.

Swartz JR, Burgoyne K, Smith M, et al. (1997). Tardive dyskinesia and ethnicity: review of the literature. *Ann Clin Psychiatry* 9,53–59.

Swedo SE, Rapoport JL, Cheslow DL, et al. (1989). High prevalence of obsessive-compulsive symptoms in patients with Sydenham's chorea. *Am J Psychiatry* 146,246–249.

Tarazi FI, Florijn WJ, Creese I (1995). Distinct localization and regulation of dopamine D3 receptors: autoradiographic studies. *Schizophr Res* 15,168.

Tarsy D, Baldessarini RJ (1977). The pathophysiologic basis of tardive dyskinesia. *Biol Psychiatry* 12,431–450.

Van Hartesveldt C (1997). Temporal and environmental effects on quinpirole-induced biphasic locomotion in rats. *Pharmacol Biochem Behav* 58,955–960.

Waddington JL, Youssef HA (1988). The expression of schizophrenia, affective disorder and vulnerability to tardive dyskinesia in an extensive pedigree. *Br J Psychiatry* 153,376–381.

Waldman ID, Robinson BF, Feigon SA (1997). Linkage disequilibrium between the dopamine transporter gene (DAT1) and bipolar disorder: extending the transmission disequilibrium test (TDT) to examine genetic heterogeneity. *Genet Epidemiol* 14,699–704.

Weinhold P, Wegner JT, Kane JM (1981). Familial occurrence of tardive dyskinesia. *J Clin Psychiatry* 42,165–166.

Williams J, Spurlock G, Holmans P, et al. (1998). A meta-analysis and transmission disequilibrium study of association between the dopamine D3 receptor gene and schizophrenia. *Mol Psychiatry* 3,141–149.

Willner P (1995). Dopaminergic mechanisms in depression and mania. In: *Psychopharmachology: the Fourth Generation of Progress*, Bloom FE, Kupfer DJ, eds. New York: Raven, pp. 921–931.

15.

Dopaminergic Systems and Motor Control

Lamine Gueye, Ibrahima Pierre Ndiaye, and Elisabeth Trouche

ABSTRACT

The dopaminergic system is one of the most important systems of the basal ganglia.. Most of our current knowledge about the involvement of the dopaminergic system in motor functions has been derived from the study of human disorders, in particular Parkinson's disease, and from animal models mimicking this disease. Research during the past three decades suggests that the dopaminergic system modulates activity of the excitatory and inhibitory systems of the basal ganglia. The motor circuit (in the basal ganglia) might be seen as playing a dual role in the modulation of motor patterns initiated at cortical levels by both reinforcing the currently selected pattern via the direct pathway of the basal ganglia and suppressing potentially conflicting patterns via the indirect pathway. Overall, this could result in the focusing of neural activity underlying each cortically initiated movement in a fashion analogous to the "inhibitory surround" seen in various sensory systems. Thus, motor circuits of basal ganglia are considered in preparation and execution of normal movement generated in the cerebral cortex. Furthermore, recent findings have demonstrated dopaminergic system involvement in motor learning. However, during the last decade, despite many findings about the functional organization of the basal ganglia, the proper role of the dopaminergic system in motor behavior is still unclear.. This review is focused on the role of the dopaminergic system in motor control and the pathophysiological mechanisms of parkinsonism.

INTRODUCTION

Most of our current knowledge about the involvement of the dopaminergic system in motor functions has been derived from the study of human disorders, in particular Parkinson's disease, and from animal models mimicking this disease. Thus, the disturbed movements seen in disorders of the dopaminergic system, such as parkinsonism, emphasize the importance of the dopaminergic system for normal motor control. The dopaminergic system is one of the most important systems of the basal ganglia, which is comprised of brain structures that are key in motor functions and limbic and cognitive processes. Research during the past three decades suggested that the dopaminergic system modulates the activity of the basal ganglia output structures. Accurate knowledge of the anatomical and functional organization of the dopaminergic system is essential to improve our understanding of how motor and cognitive functions operate in the normal brain. There is also a fundamental need to clarify the consequences of the pathophysiological changes that occur in Parkinson's disease and other disorders of the dopaminergic system. Despite many findings about the functional organization of the basal ganglia, the precise role of the dopaminergic system in motor control is still unclear.

ANATOMICAL BACKGROUND

The basal ganglia is a group of anatomically and functionally related nuclei located in the telencephalon, diencephalon, and mesencephalon. This group includes the striatum (formed by caudate nucleus and putamen), globus pallidus, substantia nigra, and subthalamic nucleus. The nucleus acumbens and olfactory tubercle are considered to be ventral extensions of the striatum because of their morphological and anatomical similarities (DeLong and Geourgopoulos, 1981).

The striatum is generally regarded as the major receptive portion of the basal ganglia. Corticostriatal fibers arise from all areas of the neocortex. The striatum of primates and carnivores is separated by the internal capsule into two parts: a dorsomedial portion (caudate nucleus) and ventrolateral portion (putamen). The projections of the sensorimotor cortex are organized somatotopically (Parent and Hazrati, 1995a,b). The striatum projects to the pallidum (globus pallidus) and substantia nigra pars reticulata.

The pallidum is a composite structure formed by the external segment of the globus pallidus (GPe) and an internal segment (GPi). The substantia nigra is also a composite structure formed by a conspicuously pigmented and cellular dorsomedial portion [substantia nigra compacta (SNc)] and a less dense nonpigmented ventrolateral portion [substantia nigra pars reticulata (SNpr)]. The pallidum (GPi) and the SNpr send projections to the thalamus, which sends return projections to the neocortex (Alexander and Crutcher, 1990). The GPe projects mainly to the subthalamic nucleus (STN). The SNc sends dopaminergic ascending projections to the striatum. Projections from the SNc terminate topographically on the striatum, forming the nigrostriatal dopaminergic system.

Other dopaminergic-containing terminals originate from the neighboring ventral tegmental area and give rise to the mesolimbic dopamine system, which projects to the nucleus accumbens, olfactory tubercle, and central nucleus of the amygdala. These latter dopamine-containing neurons lie medial and dorsal to the substantia nigra. A dopamine projection to portions of the frontal cortex arises from neurons intermingled with cells of the other dopamine systems (Parent and Hazrati, 1995a).

A persuasive theme explored by many authors is the concept of two separate systems within the motor circuit of the striatopallidal complex (Albin et al., 1990; Alexander and Crutcher, 1990; Delong, 1990) (Fig. 15-1). First, there is a direct putaminomedial pallidal (GPi) γ-aminobutyric acid (GABA) colocalized with substance P] and GPi-thalamic (GABA) system. This pathway arises from the putamen and projects to SNpr, which is homologous to the GPi, and innervates the thalamus and brainstem. Stimulation of this "direct pathway," either by glutamatergic corticostriatal input from sensorimotor areas of the cerebral cortex or by dopaminergic excitation from SNc, results in disinhibition of the thalamic targets that project

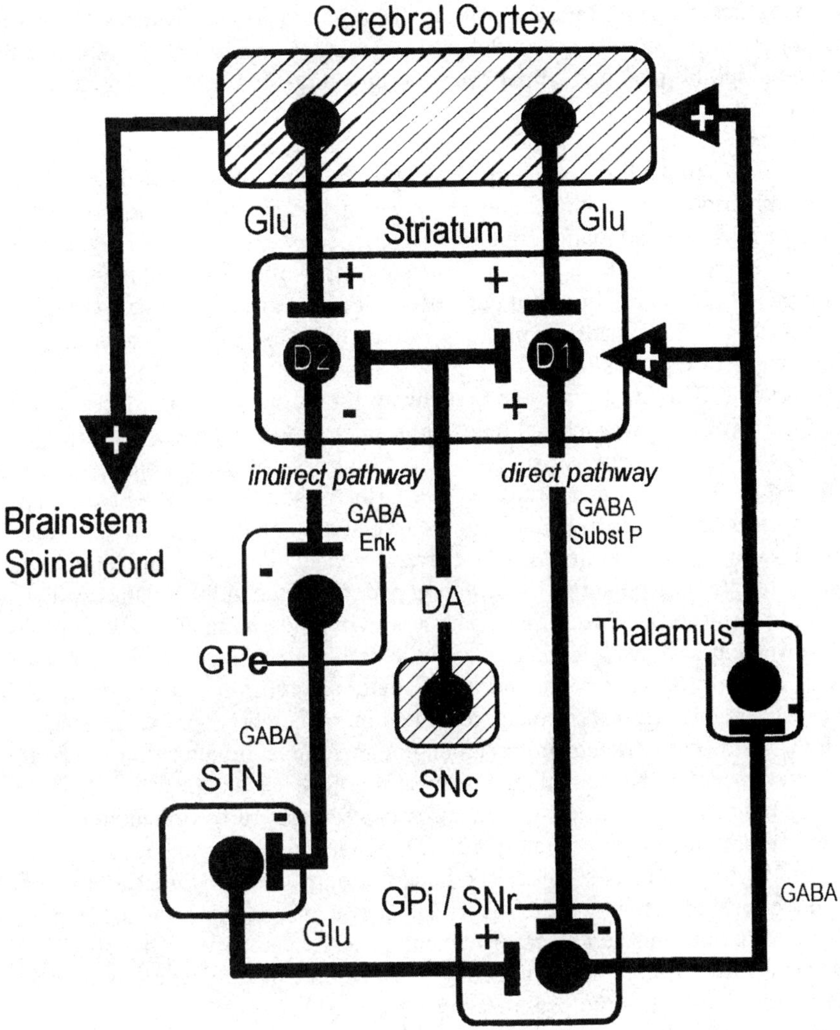

FIG. 15-1. Main anatomical connections within basal ganglia. Glu, glutamate; Enk, enkephalin; Subst P, substance P; DA, dopamine; GPe, external segment of globus pallidus; STN, subthalamic nucleus; SNc, substantia nigra compacta; GPi, internal segment of globus pallidus; SNpr, substantia nigra pars reticulata (Alexander and Crutcher, 1990).

excitatory pathways onto precentral motor fields. The net effect is considered to be facilitation of cortically initiated movement.

Second, there is an "indirect pathway" involving putaminolateral pallidal (GPe) (GABA colocalized with enkephalin), GPe-subthalamic (GABA)-subthalamo-GPi (glutamate), and GPi-thalamic (GABA) relays. Corticostriatal stimulation of this indirect system has the net effect of releasing subthalamic drive to medial pallidum, leading to increased GPi inhibition of the thalamic targets and reduced thalamocortical input to precentral motor fields. Dopaminergic nigrostriatal input is thus believed to inhibit this indirect pathway and in contrast to exert an excitatory action on the direct system.

In summary, the direct pathway provides positive feedback to precentral motor fields, whereas the indirect pathway contributes to a negative feedback. Deprivation of dopaminergic nigrostriatal input (such as in Parkinson's disease or MPTP, a selective toxin for the dopaminergic system) exposure reduces the positive feedback to the cortex via the indirect system. Thus the overall effect of dopamine loss in the striatum could be an inhibition of cortically initiated movements, which may cause akinesia (loss of movement), hypokinesia (reduction of movement), and bradykinesia (slowness of movement).

The overall functions of these two pathways in motor behavior are conceived as follows. The direct pathway facilitates appropriate cortically initiated movements, whereas the indirect pathway suppresses conflicting unwanted motor patterns. As expressed by Alexander and Crutcher (1990), the motor circuit in the basal ganglia might be seen as playing a dual role in the modulation of motor patterns initiated at cortical levels by both reinforcing the currently selected pattern via the direct pathway and suppressing potentially conflicting pattern via the indirect pathway. Overall this could result in the focussing of neural activity underlying each cortically initiated movement in a fashion analogous to the "inhibitory surround" seen in various sensory systems. Motor circuits of basal ganglia are considered key in preparation and execution of normal movement generated in the cerebral cortex.

However, recent advances in basal ganglia anatomical organization (Levy et al., 1997) proposed that the subthalamic nucleus is not merely a relay along the indirect pathway but can likely be considered an input structure from cortical and thalamic influences, bringing major excitatory afferent inputs into the basal ganglia (Fig. 15-2). Its excitatory influence is considered crucial not only for the GPi/SNpr but also for the GPe neuronal activity, which likely appears under the antagonistic control of both the striatum and subthalamic nucleus. The overactivity of the subthalamic nucleus resulting from removal of the nigrostriatal dopaminergic input is considered crucial in the pathophysiological mechanism of parkinsonism.

MOTOR EFFECTS OF LESIONS OF DOPAMINERGIC SYSTEM

The substantia nigra is a composite structure formed by the dopamine-containing cells of the pars compacta and the more widely dispersed cells of the pars reticulata. It is impossible to make selective lesion of the SNc by coagulative methods. It is possible to lesion more selectively the ascending dopamine projections of the pars compacta and other dopamine systems using 6-hydroxydopamine and more recently MPTP injections.

The first direct experiment on the substantia nigra was conducted by von Bechterew, who stimulated and lesioned this structure in dogs (von Bechterew, 1909). Bilateral lesions into animals resulted in profound immobility that could not be explained on the basis of an elementary sensory or motor impairment. Both ani-

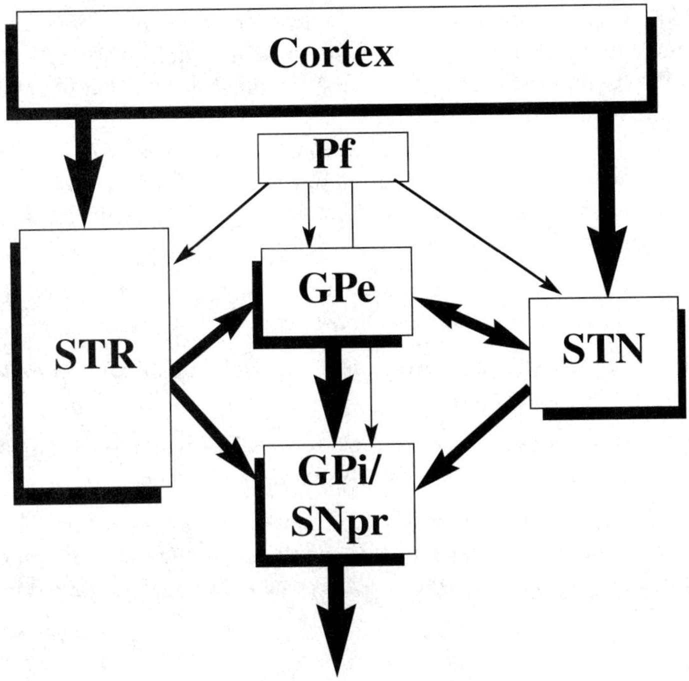

FIG. 15-2. New model of organization of basal ganglia based on novel anatomical, neurochemical, and physiological data. Findings imply that GPe and STN display broad projections to more structures than those predicted by the "direct/indirect" model. Striatum (STR) and STN are both considered input structures for basal ganglia. They both distribute cortical information: the striatum (from broader cortical areas) and STN (from more restricted cortical areas) to the same targets, i.e., GPe and GPi/SNpr, where they converge into the same groups of cells. Conversely, output structures (GPi/SNpr) are under the antagonistic effect of both input stations and a strong GABAergic input from GPe. Moreover, although not shown, all these structures are modulated by a direct dopaminergic projection from the substantia nigra pars compacta. Pf, parafascicular nucleus of thalamus. See Fig. 15-1 for other abbreviations (Levy et al., 1997).

mals died some days later, after refusing to take any nourishment. Carey and DeJong (1954) described unilateral lesions in one monkey and bilateral lesions in another that resulted in only mild hypotonia. However, Carpenter and McMaster (1964) observed that monkeys with unilateral damage to the substantia nigra showed no abnormality. Stern (1966), in a study of the nigral lesion in the primate, observed that bilateral lesions resulted in hypokinesia, with a general poverty and slowness of the movements and tendency to assume fixed postures.

In all these studies, the lesions involved both the pars reticulata and the pars compacta of the substantia nigra. More selective lesion of the ascending dopamine fiber systems were accomplished with 6-hydroxydopamine. In the rat and monkey, local unilateral injection of 6-hydroxydopamine into the ascending dopamine system results in a profound disturbance of posture, bradykinesia, and contralateral neglect (Schultz et al., 1989; Spirduso et al., 1985; Ungerstedt and Arbuthnott, 1970; Viallet et al., 1984). These symptoms are rapidly reversed by apomorphine, a directly acting dopamine agonist. In the primates, systemic injection of MPTP results in akinesia and rarely tremor. Severity of these symptoms is correlated with the degree of the dopamine depletion in the striatum.

Clinical studies in humans have demonstrated that focal lesions in the other structures of the basal ganglia caused motor disorders. Based on a meta-analysis of 204 cases with lesions in the basal ganglia, Bhatia and Marsden (1994) have drawn the following general conclusions.

- Lesions of the caudate nucleus infrequently cause motor disorders. If they do, it usually is chorea or dystonia and almost never parkinsonism.
- Lesions of lenticular nucleus (putamen and globus pallidus) commonly cause dystonia and rarely cause chorea.
- Bilateral lesions of the lenticular nucleus, usually involving the globus pallidus, infrequently cause parkinsonism or dystonia-parkinsonism.

Although not exhaustive, this study shows motor effects of the lesions of dopaminergic systems and/or other basal ganglia areas and suggests that the ascending dopamine projections from the pars compacta are largely involved in control of motor behavior.

PLANNING, INITIATION, AND EXECUTION OF MOVEMENT AND MOTOR LEARNING

Several physiological and anatomical findings imply that distinct input-output subsystems in the striatum modulated by different sets of dopaminergic neurons may participate in the neural processing related to movement control. According to suggestions by Mink and Thach (1993), the dopaminergic system may be more concerned with selection of the appropriate movements. Neurons recorded in primate putamen, caudate nucleus (Kermadi and Joseph, 1995), and globus pallidum (Brotchie et al., 1991) discharge in relation to the various phases of a movement sequence and of a single movement. On the basis of the architecture of the basal ganglia circuits, Gentilucci and Negrotti (1999) suggest that discharge of the neurons could be involved in controlling the execution of the action and in signaling the normal course of the motor programs to premotor areas. According to all these findings, some authors have proposed that the basal ganglia are a store in which the motor program is placed during its execution (Gentilucci and Negrotti, 1999; Viallet et Trouche, 1990). Their function can be to command the execution of the various phases of movement, releasing higher motor centers from directly controlling their execution.

Several attempts have been made to analyze and measure the motor disorders caused by dopaminergic system deficits in humans. Almost all motor behavioral studies have been performed in parkinsonian patients. Diverse aspects of motor performance, including reaction time, movement time, and velocity, have been examined with the view of elucidating the motor functions of the dopaminergic system.

Because of the pioneering study by Wilson (1925), a large body of data on the overall slowing of the reaction time that occurs in Parkinson's disease has been collected. Comparison of performance of simple and choice reaction time tasks yielded some discrepancies. Some authors observed that the reaction time likely reflecting central delay for the treatment of information used in the paradigm was shorter in these patients compared with normal subjects (Bloxham et al., 1984; Evarts et al., 1981; Goodrich et al., 1989; Pullman et al., 1988; Sheridan et al., 1987). However, others stressed the fact that the parkinsonian patients' delay was equivalent to that of controls (Girotti et al., 1986; Jordan et al., 1992; Mayeux et al., 1987) or even longer (Gueye et al., 1998a,b; Jahanshahi et al., 1992; Lichter et al., 1988; Reid et al., 1989). It was therefore difficult to propose a global interpretation from these central delay studies.

The most simple explanation focuses, however, on the slowness of parkinsonian patients' response initiation, a stage of processing that is common to both reaction time studies (Gueye et al., 1998b). In contrast, concerning movement execution, it is generally agreed that movement times of parkinsonian patients are longer than those of healthy subjects (Gueye et al., 1998a,b; Marsden, 1989; Pullman et al., 1988; Sheridan et al., 1987). It thus appears from these studies of motor behavior in Parkinson's disease that the dopaminergic system is involved in the preparatory and executing phases of motor activities.

Using positron emission tomography, Jueptner and Weiller (1998) observed that the prefrontal loop of the motor system (motor), i.e., dorsolateral prefrontal cortex and striatum, is engaged when normal subjects attend to the performance of an automatic (overlearned) task. During the last decade, work with positron emission tomography (Grafton et al., 1992; Jahanshahi et al., 1995; Jenkins et al., 1994; Jueptner and Weiller, 1998) has suggested that 1) the dopaminergic system and striatum are activated during selection of movements, 2) dopamine is engaged when subjects improve their motor performance, 3) dopamine is less active when movements were optimized using sensory feedback (visuomotor coordination), and 4) there is no activation of the basal ganglia when passive movements are examined.

According to all these findings, the dopaminergic system is considered key in preparation and execution of normal movement generated in the cerebral cortex. Thus the dysfunction of such systems can produce pronounced disturbance of volitional movement.

Furthermore, recent findings have demonstrated that the dopaminergic system could also be involved in motor learning. Single cell recording in primates has shown that the class of striatal neurons known as tonically active neurons (TAN) may contribute to temporal coordination in motor activity by undergoing dopamine-sensitive changes in their response properties (Apicella et al., 1997; Graybiel et al., 1994). In the striatum, TANs, considered the striatal cholinergic interneurons, are rare neurons that fire "spontaneously" at low frequency (2–10 Hz). TANs undergo changes in responsiveness during motor conditioning. The response of TANs to conditioned stimuli fits well with the idea that the striatum is involved in predictive motor control. Their change in responsiveness is also compatible with the idea that the striatum is involved in some aspects of sensorimotor learning (Graybiel et al.,

1994). Because modulation of TANs discharge is controlled by dopamine, such an idea is compatible with a teaching role for reward-related nigrostriatal dopaminergic input (Apicella et al., 1997), and it may help in understanding the remarkable success of dopamine replacement therapies in facilitating the movements of patients with Parkinson's disease.

MECHANISMS RESPONSIBLE FOR PARKINSONISM

The pathophysiological mechanism of parkinsonism is still unclear. Degeneration of the pigmented neurons in the SNc leads to profound loss of the dopaminergic innervation in the striatum, particularly in the putamen, which receives major input from the premotor and sensorimotor cortex. Neuronal loss is thought to have reached 70% when the first symptoms appear (Bernheimer et al., 1973; Riederer and Wuketich, 1976). However, the impact of striatal dopamine depletion is complex. A currently accepted model of the pathophsysiologal mechanism of Parkinson's disease was proposed by Albin et al. (1989) and DeLong (1990).

According to this scheme, dopaminergic drive is thought to enhance thalamocortical support of premotor cortical areas by its actions on both the direct and indirect striatopallidal (nigral) systems. Dopaminergic striatal denervation in Parkinson's disease, causing loss of both its excitatory effect on the direct striatopallidal (nigral) pathway and its inhibitory effect on the indirect pathway, thus withdraws striatopallidothalamocortical support of cortically generated movement. According to this model, dopaminergic striatal denervation in parkinsonism leads to an overactivity of the output station of the basal ganglia, namely the GPi/SNpr. This pathological hyperactivity of the GPi/SNpr has been interpreted as being the result of a reduced inhibitory input from the striatum and increased excitatory input from the STN. Enhanced activity of the STN neurons is considered the direct consequence of a release from the tonic inhibitory control normally exerted by the GABA-containing neurons of the GPe on STN neurons, but this hypothesis is highly discussed.

Nevertheless, according to the established model, the possible hypoactivity of the GPe could result in increased STN activity, which in turn (in addition to the diminished influence of the direct striatal GABAergic input) could induce the pathological overactivity of GPi/SNpr. Subsequently new therapeutic approaches to Parkinson's disease were proposed, such as high frequency stimulation (to block neuronal activity), lesions of GPe or STN, or use of agonists of GABA.

Levy et al. (1997) failed to prove a GPe hypoactivity from GABAergic and metabolic activity markers either in MPTP-intoxicated monkeys or Parkinson's disease patients. This would indicate that the inhibitory neurotransmission (GABAergic) provided by GPe neurons to subthalamic neurons is not quantitatively altered in parkinsonism. Thus GPe does not appear to be responsible for the well-documented STN overactivity observed in Parkinson's disease. According to Levy et al. (1997), the STN receives projections from three afferent systems that may represent potential candidates to explain its hyperactivity in parkinsonism (Fig. 15-2): 1) glutamate-excitatory projections from the cerebral cortex, 2) glutamate-excitatory projections from parafascicular nucleus of the thalamus, and 3) dopaminergic pathway from the substantia nigra pars compacta and ventral tegmental area.

The increase in STN activity should be due either to an increase in the excitatory effect produced by the cortex and/or the parafascicular nucleus or a decrease in the regulatory control exerted by dopaminergic neurons. However, little is known about the pathological modifications that might occur in these circuits in MPTP-intoxicated monkeys and in Parkinson's disease. It is well-established that the dopaminergic nigrostriatal projection is markedly altered in MPTP-intoxicated monkeys (Parent and Lavoie, 1993). However, the effect of the release from this dopaminergic innervation remains controversial. Thus the precise influence of each of these afferent systems on the STN remains to be determined in normal and parkinsonian brains.

Furthermore, based on classical anatomical data, the GPe was, until recently, considered almost exclusively a structure that regulates the output neurons from the GPi and SNpr indirectly through its projections to the STN. However, direct GABA-containing projections from GPe to GPi, SNpr, and reticular thalamic nucleus have recently been described in rats and primates (Chesselet and Delfs, 1996; Parent and Hazrati, 1995b). Therefore the GPe may exert a more widespread effect on output of the basal ganglia than just by controlling activity of the STN.

CONCLUSIONS

A new model of the basal ganglia circuitry in healthy and parkinsonian brains emerges. In this picture, the GPe, with its widespread projections, and the STN, with its multiple inputs/outputs, are more centrally involved in basal ganglia circuitry than previously appreciated. Although these novel data do not challenge the general view that dopamine depletion induces an increased inhibitory output from the basal ganglia to the thalamus, they suggest new targets for therapeutic approaches to counteract the effects of neuronal loss at the level of neurotransmitter production, release, or action.

REFERENCES

Albin RL, Young AB, Penney JB (1989). The functional anatomy of basal ganglia disorders. *Trends Neurosci* 12,366–375.

Alexander GE, Crutcher MD (1990). Functional architecture of basal ganglia circuits: neural substrates of parallel processing. *Trends Neurosci* 13,266–271.

Apicella P, Legallet E, Trouche E (1997). Responses of tonically discharging neurons in the monkey striatum to primary rewards delivered during different behavioural states. *Exp Brain Res* 116,456–466.

Bernheimer H, Birkmayer W, Hornykiewicz O, et al. (1973). Brain dopamine and the syndromes of Parkinson and Huntington. Clinical, morphological and neurochemical correlations. *J Neurol Sci* 20,415–455.

Bhatia KP, Marsden CD (1994). The behavioural and motor consequences of focal lesions of the basal ganglia in man. *Brain* 117,859–876.

Bloxham CA, Mindel TA, Frith CD (1984). Initiation and execution of predictable and unpredictable movements in Parkinson's disease. *Brain* 107,371–384.

Brotchie P, Iansek R, Horne MK (1991). Motor function of the monkey globus pallidus. 2. Cognitive aspects of movement and phasic neuronal activity. *Brain* 114,1685–1702.

Carey JH, DeJong RN (1954). Preliminary studies on the production of Parkinson's syndrome. *Trans Am Neurol Assoc* 79,28–35.

Carpenter MB, McMaster RE (1964). Lesions of the substantia nigra in the rhesus monkey. Efferent fibers degeneration and behavioral observations. *Am J Anat* 114,293–320.

Chesselet MF, Delfs JM (1996). Basal ganglia and movement disorders: an update. *Trends Neurosci* 19,417–421.

DeLong MR (1981). Motor functions of the basal ganglia. In: *Handbook of Physiology, The Nervous System II: Motor Control*, Brookhart JM , Mouncastle VB, Brooks VB, eds. Bethesda MD: American Physiological Society, pp. 1017–1061.

DeLong MR (1990). Primate models of movement disorders of basal ganglia origin. *Trends Neurosci* 13,281–285.

Evarts EV, Teräväinen H, Calne DB (1981). Reaction time in Parkinson's disease. *Brain* 104,167–186.

Gentilucci M, Negrotti A (1999). Planning and executing and action in Parkinson's disease. *Mov Disord* 14,69–79.

Girotti F, Carella F, Grassi MP, et al. (1986). Motor and cognitive performances of patients in the on and off phases of the disease. *J Neurol Neurosurg Psychiatry* 49,657–660.

Goodrich S, Henderson L, Kennard DC (1989). On the existence of an attention-demanding process peculiar to simple reaction time: converting evidence from Parkinson's disease. *Cogn Neuropsychol* 6,309–331.

Grafton ST, Mazziotta JC, Presty S, et al. (1992). Functional anatomy of human procedural learning determined with regional cerebral blood flow and PET. *J Neurosci* 12,2542–2548.

Graybiel AM (1990). Neurotransmitters and neuromodulators in the basal ganglia. *Trends Neurosci* 13,244–254.

Graybiel AM, Aosaki T, Flaherty AW, et al. (1994). The basal ganglia and the adaptative motor control. *Science* 265,1826–1830.

Gueye L, Viallet F, Legallet E, et al. (1998a). Effets de l'information préalable donnée par des indices sensoriels sur la durée et la précision d'un mouvement de pointage dans la maladie de Parkinson. *Dakar Méd* 43,49–53.

Gueye L, Viallet F, Legallet E, et al. (1998b). The use of advance information for motor preparation in Parkinson's disease: effects of cueing and compatibility between warning and imperative stimuli. *Brain Cognition* 38,66–86.

Jahanshahi M, Brown RG, Marsden CD (1992). Simple and choice reaction time and the use of advance information for motor preparation in Parkinson's disease. *Brain* 115,539–564.

Jahanshahi M, Jenkins IH, Brown RG, et al. (1995). Self-initiated versus externally triggered movements. I. An investigation using measurement of regional cerebral blood flow with PET and movement-related potentials in normal and Parkinson's disease subjects. *Brain* 118,913–933.

Jenkins IH, Brooks DJ, Nixon PD, et al. (1994). Motor sequence learning: a study with positron emission tomography. *J Neurosci* 14,3775–3790.

Jordan N, Sagar HJ, Cooper JA (1992). Cognitive components of reaction time in Parkinson's disease. *J Neurol Neurosurg Psychiatry* 55,658–664.

Jueptner M, Weiller C (1998). A review of differences between basal ganglia and cerebellar control of movements as revealed by functional imaging studies *Brain* 121,1437–1449.

Kermadi I, Joseph JP (1995). Activity in the caudate nucleus of monkey during spatial sequencing. *J Neurophysiol* 74,911–933.

Langston JW, Forno LS, Rebert CS, et al. (1984). 1-Methyl-phenyl-1,2,3,6-tetrahydropyridine causes selective damage to the zona compacta of the substantia nigra in the squirrel monkey. *Brain Res* 292,390–394.

Levy R, Hazrati L-N, Herrero M-T, et al. (1997). Re-evaluation of the functional anatomy of the basal ganglia in normal and parkinsonian states. *Neuroscience* 76,335–343.

Lichter DG, Corbett AJ, Fitzgibbon GM, et al. (1988). Cognitive and motor dysfunction in Parkinson's disease: clinical performance and computed tomographic correlations. *Arch Neurol* 45,854–860.

Marin O, Wilhelmus JA, Smeets WJ, et al. (1998). Evolution of the basal ganglia in tetrapods: a new perspective based on recent studies in amphibians. *Trends Neurosci* 21,487–494.

Marsden CD (1989). Slowness of movement in Parkinson's disease. *Mov Disord* 4,26–37.

Marsden CD, Obeso JA (1994). The functions of the basal ganglia and the paradox of stereotaxic surgery in Parkinson's disease. 117,878–897.

Mayeux R, Stern Y (1983). Intellectual dysfunction and dementia in Parkinson's disease. In: *Advances in Neurology*, Mayeux R, Rosen WC, eds. New York: Raven, vol. 38, pp. 211–227.

Mink JW, Thach WT (1993). Basal ganglia intrinsic circuits and their role in behavior. *Curr Opin Neuriobiol* 3,950–957.

Parent A, Hazrati LN (1995a). Functional anatomy of the basal ganglia. I. The cortico-basal ganglia-thalamo-cortical loop. *Brain Res Rev* 20,91–127.

Parent A, Hazrati LN (1995b). Functional anatomy of the basal ganglia. II. The place of subthalamic nucleus and external pallidum in basal ganglia circuitry. *Brain Res Rev* 20,128–154.

Pullman SL, Watts RL, Juncos JL et al. (1988). Dopaminergic effects on simple and choice reaction time performance in Parkinson's disease. *Neurology* 38,249–254.

Reid WG, Broe GA, Hely MA, et al. (1989). The neuropsychology of de novo patients with idiopathic Parkinson's disease: the effects of age of onset. *Int J Neurosci* 48,205–217.

Riederer P, Wuketich S (1976). Time course of nigrostriatal degeneration in Parkinson's disease. *J Neural Transm* 38,277–301.

Schultz W, Studer A, Romo R, et al. (1989). Deficits in reaction times and movement times as correlates of hypokinesia in monkeys with MPTP-induced striatal dopamine depletion. *J Neurophysiol* 61,651–668.

Sheridan MR, Flowers KA, Hurrel J (1987). Programming and execution of movement in Parkinson's disease. *Brain* 110,1247–1271.

Spirduso WW, Gillam PE, Schallert T, et al. (1985). Reactive capacity: a sensitive behavioural marker of movement initiation and nigro-striatal dopamine function. *Brain Res* 335,45–54.

Stern GM (1966). The effects of lesions in the substantia nigra. *Brain* 89,449–478.

Ungerstedt U (1970). Quantitative recording of rotational behavior in rats after 6-hydroxydopamine lesions of the nigrostriatal system. *Brain Res* 24,485–493.

Viallet F, Trouche E (1991). Troubles de l'initiation du mouvement chez le parkinsonien. III. Actualitè de la maladie de Parkinson. *JAMA* (suppl),37–41.

Viallet F, Trouche E, Nieoullon A, et al. (1984). Unilateral electrolytic and 6-OHDA lesions of the substantia nigra. *Exp Brain Res* 65,399–410.

von Bechterew U (1909). *Die Functionen der Nervencentra.* Jena: Fischer, vol. 2, pp. 1232–1255.

Wilson SAK (1925). Some disorders of motility and of muscle tone, with special reference to the corpus striatum. *Lancet* 2,169–178.

INDEX

In this index, page numbers in *italics* designate figures; page numbers followed by the letter "t" designate tables. *See also* cross-references designate related topics or more detailed subentries.

E

F

G

H

I

J

K

L

M

N

O

P

Q

R

S

T